Art for Children Ex
Psychological Trauma

Art for Children Experiencing Psychological Trauma aims to increase understanding of art's potential to enhance learning for children living in crisis. In this groundbreaking resource, the first of its kind to focus specifically on the connection between art education and psychological trauma in youth populations, readers can find resources and practical strategies for both teachers and other school-based professionals. Also included are successful models of art education for diverse populations, with specific attention to young people who face emotional, mental, behavioral, and physical challenges, as well a framework for meaningful visual arts education for at-risk/in-crisis populations.

Adrienne D. Hunter, MEd, has over 35 years of experience teaching art to at-risk, in-crisis, and/or incarcerated youth. She is a national presenter, a past president of the interest group on Special Needs in Art Education (SNAE) within the National Art Education Association, and a past membership co-chair for the Council for Exceptional Children's Division of Visual and Performing Arts Education (DARTS).

Donalyn Heise, EdD, is founder and co-director of Teacher Effectiveness for Art Learning (TEAL), and is a leader at the local, state, and national levels. She is a researcher, author, national presenter, and award-winning educator with more than 30 years of experience teaching art to youth who have experienced psychological trauma.

Beverley H. Johns, MS, is a professional fellow at MacMurray College. She has worked in public schools with students with significant behavioral problems for more than 33 years, presented international workshops, and authored more than 20 special education books.

Art for Children Experiencing Psychological Trauma

A Guide for Art Educators and
School-Based Professionals

**Edited by Adrienne D. Hunter,
Donalyn Heise, and Beverley H. Johns**

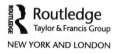
Routledge
Taylor & Francis Group

NEW YORK AND LONDON

First published 2018
by Routledge
711 Third Avenue, New York, NY 10017

and by Routledge
2 Park Square, Milton Park, Abingdon, Oxon, OX14 4RN

Routledge is an imprint of the Taylor & Francis Group, an informa business

© 2018 Taylor & Francis

The right of Adrienne D. Hunter, Donalyn Heise, and Beverley H. Johns to be identified as the authors of the editorial material, and of the authors for their individual chapters, has been asserted in accordance with sections 77 and 78 of the Copyright, Designs and Patents Act 1988.

Library of Congress Cataloging-in-Publication Data
Names: Hunter, Adrienne D., editor.
Title: Art for children experiencing psychological trauma : a guide for art educators and school-based professionals / Adrienne D. Hunter, Donalyn Heise, and Beverley H. Johns, editors.
Description: New York, NY : Routledge, 2018. | Includes bibliographical references.
Identifiers: LCCN 2017052876 (print) | LCCN 2017054105 (ebook) | ISBN 9781315301358 (eBook) | ISBN 9781138236943 (hbk) | ISBN 9781138236950 (pbk) | ISBN 9781315301358 (ebk)
Subjects: LCSH: Art therapy for children. | Psychic trauma in children—Treatment. | Art in education—Therapeutic use.
Classification: LCC RJ505.A7 (ebook) | LCC RJ505.A7 A75 2018 (print) | DDC 618.92/891656—dc23
LC record available at https://lccn.loc.gov/2017052876

ISBN: 978-1-138-23694-3 (hbk)
ISBN: 978-1-138-23695-0 (pbk)
ISBN: 978-1-315-30135-8 (ebk)

Typeset in Bembo
by Swales & Willis Ltd, Exeter, Devon, UK

Dedication

This book is dedicated to all students who have experienced psychological trauma, and to all art educators who nurture the strengths, talents, and hopes of all students.

Contents

Biographies of Editors and Contributors

Adrienne D. Hunter, MSEd, Special Education, is a pioneer in teaching art to in-crisis, at-risk, and incarcerated students. Recently retired, she was an art teacher in the Allegheny Intermediate Unit Alternative Education Program in Pittsburgh, Pennsylvania, for over 35 years. Ms. Hunter designed and implemented fully inclusive art curriculums for students aged 6 to 21, from homeless shelters, crisis centers, alternative education high schools, and maximum-security institutions. Through her sensitive and innovative curricula, she has addressed within her classroom the issues of gangs, domestic violence, homelessness, substance abuse, mental illness, and death. At the same time, she created a safe haven for inner-city youth through art. Ms. Hunter's commitment to education and advocacy extends far beyond the workplace. She has reached across racial, generational, economic, and community boundaries to form partnerships with colleges and universities, senior citizen centers, day care centers, local merchants, and community agencies throughout Allegheny County. Her students have created quilts for children with AIDS; murals that decorate schools, senior centers, and juvenile detention centers; and poetry and art books to help students on their journeys toward healing. Ms. Hunter has regularly enlisted local newspapers and merchants to gain publicity for her students' positive contributions to their communities. In addition, as an advocate for art education for alternative education and for gifted education, she has spoken at Pennsylvania state legislature hearings. Her professional training reflects her interests in both art education and special education. Ms. Hunter co-authored "Identifying the Visually Gifted: A Case Study" in *Art, Science, and Visual Literacy* and the "Teacher's Assessment Resource Booklet" for the Pennsylvania Art Education Association (PAEA). She also co-authored "Students with Emotional and/or Behavior Disorders" in National Art Education Association's (NAEA) *Reaching and Teaching Students with Special Needs through Art*. She is a nationally recognized presenter and an internationally exhibited fiber artist and is the recipient of numerous awards and grants, including a Fulbright Memorial Fund Teacher Scholarship to study art and education in Japan. In 2016, she was awarded the NAEA, VSA,[1]

Council for Exceptional Children, Beverly Levett Gerber Special Needs Art Educator Lifetime Achievement Award. In 2008, she became the first recipient of the NAEA/Special Needs Art Educator of the Year Award. In 1996, she was awarded the PAEA Outstanding Secondary Art Educator of the Year Award. Ms. Hunter is a Past- President of the NAEA/Special Needs Art Educators. She holds a Bachelor of Fine Arts from Pratt Institute, Brooklyn, New York, and a Master of Education from Duquesne University, Pittsburgh, Pennsylvania, and continues post-graduate work in art education.

Donalyn Heise, EdD, is the Founder and Co-Director of Teacher Effectiveness for Art Learning, an affiliate of Advanced Learning, Inc., and retired Associate Professor of Art Education at the University of Memphis, Tennessee. She has been an artist and educator for more than 30 years and has taught art in K-12 public and private schools and several universities. Her research focuses on art teacher preparation, art and resilience, and community art collaborations. Dr. Heise has designed and conducted over a hundred professional development workshops and presentations at the state, regional, and national levels. She served as Director of the Center for Innovation in Art Education, Director of the Paul R. Williams Project Education, President of the Tennessee Art Education Association, President of the Nebraska Art Teachers Association, and founding board member of the Nebraska Alliance for Art, and Education Advisory Committee of the Dixon Gallery and Gardens. As Art and Technology Coordinator for ConferNet, she designed, implemented, and evaluated professional development for six school districts, and coordinated one of the nation's first virtual art-based academic K-16 conferences funded by the United States Department of Education. Awards and accomplishments include the 2013 Tennessee Special Needs Art Educator of the Year Award; 2010 Tennessee Art Educator of the Year; 2010 NAEA Southeastern Region Higher Education Award; 2009 National Art Education Association, VSA, Council for Exceptional Children, Beverly Levett Gerber Special Needs Lifetime Achievement Award; 2007 Tennessee Higher Ed Art Educator of the Year; and 1997 Nebraska Art Teachers' Association Supervisor/ Administrator of the Year Award. Selected publications include: "Preparing Competent Art Teachers for Urban Schools," "The Indispensable Art Teacher," "Differentiation of Instruction," "Anticipatory Sets for Art Instruction," "Perspectives on the Use of Internet in Art Classrooms," "Creating Interaction in an Online Distance Learning Environment," "Best Practices in Classroom Management," "Implementation of a Combination of Traditional and Online Professional Development to Improve Teacher Competencies in the Use of Computer Technology," "Steeling and Resilience in Art Education," "Fostering Resilience through Art," and "Fostering Resilience in an Intergenerational Art and Literacy Program in a Shelter for Families Who Are Homeless."

Beverley H. Johns, MSEd, Special Education, is a learning and behavior consultant and Professional Fellow for MacMurray College, Jacksonville, Illinois, where she teaches courses on Special Education Law, Adaptations for the General Education Classroom, emotional behavioral disorders (EBD), and Diverse Learners. She has 40 years' experience working with students with learning disabilities (LD), and/or EBD within the public schools. She supervised LD and EBD teachers in 22 school districts; was the founder and administrator of the Garrison Alternative School for students with severe EBD in Jacksonville, Illinois; and later coordinated staff development for the Four Rivers Special Education District. Johns is the lead author of 15 books (and co-author of four others). She is co-author with Janet Lerner of the seminal college LD text book, *Learning Disabilities and Related Disabilities* (13th edition). She is the 2000 recipient of the International Council for Exceptional Children (CEC) Outstanding Leadership Award, Past International President of the Council for Children with Behavioral Disorders, Past President of the CEC Pioneers, Past Secretary and Governmental Relations Chair for the Division for Learning Disabilities, and the 2007 Recipient of the Romaine P. Mackie Leadership Service Award. She is listed in Who's Who in America, Who's Who of American Women, Who's Who in American Education, and Who's Who among America's Teachers. She has presented workshops across the United States and Canada; in San Juan, Puerto Rico; Sydney, Australia (keynote); Warsaw, Poland; Wrocław, Poland (keynote); Hong Kong, China; Lima, Peru; and Riga, Latvia. She is a graduate of Catherine Spalding College in Louisville, Kentucky, and received a fellowship for her graduate work at Southern Illinois University (SIU) in Carbondale, Illinois, where she received a Master of Science in Special Education. She has done post-graduate work at the University of Illinois, Western Illinois University, SIU, and Eastern Illinois University.

Darla Dawn Absher, PsyD, LPC–S, is a Doctor of Psychology and a Licensed Professional Counselor-Supervisor and currently works as director of admissions for a large psychiatric hospital. She also has a successful private practice in Austin, Texas. Dr. Absher performs *pro bono* work around Austin, providing education on suicide awareness, suicide prevention, and crisis negotiations. She earned her Bachelors in Psychology, Master of Arts in Counseling, and a Master of Arts in Human Services all from St. Edward's University, Austin. She earned her Doctor of Clinical Psychology from Argosy University in Dallas, Texas.

Matthew Adams, MA, Geography, currently conducts policy research for the Fire Department of New York City. He worked for seven years as a Principal Policy Analyst at the Institute for Children, Poverty, and Homelessness, where he led a research team that analyzed public policies impacting homeless families and their children across the United States. Mr. Adams specializes in spatial analysis and statistics and holds a Master of Arts in Geography from Boston University, Massachusetts, and a Bachelor of Arts in Geography from Clark University, Worcester, Massachusetts.

Dona Anderson, MPA, Environmental Science and Policy, is the Deputy Executive Director at the New York Early Childhood Professional Development Institute, where she is responsible for programmatic and operational oversight, as well as communications. She coordinates the Institute's internal data collection and evaluation efforts and represents the Institute at community and university events. Prior to her work at the Institute, she was the Director at the Institute for Children, Poverty, and Homelessness, where she led a team of researchers in exploring the impacts of poverty and homelessness on children, students, and families in New York City and across the United States. She also supervised early childhood care and education programs, after-school programs, residential summer camps, and a family support program as the Director of Programs and Development at Homes for the Homeless, a homeless services provider. Ms. Anderson has presented at national conferences and co-authored a variety of public policy reports on the topics of child poverty, homelessness, early childhood, and trauma. She holds a Master in Public Administration from Columbia University's School of International and Public Affairs and a Bachelor Degree from Claremont McKenna College, Claremont, California.

Laura Bailey Saulle, BFA, Printmaking, has held a variety of roles in the fields of education and youth development, with a focus on homeless and unaccompanied youth. She currently works in the field of youth workforce development. For several years, Ms. Bailey served as Program Director and then Assistant Executive Director at the Homeless Children's Education Fund, where her responsibilities included creating and managing out-of-school-time arts and enrichment programs for homeless children and youth living in the Greater Pittsburgh region. After earning a BFA in printmaking from The Pennsylvania State University, University Park, Laura completed a Fulbright teaching fellowship in Italy and taught youth art classes at the Carnegie Museum of Art in Pittsburgh.

Kari Caddell, MS, Art Therapy, is a registered and board-certified art therapist at the Integrated Learning Program in Omaha Public Schools (OPS), Nebraska, an alternative program for children with special educational needs in the areas of learning and behavior. She has worked in OPS since 2002. She is a licensed mental health practitioner for the state of Nebraska and a licensed Professional Counselor. Ms. Caddell has experience working with adults, adolescents, and children in groups and individually. She is a practicing visual mixed-media artist.

Robin Crawford, BA, is a skilled fiber artist with a background in social work, youth counseling, and teaching artists. She is presently sharing her love for art while working at The Maker's Clubhouse, an out-of-school-time program for elementary students in Pittsburgh, Pennsylvania. She received a Bachelor of Arts with a minor in psychology and a certificate in counseling from Carlow University, Pittsburgh, Pennsylvania. Ms. Crawford received a grant from the Pittsburgh Foundation-Howard Heinz Endowments Multicultural Arts Initiative to support a month-long exhibit at the Kingsley Association. Her quilts were included in the Senator John Heinz History Center's 2003 exhibit, "Bold and Improvisation: 120 Years of African American Quilts." She also was one of 20 contemporary quilters selected that year for the highly acclaimed traveling exhibit, "African American Quilters and Preservation of Western Pennsylvania."

Juliann B. Dorff, MA, Teaching, is a senior lecturer teaching art education in the School of Art at Kent State University. She is the 2015 Ohio Higher Education Division Award winner presented by the Ohio Art Education Association (OAEA) and a 2014 Outstanding Art Educator for the Northeast Region of the OAEA. Ms. Dorff was an invited participant at Examining the Intersection of Arts Education and Special Education: A National Forum, sponsored by the Kennedy Center in the summer of 2012, and has a white paper published in the resulting work: *The Intersection of Arts Education and Special Education: Exemplary Programs and Approaches.* She has presented extensively at the OAEA, National Art Education Association (NAEA), and the Council for Exceptional Children conferences. She is a contributing author in the book *Understanding Students with Autism through Art* (2010) published by NAEA,

Barbara Duffield, BS, Political Science, is a founder and Executive Director of SchoolHouse Connection. She is the former Policy Director for the National Association for the Education of Homeless Children and Youth (NAEHCY). NAEHCY, a national membership association, serves as the voice and the social conscience for the education of children and youth in homeless situations. Ms. Duffield's involvement in homeless issues began in 1990 as a tutor for homeless children in Washington, D.C. She subsequently joined the National Coalition for the Homeless (NCH) and served as Director of Education for NCH from 1994 to 2003, working closely with educators, service providers, federal agencies, and Congressional offices to strengthen policy and practice on children's issues. Ms. Duffield has conducted hundreds of trainings around the United States for school districts, community organizations, and local, state, and national groups to assist in the implementation of the McKinney-Vento Act.

Amanda Ferrara, **BS, Psychology; BA, Philosophy,** has been conducting cognitive and educational research for nearly a decade. She has worked as a public school teacher as well as a research assistant benefiting pre-service teachers and military families. She is currently a doctoral student in the educational psychology program at the Pennsylvania State University, University Park. Ms. Ferrara earned a Bachelor of Science in Psychology and a Bachelor of Arts in Philosophy from the University of Pittsburgh, Pennsylvania.

Peter J. Geisser, HonD, Fine Arts, teaches art education majors at the University of Massachusetts, Dartmouth, and gives workshops and lectures on art and special education nationally. He was the K-12 art teacher at the Rhode Island School for the Deaf from 1973 to 2003. He co-authored, with Maura Geisser, a chapter in the National Art Education Association's best-selling publication *Reaching and Teaching Students with Special Needs through Art*. Mr. Geisser created and directed the award-winning "Circle of Clay" project for VSA Arts Rhodes Island at the Hasbro Children's Hospital, Providence, and his stained glass commissions are in churches, hospitals, homes, and buildings around New England.

Elizabeth Hlavek, MA, Art Therapy; ATR-BC; and LCPAT, is an art therapist practicing in Annapolis, Maryland; an adjunct instructor in psychology at Anne Arundel Community College; and a doctoral candidate in art therapy at Mount Mary University. In her clinical practice, she works primarily with adolescents and adults struggling with eating disorders and body image concerns. Her academic research explores the relevance of art work created in the Holocaust to art therapy theory and practice. In 2012, she worked with state legislators to develop the first clinical art therapy license in Maryland and previously sat on the Maryland Board of Professional Counselors and Therapists. Ms. Hlavek is an active member of the American and Maryland Art Therapy Associations. She completed her Master in Art Therapy at Pratt Institute, Brooklyn, New York, and earned a BFA from Carnegie Mellon University, Pittsburgh, Pennsylvania.

Lynne J. Horoschak, MAEd, earned her Master in Education, plus sixty credits from Temple University; University of the Arts, Philadelphia, Pennsylvania; and University of Alaska, Fairbanks. She has been the distinguished Professor and Program Manager of Master in Art Education with an Emphasis in Special Populations, and Professor and Chair of Art Education at Moore College of Art and Design, Philadelphia, Pennsylvania. She has received many honors throughout her career, including: The Bob and Penny Fox Distinguished Professor Award for Moore College of Art and Design; the Kassandara Madison Art Education Leadership and Inspiration Award from the Picasso Project; the Pennyslvania Art Education Association Award for Outstanding Art Educator in Higher Education, 2008; and The Educators 3E Award from West Chester University for Educational Excellence and Entrepreneurship. From 2013 to 2014, she was the President of the National Art Education Association/

Special Needs Art Education. She is a founding officer of the DARTS Division of the Council for Exceptional Children.

Oriana C. Hunter, MD, PhD, is currently completing her residency in General Surgery at Lehigh Valley Health Network in the Department of Surgery, where she often cares for victims of traumatic child abuse. Previously, she worked at the University of Pittsburgh Medical Center's (UPMC) Artificial Heart Program as a clinical biomedical engineer and she performed research at the UPMC Hillman Cancer Institute. She has lectured nationally and written numerous scientific publications. She has taught the principles of adult and pediatric mechanical circulatory support and the history of artificial organs at the collegiate and professional level. She has volunteered at the Children's Hospital of Pittsburgh of UPMC's Child Life Program. Dr. Hunter's awards include the 2007 UPMC ACES Award for Commitment and Excellence in Service. Dr. Hunter graduated from the Massachusetts Institute of Technology with her Bachelor of Science in mechanical engineering, before going on to earn her doctorate in bioengineering from the University of Pittsburgh and her M.D. from the University of Pittsburgh School of Medicine.

Lisa Kay, EdD, Art Therapy, is Assistant Professor and Art Education Area Head, and Graduate Coordinator at the Tyler School of Art/Center for the Arts at Temple University in Philadelphia, Pennsylvania. In addition to teaching undergraduate and graduate art education at Tyler, Dr. Kay has taught art therapy at the School of the Art Institute of Chicago. In 2011–2012, she was awarded a Fulbright Interdisciplinary Research/Teaching Fellowship in Hungary that combined art therapy, art education, and arts-based qualitative research. A board-certified art therapist, Dr. Kay's research and publications concern the intersections and collaborations between contemporary art education and school art therapy, with special attention to students with special needs, symbols and metaphors of beauty and ugliness in adolescents' drawings, and the use of creative arts and visual imagery as qualitative research methods.

Steven Kelly, MSW, currently serves as a CEO for a large psychiatric hospital. Prior to that, he worked as Vice President of Customer Relations for Beacon Behavioral Health in Baton Rouge, Louisiana. For the last 26 years Mr. Kelly has worked in the field of psychiatry, with the majority of his experience in acute psychiatric mental health systems, as a mental health technician, social worker, community liaison, or management. He earned his Bachelor of Arts degree in Psychology from Louisiana State University, and his Master of Social Work from the University of Nebraska at Omaha.

Joseph Lagana, EdD, is the founder and CEO of the Homeless Children's Education Fund, a 501(c)3 not-for-profit organization, whose mission is to provide advocacy, community engagement, and direct service programs that support the education of children and youth experiencing homelessness in Allegheny County, Pennsylvania. In his long career as an educator in the Penn Hills and North Allegheny school districts, Dr. Lagana was a classroom teacher, counselor, and administrator before becoming superintendent of the Northgate School District. From 1992 to 1999, he was Executive Director of the Allegheny Intermediate Unit (AIU) comprised of 42 school districts. Upon his retirement from the AIU, he was named Executive Director Emeritus.

Susan D. Loesl, MA, ATR–BC, has been an adaptive arts specialist/ art therapist for the Milwaukee Public Schools, Milwaukee, Wisconsin, for the past 26 years. She has also worked in nursing homes with developmentally disabled adults, with adjudicated youth in prison, and with adolescent males and females in residential treatment centers. Ms. Loesl is an Art Therapy and Graduate Education Adjunct Faculty at Mount Mary University, Milwaukee, Wisconsin, and a presenter at many national conferences related to persons with disabilities and adaptations of the arts. Ms. Loesl is currently working on her own book on adaptive arts strategies, tools, and techniques.

Carlomagno Panlilio, PhD, Human Development, is currently investigating the important role that teachers can play in promoting the academic achievement for students with a history of maltreatment. Also, using a longitudinal latent variable framework, his research focuses on understanding the developmental trajectories of school readiness domains (i.e., emotion regulation and language) across the preschool years for maltreated children. He is studying how child welfare-specific contextual factors of placement stability and caregiver quality at different time points influence development, and how these different developmental trajectories predict later academic achievement. Additionally, Dr. Panlilio is interested in examining how maltreatment alters students' motivation and engagement in the classroom at later ages, and how these domains influence academic performance. Dr. Panlilio received his doctorate at the University of Maryland, College Park, with a specialization in Developmental Science and a Certificate in Measurement and Statistics.

Joseph A. Parsons, BFA, MSEd, Guidance and Counseling, has been a classroom and art teacher exclusively of severely emotionally/behaviorally-disabled (ED/EBD) students for 37 years. He has worked in both residential and day treatment programs for ED/EBD students in Des Moines, Iowa, and Broward County, Florida. He has been a guest speaker for professors at Broward Community College and Florida Atlantic University. He has also presented numerous workshops in his schools, as well as being a presenter in Iowa and at the National Art Education Association's national conventions. He is a long-time member of Special Needs in Art Education, and has served as an elected officer in the organization.

Athena Petrolias, MA, Teaching, is the Director of the Alternative Education Program (AEP) at the Allegheny Intermediate Unit, an educational service agency located in Homestead, Pennsylvania. The AEP, operating for over 54 years, is responsible for educating youth at the Allegheny County Jail, Shuman Detention Center, Auberle Inc., and at three Pennsylvania Department of Education approved alternative schools for disruptive youth. She serves as a seven county Regional Coordinator for Alternative Education for Disruptive Youth for the Pennsylvania Department of Education and has been a board member of the Pennsylvania Academic and Career/Technical Training Alliance. She is also responsible for a Truancy Prevention Program in collaboration with local school districts, the Allegheny Department of Human Services, Juvenile Probation, and the Pennsylvania Truancy Round Table.

Mindi Rhoades, PhD, is an Assistant Professor in the Department of Teaching and Learning in the College of Education at the Ohio State University, Columbus, Ohio. Her research includes collaborations with colleagues, teachers, and artists on interdisciplinary arts-based research, teaching, learning, and activism. Dr. Rhoades combines interests in multimedia art-making with a passion for issues of equity, diversity, and social justice. Her previous research and activism includes working with digital video artist Liv Gjestvang and a group of LGBTQ youth in Columbus, Ohio. They planned, produced, and distributed a documentary, *20 Straws: Growing Up Gay in the Midwest*. In *20 Straws*, LGBTQ youth tell their own stories, in contrast to LGBTQ adults reflecting on stereotypes, fears, and mostly negative experiences.

AnneMarie Swanlek, MA, Teaching and K–12 Public School Principal, is a leader in education administration for incarcerated youth and incarcerated adult students. For the past 16 years, she has been employed with the Pennsylvania Department of Corrections, and currently is the Education Administration Manager for the Bureau of Corrections Education. While employed in corrections, she was the school principal at the State Correctional Institution (SCI) Somerset (which has both young and adult male inmates), SCI Laurel Highlands (which has geriatric and terminally ill male inmates), and SCI Cresson (adult male inmates and those with mental health issues). She was also a teacher at SCI Pine Grove (male young adult offenders). She has completed the Pennsylvania Inspired Leadership program and the Pennsylvania Commonwealth Mentor Program.

Note

1 Founded in 1974, and named Very Special Arts in 1985, the organization was renamed VSA in 2010. In 2011, it merged with the Kennedy Center's Office on Accessibility to become the Department of VSA and Accessibility at the John F. Kennedy Center for the Performing Arts.

Acknowledgments

The idea for this book emerged from years of struggling to meet the needs of all students. With so few resources available in print form on art for young people who have experienced psychological trauma, we looked to each other, as professionals in the field, to share effective, successful ideas and strategies.

We appreciate the opportunity given to us by Taylor & Francis/ Routledge, to extend the benefits of our successful, innovative teaching strategies to a much wider audience.

Sincere thanks to our contributing authors, who graciously shared their insights.

Our appreciation to Joe Lagana for reminding us of the disconnection between research and classroom practice.

A special thanks to Beverly Gerber, who brought the three of us together to make this book a reality.

We can never thank Cathy Gerhold enough for completing the overwhelming job of copyediting. Not only was she thorough but consistently demonstrated kindness, compassion, and encouragement.

Thank you to Mike Podlipsky for his IT assistance.

Part I

Overview of Behaviors

Who Are the Children in Crisis?
Definitions and Demographics

1   Introduction and Purpose of this Book

Adrienne D. Hunter, Donalyn Heise, and Beverley H. Johns

Many children are living in crisis, struggling with trauma from natural or environmental disasters, domestic or societal violence, bullying, homelessness, human trafficking, or from lack of acceptance of sexual preference. Those who have experienced trauma may have been in the criminal justice system or have family members who are incarcerated. Children who have experienced trauma are less likely to succeed in school and are at risk of dropping out of school altogether (Steele & Kuban, 2002).

Children may suffer different types of trauma, including simple, or single-incident, trauma or exposure to repeated traumatic experiences over a prolonged period of time (Lawson & Quinn, 2013). More than one-quarter of children between birth and the age of five who have entered the child welfare system exhibit trauma symptoms. In 2011, 3.4 million referrals alleging child abuse were made to the child welfare system (Fusco & Cahalane, 2014). Childhood trauma results in a child feeling an overwhelming sense of terror and powerlessness (Steele & Kuban, 2002).

The number of children who are homeless is staggering. In 2009, the National Center on Family Homelessness reported that 1.6 million children a year were homeless, and the average age of a homeless child was 7 years; 59% of homeless people living in shelters are under age 18 (Substance Abuse and Mental Health Services Administration [SAMHSA], 2011). At least 7% of all fifth-graders have lived in a shelter or car at some point in their young lives. Children who are homeless are often at risk of poor health and negative academic and social outcomes (Moore & McArthur, 2011). They are often exposed to other traumatic circumstances such as domestic violence, community crime, and weak family structures. They are subjected to repeated traumatic experiences. Many have family members who struggle with mental health issues. Children who are homeless often lack the transportation and resources necessary for full participation in school.

Racial minorities and students with disabilities are disproportionately represented in incarceration. Students with disabilities comprise 8.6% of public school children, yet make up about 32% of youth in juvenile detention centers (Elias, 2013); 15% of jail inmates were homeless at some point in the year prior to their incarceration (SAMHSA, 2011), and 49% of homeless adults reported spending five or more days in a city or county jail.

It is critical that educators be trauma-informed and understand the impact that trauma has on childhood development and behavior. Whatever the type of school setting the child is in, art educators have the capacity to meet the needs of children who have suffered trauma.

Children who have experienced trauma may act out and may exhibit other behaviors such as withdrawal, fear, or agitation. Their behavior communicates the reality of their world and the experiences they have encountered.

The arts can play a vital role in the education of children who have suffered trauma, are at-risk, homeless, and/or incarcerated. Effective interventions involve children in their own healing so they can feel safe and empowered (Steele & Kuban, 2002). Yet many teachers feel ill-prepared to address the needs of these vulnerable populations. Those who are working with children need to understand effective interventions to help children heal (Walkley & Cox, 2013). This book provides an array of teaching techniques throughout, and each chapter features a summary of teaching tips.

Currently, very few resources exist relevant to art education for children who have suffered psychological trauma. This book provides insights for understanding and offers research-based best practices for enhancing the academic potential of this growing population.

The purposes of this book are to:

- increase understanding of the role of visual art education for enhancing learning for children living in crisis;
- provide resources for pre-service teacher candidates and professional development for art teachers, general educators, school counselors, and social workers;
- help art educators improve their ability to recognize students living in turmoil, and design effective, appropriate instruction, and classroom management, to meet their needs;
- contribute to the field of art education situated within social-cultural contexts;
- offer successful models of visual art education for diverse K-12 classrooms with specific attention to youth who face emotional, mental, behavioral, and physical challenges;
- describe a framework for meaningful visual art education for at-risk populations; and
- share the expertise of art educators, building on their experiences and best practices.

This book is organized in three sections: Part I gives an overview of behaviors, including definitions and demographics of children who have experienced trauma. It provides a framework of information for understanding children who are homeless or highly mobile, children who have suffered abuse, the human trafficking of children, and children who are incarcerated. An additional chapter provides recent brain research and implications for working with children exposed to trauma. Part II highlights art education in practice, offering strategies for creating a safe and supportive environment in the art room, as well as successful techniques for teaching art to children living in crisis. Part III identifies future directions for meeting the needs of all students, and includes information for successful collaborations and community-based art programs. We conclude with stories of success and how art teachers can make a difference in the lives of students who have suffered trauma.

References

Elias, S. (2013). *An after school program for at-risk youth: A grant proposal project* (unpublished doctoral dissertation, California State University, Long Beach).

Fusco, R. & Cahalane, H. (2014). Young children in the child welfare system: What factors contribute to trauma symptomology? *Child Welfare, 92*(5), 37–58.

Lawson, D. & Quinn, J. (2013). Complex trauma in children and adolescents: Evidence-based practice in clinical settings. *Journal of Clinical Psychology: In Session, 69*, 497–509.

Moore, T. & McArthur, M. (2011). 'Good for Kids': Children who have been homeless talk about school. *Australian Journal of Education, 55*(2), 147–160.

National Center on Family Homelessness, Substance Abuse and Mental Health Services Administration (2011). Current statistics on the prevalence and characteristics of those experiencing homelessness in the United States.

Steele, W. & Kuban, C. (2002). Healing trauma, building resilience: SITCAP in Action. *Reclaiming Children and Youth, 22*(4), 18–20.

Walkley, M. & Cox, T. (2013). Building trauma-informed schools and communities. *Children and Schools, 35*(2), 123–126.

2 Children Exposed to Trauma

Children in Crisis

Lisa Kay

This chapter provides an overview of information relevant to art educators concerning children exposed to traumatic events or who are in crisis, including different types of trauma and children's reactions to trauma. The at-risk spectrum is discussed, including definitions of the term as well as approaches to and alternative models for viewing students with such a label. A comparison of practices of an art teacher and art therapist who may work with children exposed to trauma is also covered. The chapter concludes with what art education can offer and what art teachers can do to assist children exposed to trauma or in crisis.

Introduction

When we think about children, trauma, and crisis, many word associations may come to mind: divorce, neglect, abuse, severe accidents, violence, homelessness, poverty, fire, and even death. Children are typically exposed to at least one traumatic event by age 16, but many will experience multiple traumatic events by that age (American Psychological Association, 2008; Costello, Erkanli, Fairbank, & Arnold, 2002). Some of these students may be homeless, in-crisis, or at-risk; often these students have had traumatic experiences that affect their ability to learn and function in social settings like schools and art rooms. Similar to children who experience war, Garbarino, Kosteiny, and Dubrow (1991) report that a high percentage of urban youth exposed to violence and living in poverty develop post-traumatic stress disorder (PTSD). They may also exhibit "fight or flight behavior" as a result of adverse childhood experiences, recurring trauma, or toxic stress.

Unfortunately, trauma exists in our lives, and surviving traumatic events is often scary. The term "trauma" is broad and complex. It can describe a wide range of experiences and events that can have a profound impact on students' social, emotional, and cognitive learning. Traumas range in severity, duration, and reactions and can include serious accidents, like a car wreck; illness; sexual or physical assault and abuse; violence (community, school shooting, terrorism, war); or a natural disaster like a fire, tornado, hurricane, or earthquake (National Center for PTSD, 2013). A trauma could be one event like the death of a special pet for a young student, the loss of a sibling for a middle school student, or the suicide of a peer for a high school student. According to the U.S. Centers for Disease Control (2003), a traumatic event is "marked by a sense of horror, helplessness, serious injury, or the threat of serious injury or death" (p. 1). These events are coupled with an overpowering inability to cope (van de Kolk, Bessel, & Fisher, 1995, as cited in Eisen & Goodman, 1998).

What Is Trauma?

The National Child Traumatic Stress Network (NCTSN, 2013) outlines different types of psychological or physical trauma, including early childhood trauma, traumatic stress, traumatic grief, complex trauma, toxic stress, and PTSD. Early childhood trauma is a traumatic experience that occurs between birth and age 6. Depending on what has occurred, the traumatic experience can have long-range impact on a child's health, education, and life. Traumatic stress can occur as a result of a painful medical treatment or the sudden loss of a loved one. Grief becomes traumatic when the trauma symptoms interfere with the child's ability to experience a typical process of bereavement. The combination of trauma plus grief symptoms can be so unrelenting that painful reminders can create scary thoughts, images, and/or memories for the child. Complex trauma refers to a child's response to multiple or prolonged traumatic events and the impact of this exposure in their development (NCTSN, 2013). The Center on the Developing Child at Harvard University (2013) refers to this type of trauma as a toxic stress. Toxic stress can be physical or emotional abuse, longstanding neglect, substance abuse or mental illness of a main caregiver, constant exposure to violence, and/or poverty. One of the key factors in toxic stress is the lack of adequate adult support in a child's life (National Scientific Council on the Developing Child, 2007). Toxic stress is pervasive and recurrent. Many children living in poverty experience this type of stress.

What Do Art Educators Need to Know about Trauma Reactions?

Children's reactions to trauma may be difficult to understand and/or confusing. Some behavioral reactions may not seem to connect directly with the trauma. Art teachers can help students through difficult times by understanding how children react to traumatic life events. It is important to note that children respond differently to traumatic events depending on their age and cognitive and emotional developmental levels. As a result, elementary, middle, and high school students may exhibit different behavioral reactions to trauma. For example, elementary students may appear nervous and afraid, worried about their own safety or others' safety, or become clingy with a teacher or parent. A minor incident may cause a huge upset. They may feel guilty, ashamed, or startle easily. Young students may retell the story of a traumatic event repeatedly and may worry that the event will happen again. Children may have difficulty expressing their feelings or concentrating. They also may have trouble sleeping (NCTSN, 2013; Zubenko, 2002). An art teacher may see changes in the student's overall school performance or projects, such as in art work.

Middle and high school children may appear or feel depressed, alone, and different from their peers. They may report that their life is out of control. Older students may discuss the specific details of the traumatic event and avoid places that remind them of the event. Students who have experienced trauma may show changes in behavior; develop eating disorders, begin self-harming behaviors like cutting or hair pulling; or start using or abusing alcohol or drugs. They may become sexually active or engage in risky behaviors (Zubenko, 2002). They may say that they feel nothing about what has happened (Lubit et al., 2003, as cited in Wolfe et al., 2006). Like younger children, adolescents may experience sleep disturbances (NCTSN, 2013). Traumatic stress can impact many levels of functioning—the psychological, physiological, social, emotional, and cognitive. Students may appear oppositional, defiant, hyperactive, uncooperative, and/or inattentive. Students may show signs of depression, anxiety, or seem withdrawn; have social conflicts with peers; exhibit angry outbursts; and act-out trauma via art work, stories, or through play.

What Do Educators Need to Know about PTSD?

When traumatic stress becomes disabling and lasts for an inordinate amount of time, children can develop a more serious disorder, like PTSD. PTSD is characterized by hypervigilance, exaggerated startle response, sleep disturbances accompanied by nightmares, chronic fears for safety, irritability and angry outbursts, difficulty concentrating, and repeated or perceived threats of harm. These behavioral, psychological, and physiological symptoms are often triggered by memories of severe trauma. Researchers report that rates of PTSD are higher in identified at-risk groups such as youth in foster care or abused and neglected children (McCloskey & Walker, 2000; Shumow & Perry, 2006).

According to Shumow and Perry (2006), students with PTSD live in a persistent state of vigilance, which is due to changes in the central nervous system.[1] Behavioral responses may manifest as inattentiveness, lack of focus, or oversensitivity to perceived environmental threats. Often, signs of hypervigilance are misunderstood and students are labeled as being oppositional, resistive, and uncooperative or are misdiagnosed and treated for other disorders, like attention deficit/hyperactivity disorder or anxiety, when in fact the symptoms are emotional reactions to trauma. In addition, "youth [at-risk] in urban schools who have sustained severe and repeated traumatization may have strong concerns about their own humanness, may appear frozen in a heightened state of arousal and [may] have great difficulty processing information verbally" (Steele, 2002, p. 1).

It is important for art educators to know that students who have experienced traumatic stress or who are diagnosed with PTSD may not have conscious control of their behavior. Some students have exaggerated fears for their safety and the safety of others. Teachers often misunderstand that these behavioral, psychological, and physiological symptoms are often triggered by memories of severe trauma. Shumow and Perry (2006) explain that students with PTSD and traumatic stress may appear inattentive, lack focus, or seem oversensitive to perceived threats in their environment. They may be in a persistent state of vigilance, watchfulness, or alertness caused by changes in their central nervous system. These students may also appear "more likely to engage in traumatic reenactment in which they incorporate aspects of the trauma into their daily lives and exhibit impulsive and aggressive behaviors" (Hamblen, 2005, p. 2), which may be troublesome or perplexing to educators. Students may have difficulty expressing their feelings and have trouble getting along with other students. Their behavior may be unpredictable; they hold their emotions in or lash out at others. While students' actions may appear deliberate, their behavior may not be intentional, and "ordinary" education is not always effective. However, art education, as subsequent chapters in this volume will illustrate, may provide a complementary approach.

Defining At-Risk

Students who have been exposed to trauma may be labeled "at-risk." At-risk, according to the *Merriam-Webster Online Dictionary* (2013), is defined as "endangered, troubled and in potentially dangerous situations or exposed to danger or harm of some kind." Hixson and Tinzmann contend that defining who students at-risk are can be controversial. Historically, students at-risk have been those students "whose appearance, language, culture, values, communities, and family structures did not match those of the dominant white culture that schools were designed to serve and support" (1990, p. 11). Traditionally, students who are labeled "at-risk" have been categorized using many terms, including educationally disadvantaged, culturally deprived, low income, drop out, alienated, marginalized, handicapped, disenfranchised, homeless, disabled, impoverished, underprivileged, low-achieving, and low-performing. "At-risk" describes multiple types of individuals, who for numerous reasons have experienced "failure in their careers as learners" (Presseison, 1991, p. 5).

According to Frostig and Essex (1998), students at-risk are children and adolescents prone to academic failure due to a variety of risk factors that include emotional disturbance and/or social adjustment problems that can be further compounded by family issues of neglect, violence, and/or poverty. Art educators O'Thearling and Bickley-Green explain the dissonance that may exist within the skill sets of students who are labeled at-risk:

From a social constructionist point of view, at-risk youths have assembled a reality that is dissonant with the general social structure. Within their cohort they may display social talents, skills, and knowledge that are as highly developed as those of more conventional students. Nevertheless, the at-risk apply these talents in an apparently contrary manner, and as a result they are marginalized.

(1996, p. 20)

Approaches for Working with Students At-Risk

There are no simple descriptors or categories that define this growing population of students (Presseison, 1991). Scholars McCann (1991) and Hixson and Tinzmann (1990) offer different perspectives. McCann's approach suggests that individual student characteristics, environmental circumstances, student abilities, and student behaviors define students at-risk. This approach emphasizes negative qualities: student deficiencies, deficient environments, self-destructive behaviors, and failure to meet educational standards. McCann adds that "these multiple definitions, with their multiple components have led to fragmentation in educational delivery systems" (1991, p. 15). Instead, Hixson and Tinzmann (1990) describe four approaches to identify students at-risk: predictive, descriptive, unilateral, and school factors. The predictive and descriptive approaches, which are the most common, focus on students' deficits, paralleling McCann's approach. The unilateral approach suggests that "all students are at risk in some way or another" (p. 13). School factors may include rigid scheduling, narrow curricula, emphasis on basic skills, unsuitable teaching materials and/or curricular decisions, tracking, isolated pull-out programs, inappropriate placement, controlling environments, and/or teacher/administrators' attitudes toward students at-risk and toward their parents.

The Spectrum of At-Risk

Few scholars, teachers, administrators, or students tagged with the label agree on a single definition of at-risk, yet most people have a preconceived notion of its meaning. Some art educators approach their work with students at-risk positively (Anderson, 1984; Losel, 2007; Metcalf, Gervais, Dase, & Griseta, 2005), while others consider the inclusion of students at-risk in their classrooms as an educational and professional dilemma (Poelstra, 1996). When there is no clear understanding of the term, confusion abounds. Students and their teachers, including art educators, are at a disadvantage. With the increasing preponderance and complexity of issues faced by contemporary youth, Hixson and Tinzmann (1990) offer clarity with their ecological approach, which is a unilateral model, that is, proactive, democratic, and does not assign sole responsibility or place blame on any one entity (student, parent, school, environment, community).

Art Teachers and Art Therapists Working with Children Exposed to Trauma

Art-making in an educational context with a supportive art teacher can foster some of these protective factors in students who have experienced psychological trauma and/or traumatic stress. Art educators are not art therapists; however, they can be role models who help students cope, gain mastery over some life experiences, and make sense of their world. Art educators can engage the students in art-making that focuses on the exploration of personal and social ideas and/or identities in visual form. They can provide opportunities for students in crisis to create art in a social context that provides support. Art education can offer students alternative ways to communicate and express feelings, develop a greater sense of who they are as individuals, and assist them in making positive connections with others (Kay, 2008). Specifically, transformational art education programs with students who struggle with issues of self-esteem, mental health, and past traumas can have healing value and will be discussed later in the book.

Both art educators and art therapists are concerned for the social and emotional well-being of their students. Art teachers teach students who have been exposed to trauma; art therapists treat children and adolescents who have been exposed to trauma. Both educators and therapists develop plans with goals and objectives for lessons or treatment plans and keep ongoing records of students' progress.

Conclusion

The good news is there is hope; things can change. Children's brains are amazingly pliable; children are resilient. There is a "window of opportunity" until the ages of 25 to 30 for damage to brain pathways to rebuild (Bloome, 2015). Scholars Southwick and Charney (2012) outline ten factors that can contribute to the development of resilience. Several of these include optimism, confronting fears, meaning and purpose, social support, role models, and cognitive and emotional flexibility. Other protective factors that help children develop resilience include at least one stable, caring, supportive relationship; gaining mastery over experiences; making sense of their world; learning coping skills; learning to regulate emotions; and affirming one's faith or cultural traditions (Bloome, 2015).

This chapter presented important information regarding different types of trauma, children's reactions to traumatic events, and an overview of the spectrum of "at-risk." The differences between educational and therapeutic practices of an art teacher and art therapist practice were compared. As art teachers consider the impact of trauma on students in their teaching settings, the following ten tips may help guide their pedagogy and practice when working with children who have been exposed to psychological trauma and children in crisis.

Ten Teaching Tips

1 Understand how traumatic events impact children's growth, development, and learning.
2 Recognize students' responses to trauma are based on their age and developmental levels.
3 Help restore a sense of balance in students' lives when they are faced with a traumatic event.
4 Know the boundaries of your practice as an art educator when working with students who have been exposed to trauma or who are in crisis.
5 Reassure students (if you can) that an event is over and they are safe.
6 Develop strong supportive relationships with students.
7 Help students verbalize and control emotions so they do not feel isolated.
8 Talk to the classroom teacher, counselor or principal, parents or caregivers if you have concerns about a student's thoughts that appear to be impeding their ability to focus or learn.
9 Provide opportunities for individual's creative expression within a social context.
10 Advocate for your students; make referrals when needed; consult with an art therapist.

Note

1 See Chapter 10, Neurological Impact of Trauma.

References

American Psychological Association Presidential Task Force on Posttraumatic Stress Disorder and Trauma in Children and Adolescent (2008). *Children and Trauma: Update for Mental Health Professionals*. Washington, D.C.: American Psychological Association. Retrieved June 5, 2015, from APA.org.

Anderson, F. A. (1984). Mainstreaming art as well as children. *Art Education, 28(8)*, 26–29.

Bloome, S. (2015). Biological and psychological factors: Building children's capacities to improve. Paper presented at Children's Crisis Treatment Center's Panel on *Children's Recovery from Adverse Experiences: Is It Luck or Something Else?* Philadelphia, PA.

Center on the Developing Child at Harvard University (2013). Retrieved June 9, 2017, from thecenterforchilddevelopment.com/toxic-stress-and-development-in-children.

Costello, E. J., Erkanli, A., Fairbank, J. A., & Angold, A. (2002). The prevalence of potentially traumatic events in childhood and adolescence. *Journal of Traumatic Stress, 15*, 99–112.

Eisen, M. L., & Goodman, G. S. (1998). Trauma, memory, and suggestibility in children. *Development and Psychopathology, 10,* 717–738.

Frostig, K., & Essex, M. (1998). *Expressive Arts Therapies in Schools: A Supervision and Program Guide.* Springfield, IL: Charles C. Thomas.

Garbarino, J., Kostelny, K., & Dubrow, N. (1991). *No Place To Be a Child: Growing Up in a War Zone.* New York, NY: Lexington.

Hamblen, J. (2005). PTSD in children and adolescents. *A National Center for PTSD Fact Sheet.* Retrieved June 10, 2017 from https://www.ptsd.va.gov/ professional/treatment/children/ptsd_in_children_and_adolescents_overview_ for_professionals.asp.

Hixson, J., & Tinzmann, M. B. (1990). Who are the "at-risk" students of the 1990s? *North Central Regional Educational Laboratory Monograph,* 1–17. Oak Brook, IL.

Kay, L. (2008). *Art Education Pedagogy and Practice with Adolescent Students At-Risk in Alternative High Schools* (unpublished doctoral dissertation.) Northern Illinois University, DeKalb, IL.

Kay, L., & Wolf, D. (2017). Artful coalitions: Challenging adverse adolescent experiences. *Art Education 70(5),* 26–33. Alexandria, VA: National Art Education Association.

Losel, S. D. (2006). Students with physical disabilities. In B. L. Gerber & D. P. Guay (Eds.), *Reaching and Teaching Students with Special Needs through Art* (pp. 107–126). Alexandria, VA: National Art Education Association.

Merriam-Webster Online Dictionary (2007). "At-risk." Retrieved May 8, 2013, from http://www.meriam-webster.com/dictionary/at-risk.

McCann, R. A. (1991). At-risk students: Defining the problem. In K. M. Kershner & J. A. Connolly (Eds.), *At-Risk Students and School Restructuring* (pp. 13–16). Washington, D.C.: Office of Educational Research and Improvement.

McCloskey, L., & Walker, M. (2000). Post-traumatic stress in children exposed to violence and single event trauma. *Journal of the American Academy of Child and Adolescent Psychiatry, 39(1),* 108–115.

National Center for PTSD, U.S. Department of Veteran Affairs (2006). Retrieved April 10, 2006, from PTSD.va.gov.

National Child Traumatic Stress Network (2013). Age-related reactions to a traumatic event. Retrieved September 15, 2013, from ntcsn.org.

National Scientific Council on the Developing Child (2005). Excessive stress disrupts the architecture of the developing brain: Working paper no. 3. Retrieved July 15, 2013, from Developingchild.harvard.edu.

O'Thearling, S., & Bickley-Green, C. A. (1996). Art education and at-risk youth: Enabling factors of visual expression. *Visual Art Research* (pp. 20–25). Champaign Urbana, IL: Board of Trustees of the University of Illinois.

Presseison, B. (1991). At-risk students: Defining a population. In K. M. Kershner & J. A. Connolly (Eds.), *At-Risk Students and School Restructuring* (pp. 5–11). Washington, D.C.: Office of Educational Research and Improvement.

Shumow, L., & Perry, B. (2006). Literature review on trauma, stress, and its implications for the education of children in foster care. Paper presented at the Symposium on Trauma, Stress, and the Education of Children and Youth in Foster Care. Naperville, IL.

Southwick, S. M., & Charney, D. S. (2012). The science of resilience: Implications for the prevention and treatment of depression. *Science Magazine, 338(6103),* 79–82.

Steele, W. (2002). Trauma's impact on learning and behavior: A case for intervention in schools. *Trauma and Loss Journal*, *2(2)*, 1–16. Retrieved April 1, 2006, from tlcinstitute.org.

U.S. Centers for Disease Control and Prevention (2003). Coping with a traumatic event: Information for the public. Accessed April 12, 2007, from bt.cdc.gov/masscasualties.

Wolfe, D. A., Rawana, J. S., & Chiodo, D. (2006). Abuse and trauma. In D. A. Wolfe & E. J. Mash (Eds.), *Behavioral and Emotional Disorders in Adolescents* (pp. 642–671). New York, NY: Guilford.

Zubenko, W. N. (2002). Developmental issues in stress and crisis. In W. N. Zubenko & J. Capozzoli (Eds.), *Children and Disasters: A Practical Guide to Healing and Recovery* (pp. 85–100). New York, NY: Oxford University Press.

3 Who Are Homeless Children?

Dona Anderson and Matthew Adams

Homeless students face complex and interrelated challenges, which are often unique to their experiences in unstable housing situations. This chapter provides art educators interested in engaging homeless students with comprehensive information on homelessness and its effects, enabling readers to identify homeless students and help them thrive.

Due to the stigma, lack of awareness, and often hidden nature of homelessness, students experiencing homelessness can be difficult to identify. Understanding the demographics of homeless children and their families can help educators better distinguish students in need. Nationally, the typical homeless family consists of a young single mother who is a racial or ethnic minority (although this varies by locality) with one or two young children who lives doubled-up with family or friends. While many families in urban areas can access homeless shelters, families in rural locales are more likely to live doubled-up due to a dearth of available services. Homeless families often face a variety of unstable housing environments, with short stays in doubled-up situations and different housing programs common. Families who live in shelter are also at risk of being homeless multiple times. In their efforts to achieve self-sufficiency, homeless families struggle to find employment and, even when they do, must often rely upon public assistance benefits to supplement their extremely low incomes.

Family ecology significantly influences child development and well-being. Therefore, the multiple risk factors that homeless parents face are also discussed in this chapter. Homeless mothers are more likely than their housed peers to lack a high school diploma, and they experience domestic violence, mental illness, and substance abuse at higher rates. Lack of access to medical care can result in poorer health outcomes and higher rates of HIV/AIDS infection among homeless parents. Female veterans with children are more susceptible to mental health issues, placing them at increased risk of becoming homeless.

For these and many other reasons, homeless children are more likely than their housed peers to suffer from developmental delays; chronic and acute health problems; and behavioral, emotional, and mental health issues. Although homeless students are more prone to display emotional or behavioral problems and have learning disabilities, they are also less likely to receive special educational services. Moreover, homeless children suffer from poorer health even before birth, while the conditions of homelessness make them more susceptible to chronic and acute illnesses. Limited access to a nutritious diet negatively affects homeless students' classroom performance. Abuse or exposure to family and community violence is often an additional stressor. Due to an unstable childhood and a lack of safe alternatives, an older homeless student, when unaccompanied by a parent or guardian, can be more predisposed to risky behaviors than his or her housed peers. On the other end of the age spectrum, young homeless children are enrolled at lower rates in high-quality early childhood education programs than their peers, even though these programs can mitigate some of the devastating effects of homelessness.

What Is the Definition of Homelessness?

Any child or youth who lacks a fixed, regular, and adequate nighttime residence is considered by the U.S. Department of Education (ED) to be homeless (McKinney-Vento Homeless Education Assistance Improvements Act; McKinney-Vento, 2001, 2010). This includes students residing in emergency or transitional shelters, as well as those staying in substandard housing, abandoned buildings, public spaces, parks, cars, bus or train stations, or similar public or private settings that are not designated for or typically used as regular living arrangements. ED's definition also includes unstable housing situations not ordinarily perceived by the public to be forms of homelessness. These tenuous living situations include staying doubled-up with family, friends, or others due to economic hardship, loss of housing, or similar reasons. In addition, students sleeping in hotels or motels, trailer parks, or camping grounds due to the lack of alternative adequate accommodations, and children who are abandoned in hospitals are also considered to be homeless due to the temporary nature of these arrangements. Migratory children are defined as homeless if staying in any of these situations.

Federal legislation in the form of the McKinney-Vento Act contains important provisions to allow every homeless student equal access to the same free, appropriate public education as provided to children and youth in stable homes. The act disburses funds to states in order to uphold the rights of homeless students, institute an office to oversee such activities within a state educational agency, develop and implement a state plan to meet the needs of homeless students, and create professional development programs to raise awareness of and strengthen school staff's ability to respond to students' needs. The law prohibits the stigmatization of homeless students by school personnel and the segregation of homeless students into separate schools, classrooms, or programs.

Every state and local educational agency must designate a homeless liaison that can sufficiently carry out their duties to guarantee that homeless students are immediately enrolled in school despite enrollment deadlines or lack of parental consent, immunization records, or prior school or other required documentation, and that they do not face any additional barriers to success in school due to their housing status. Liaisons can provide homeless students with school supplies, clothing, pupil services or referrals to such services (including violence-prevention counseling), before- and after-school services, mentoring, and summer and other educational programs. To avoid the additional educational disruption of a school transfer, a liaison must also coordinate transportation to a homeless child's school of origin, unless it is against the wishes of the parent, regardless of the district in which the child currently resides. Liaisons also work to connect homeless students with other educational services for which they are eligible, including Head Start and other programs administered by local educational agencies, making referrals to housing, health care, dental, mental health, and related services as appropriate.

An important challenge that liaisons face is that the U.S. Department of Housing and Urban Development (HUD), which funds most emergency-housing services, uses a definition of homelessness that differs from that of ED (Homeless Emergency Assistance and Rapid Transition to Housing Act of 2009). While HUD considers families residing in places not meant for human habitation or in homeless shelters to be unconditionally homeless, its definition of who among children in doubled-up or hotel/motel situations is homeless is more limited. Students staying doubled-up may receive HUD-funded emergency housing and related services only if they are losing their living arrangement within the next 14 days. The same requirement applies to children residing in hotels or motels, unless the units are paid for by charitable or governmental organizations. Exceptions are made for families in these situations if they meet all three of the following conditions: did not hold a lease within the last 60 days; moved twice; and have either chronic disabilities or physical or mental conditions, a disabled child, histories of domestic violence or childhood abuse, substance addiction, or at least two severe barriers to employment. These complex differences in definitions between federal agencies continue to be a logistical and bureaucratic obstacle to providing services to homeless students.

What Are the Demographics of Homeless Students?

More than 1.3 million children experienced homelessness during the 2013–2014 school year. Three-fourths (75%) of homeless students lived doubled-up with family or friends, 15% resided in shelters, and 6% stayed temporarily in hotels or motels; 3%, or 45,000 students, lived unsheltered on the streets or in other places not fit for human habitation (ED, 2015b).

Over 2% of all students, or one in every 37, was homeless in the school year 2013–2014 (see Figure 3.1, ED, 2015b; National Center for Education Statistics, NCES, 2014b). Connecticut had the lowest rate of

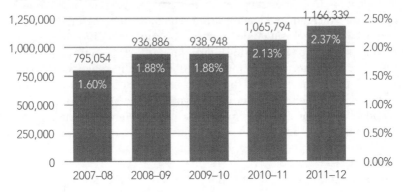

Figure 3.1 "Number and Percentage of Students Experiencing Homelessness"

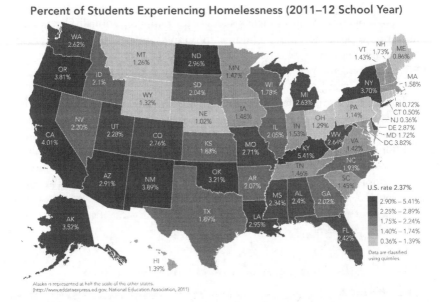

Figure 3.2 "Percentage of Students Experiencing Homelessness (2013–14 School Year)"

student homelessness at 0.5%, while at 5%, New York had the highest. California and New York accounted for one-third (33%) of all homeless students nationwide. Conversely, states in New England and the northern Mountain and Great Plains regions had both the fewest homeless students and the lowest rates (see Figure 3.2; ED, 2015b; NCES, 2014b). While city-level data are scarce, New York City had a rate (9%) three times the national average (3%) in school year 2013–2014 (NCES, 2014a; New York State Technical and Education Assistance Center for Homeless Students, 2015). Chicago's rate (6%) was double that of the nation; however, rates in other large urban areas, including Dallas (2%) and Los Angeles (2%), were less than the national average (NCES, 2014a; see also Chicago Coalition for the Homeless, 2014; Dallas Independent School District, 2014; Los Angeles Unified School District, 2014).

The rate of homelessness also differs across school grades. Younger students are more likely to be homeless than older students, as limited access to child care makes families with younger children more vulnerable to homelessness (Nunez & Adams, 2014). With the exception of slight increases in the 9th and 12th grades, the rate of student homelessness steadily decreases from a high of nearly 4% among preschoolers to a low of almost half that in the 11th grade (see Figure 3.3; ED, 2015a; NCES, 2014b).

Since school year 2007–2008, the first year of the Great Recession, the number of homeless students has increased by nearly three-fourths (71%). Led by the District of Columbia at 275%, 31 states and the District of Columbia saw an increase in student homelessness that surpassed the national rate between the 2007–2008 and 2013–2014 school years. Only two states, Louisiana and New Jersey, had decreases in the number of homeless students, the reasons for which are unknown. In general, states in

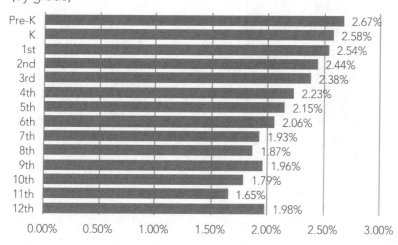

Percent of Students Homeless in School Year 2010–11
(by grade)

Grade	Percent
Pre-K	2.67%
K	2.58%
1st	2.54%
2nd	2.44%
3rd	2.38%
4th	2.23%
5th	2.15%
6th	2.06%
7th	1.93%
8th	1.87%
9th	1.96%
10th	1.79%
11th	1.65%
12th	1.98%

Figure 3.3 "Percentage of Students Homeless in School Year 2013–14 (by grade)"

Percent Change in Student Homelessness (2007–08 to 2011–12)

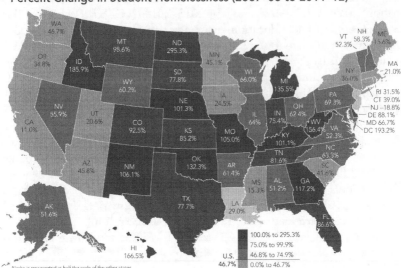

Figure 3.4 "Percentage Change in Student Homelessness (2007–08 to 2013–14)"

Percent Change in the Number of Homeless Students From Prior School Year

(by current school year)

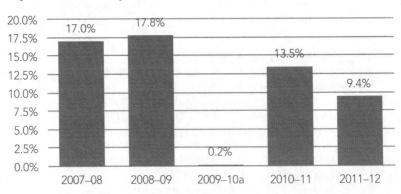

Figure 3.5 "Percentage Change in the Number of Homeless Students From the Prior School Years"

the Mountain, Midwest, and Great Plains experienced the highest increases, while states in New England and the West saw more modest upticks (see Figure 3.4, ED, 2015b).

During the two school years that coincided with the economic downturn, student homelessness increased 17% in 2007–2008 and 18% in 2008–2009 (see Figure 3.5, ED, 2015b; National Center for Homeless Education, NCHE, 2010). Even after the official end of the recession in June 2009, the number of homeless students has continued to grow. At first glance, the number of homeless students appeared to have increased only slightly during school year 2009–2010; however, California underreported its numbers that year. Excluding California, the number of homeless students actually rose by 15% (ED, 2015b; NCHE, 2010).

In a 2010 survey, two-thirds (62%) of state and local educational agencies attributed the economic downturn as the primary cause of the sharp rise in the number of homeless students reported. However, two-fifths (40%) of educators attributed the increase to improved community awareness, and one-third (33%) to a greater ability to identify students who are homeless (National Association for the Education of Homeless Children and Youth, NAEHCY, & First Focus, 2010). Educators have been particularly successful at identifying students living doubled-up with family or friends, who often do not self-identify as homeless and are more challenging to recognize. The number of homeless students living doubled-up more than doubled (104%) between 2007–2008 and 2013–2014, far outpacing the increase of students in shelters (26%) and those in hotels or motels (45%) (ED, 2015b; NCHE, 2010).

Federal funding is another significant factor in how many homeless students are identified and served. Although school districts are required by law to provide the same services to homeless students regardless of available monies, districts receiving federal McKinney-Vento dollars serve only two-thirds (64%) of all known homeless students (ED, 2015b). Only one-quarter (25%) of all school districts receive such federal funding annually (NCHE, 2015). New legislation amending McKinney-Vento seeks to remedy these financial shortfalls by increasing the authorized level of funding and making Title I, Part A monies available to serve homeless students (Every Student Succeeds Act of 2015).

What Are the Demographics of Homeless Children and Their Families?

An estimated 517,000 parents and children accessed emergency or transitional shelter over the course of 2014, representing a 9% increase since the Great Recession began in 2007 (HUD, 2015a). Although estimates vary across studies, 2.1 million family members lived doubled-up in 2008, four times more than those who entered homeless shelters over the course of that same year (National Alliance to End Homelessness, NAEH, 2010; HUD, 2015a). On a single day in January 2015, at least 20,400 family members lived unsheltered; however, enumerations of families living on the streets, under bridges, or in abandoned buildings, cars, camp sites, wooded areas, and other places not meant for human habitation are likely underestimates (HUD, 2015b). The number of homeless families who stayed temporarily in hotels or motels is not known.

Little is understood regarding the demographics of homeless families living doubled-up, in hotels or motels, or on the streets, but it can be assumed that they are similar to those of families who stay in homeless shelters. Only one-fifth (19%) of families in 2014 entered shelter directly from their own rented or owned housing; two-fifths (41%) previously lived doubled-up with family or friends. The night before entering shelter, 30% came from other shelter facilities, permanent supportive housing, or unsheltered locations, while 8% lived in other places, including hotels and motels. Only 2% of families were discharged into homeless situations directly from institutional settings, such as correctional and psychiatric facilities, foster care, and hospitals (HUD, 2015a).

The demographics of homeless families living in shelter differ from those of poor but stably housed families and those in the general family population. Parents in homeless families are much more likely to be female (78%) when compared with housed poor families (64%) and families overall (55%). Homeless parents are also younger than parents in non-homeless poor families or parents overall, although the national average or median age of homeless parents is not known (HUD, 2015a).

Homeless families in shelter have smaller household sizes than other poor families or families overall. One-quarter (23%) of homeless families consist of a single mother with one child, a rate nearly six times higher than families in the general population (4%). Homeless families are also almost half as likely as other poor families to consist of five or more people (26% versus 48%, respectively). Given the prevalence of younger mothers and smaller families within the homeless population, homeless children are more likely to be younger. Half (50%) of homeless children living in shelters are preschool-aged (under 6 years of age), while over one-third (36%) are elementary school-aged (6 to 12), and 14% are middle-school and high-school-aged (13 to 17) (HUD, 2015a).

Due to interrelated barriers to economic self-sufficiency that vary by racial and ethnic group, including generational poverty and institutionalized discrimination, minority families are more likely to experience homelessness. Facing the most severe barriers to housing stability, black and Native American or Native Alaskan families are greatly overrepresented in shelter statistics compared to their share of the general population. Hispanic families are slightly underrepresented, while white and Asian households are significantly underrepresented. In comparison to the rate at which white families experience homelessness, black, Native American or Native Alaskan, and Hispanic families are ten, seven, and three times more likely to live in homeless shelters, respectively (HUD, 2015a; Institute for Children, Poverty, and Homelessness, ICPH, 2015; U.S. Census Bureau, 2014).

Homelessness is often considered to be an urban issue, as sheltered urban families outnumber suburban and rural families two to one. Homeless families are also more likely to live in principal cities (64%), compared with poor families (35%) and families in the general population (23%). However, between 2007 and 2014, the number of homeless parents and children living in rural and suburban areas increased by half (48%), while those in urban areas decreased by 5% (HUD, 2015a). This trend is due in part to the movement of more low-income households from urban to suburban areas over the past decade (Metropolitan Policy Program at Brookings, 2010). With the majority of services centered in urban and suburban locales, lack of transportation is a significant barrier for families experiencing rural homelessness, leaving them more likely to live doubled-up with family or friends. Only 6% of homeless families access shelter in rural locations, despite those areas having higher family poverty rates than cities (ICPH, 2013).

Regardless of their geographic locale, parents and children enduring homelessness tend to face housing instability frequently. Only one-fifth (18%) of families who enter shelter lived in their prior residence for one year or more; one-third (36%) had stable housing for less than one month; with another one-quarter (24%) of families relocating between one and three months prior to shelter entry. Many families living in emergency shelter, where the average length of stay is 81 days, move into transitional housing and stay on average for an additional six months (175 days) (HUD, 2015a). Furthermore, families who live in shelter are at risk of returning after they leave (Shinn, 2013; Vera Institute of Justice, 2005).

In the pursuit of affordable housing, money represents an omnipresent struggle for homeless parents. Only one-quarter (25%) of all adults (including those who have children and those who do not) who exit shelter, supportive housing, or rental-assistance programs earn income from employment. Even when parents work, their jobs typically do not pay a living wage or provide health insurance or other benefits. As a result, homeless parents depend on benefits from the larger social safety net. However, only 17% of homeless adults receive cash income from either the federal Temporary Assistance for Needy Families or local general public-assistance programs (HUD, 2012). Two in five (39%) are enrolled in the Supplemental Nutrition Assistance Program, formerly known as food stamps, which has been shown to decrease food insecurity among homeless households (HUD, 2012; Lee & Greif, 2008). One-fifth (20%) receive Medicaid benefits, while just 1% of adults with incomes too high to qualify for Medicaid receive health care for their children through the Children's Health Insurance Program (HUD, 2012). Homeless parents are twice as likely as adults in the general family population to have a disability (21% versus 9%), and one-fifth (20%) of homeless adults are enrolled in either the Supplemental Security Income or Social Security Disability Insurance programs (HUD, 2012, 2015a). Nevertheless, due to interrelated barriers that vary by mainstream benefit programs, including complicated application processes and a lack of awareness, one-quarter (22%) of adults exit federal homelessness housing programs with no source of income (HUD, 2012). Lacking income, homeless parents are likely to continue to experience housing instability.

What Challenges Do Homeless Parents Face?

Studies estimate that between 39% and 65% of homeless mothers do not have a high school diploma or an equivalent degree, compared with 26% of poor housed mothers and 16% of all single mothers (U.S. Census Bureau, 2015; U.S. Department of Health and Human Services, HHS, 2007). Differences also exist between families at-risk of homelessness and those who experience it; one report found that half (48%) of at-risk families did not graduate from high school, compared with 60% of homeless parents (ICPH, 2011). A lower level of education often hinders parents' ability to obtain employment sufficient to support a family and maintain stable housing. Higher educational attainment is strongly correlated with increased annual earnings; workers with bachelor's degrees earn nearly twice as much as those with high school diplomas over the course of 40 years. Low educational attainment is often multigenerational, as children of parents without high school diplomas are more likely to drop out of school themselves (Civic Enterprises, 2006).

Nearly all (92%) homeless mothers experience severe physical and/or sexual abuse during their lifetimes, compared with one-quarter (26%) of all women (Bassuk et al., 1996; U.S. Department of Justice, 2000). According to a Minnesota study, one in three (31%) women cited domestic violence as a primary cause of her homelessness. Half (48%) of homeless women surveyed reported staying in abusive relationships because they had nowhere else to go (Wilder Research, 2010). Since women may attempt to leave their abusers several times before doing so successfully, their children may experience multiple episodes of homelessness. Furthermore, one in six (16%) mothers seeking housing assistance nationwide was not provided shelter on a single day in September 2015 (National Network to End Domestic Violence, NNEDV, 2016). Women facing violence also experience high rates of depression, post-traumatic stress disorder (PTSD), and substance abuse. Half (47%) of women facing domestic violence also suffer from depression, and two-thirds (64%) from PTSD. Survivors are 9 to 15 times more likely to abuse drugs and alcohol than women who have not suffered from violence (Golding, 1999; National Coalition against Domestic Violence, n.d.).

Homeless mothers have a higher lifetime rate of substance abuse than low-income housed mothers (41% versus 35%) and abuse substances at twice the rate of women overall (20%) (Bassuk et al., 1998). Poor families sometimes use drugs and alcohol as coping mechanisms; between one-third and two-thirds of all children who enter the child welfare system do so in part because of parental substance abuse (HHS, 1999a). Mothers who abuse drugs and alcohol may deliver babies with serious medical and neurobehavioral problems, and their babies have a heightened risk of low birth weight (Weinreb, 1990). Substance abuse is also linked with violence; homeless women in Los Angeles County who experienced either physical or sexual violence abused drugs and alcohol at three times the rate (24%) of women who were not victimized (8%) (Wenzel et al., 2000).

Homelessness is also associated with mental illness. Homeless mothers in Massachusetts were found to have psychiatric disabilities at a rate nearly three times higher than that of their housed peers (Buckner et al., 1993). Parents' psychological distress impacts children's emotional and behavioral health, although more research on long-term outcomes is needed. Homeless families with mentally ill parents are more likely to experience long-term homelessness and are at a greater risk of family separation. Mothers with mental illness are also more vulnerable to physical health problems, given their limited ability to maintain self-care and practice risk reduction (National Health Care for the Homeless Council, NHCHC, 2000).

For poor, uninsured families, prohibitively high medical expenses from serious injury or illness can lead to housing instability. Two-thirds (62%) of all personal bankruptcies are due to health problems (Himmelstein et al., 2009; NHCHC, 2010). Families without regular preventive and primary care are more likely to overuse expensive emergency services, which are less effective at treating long-term illnesses (National Association of Community Health Centers, 2014).

While no separate data exist for parents, homeless adults experience serious illness and injury at three to six times the rate of the general population. The risk and severity of certain medical conditions are also exacerbated by homelessness, such as heart disease, upper respiratory infections, gastrointestinal problems, hypertension, and HIV/AIDS. Proper nutrition, which can help prevent many chronic diseases, is challenging for homeless parents to maintain. Many homeless families typically eat diets high in fat, cholesterol, and sugar, due to limited income and little access to nutritious foods (NHCHC, 2010).

With limited access to screenings and preventative care, studies estimate that homeless persons are three to nine times more likely to be infected with HIV/AIDS than their housed peers (NHCHC, 2000, 2012). The effects of the disease, including the high cost of health care and loss of employment due to discrimination or extended absence, can heighten the risk of homelessness; almost 70% of persons with HIV/AIDS experience housing instability at least once (Aidala et al., 2007). Conversely, homelessness is linked with HIV-risk behaviors through substance abuse; almost one-third (31%) of HIV-positive homeless-clinic clients in Florida were injecting drug users, three times higher than the overall national rate (12%) (Hall et al., 2008; Shultz et al., 1999).

Female veterans are most at risk of homelessness when they are single parents of young children but, overall, are two to four times more likely to become homeless than the general female population (Gamache et al., 2003;

National Center on Homelessness Among Veterans, 2011). Half (53%) of homeless female veterans have at least one major mental disorder, which some research attributes to high rates (20%–48%) of sexual trauma suffered in the military (Buckner et al., 1993; U.S. Department of Labor, DOL, 2011). Three-fourths (74%) of homeless female veterans experience PTSD, which has been associated with behavioral and social problems in their children (Washington et al., 2010). One-fifth (19%) of female veterans suffer from domestic violence, while two-thirds (62%) of all Health Care for Homeless Veterans clients have substance-use disorders (DOL, 2011). However, homeless veteran families are twice as likely to have two parents present than homeless non-veteran families (54% and 22%, respectively) (HUD & U.S. Department of Veterans' Affairs, 2011).

What Are the Effects of Homelessness on Children?

Homeless students face an inordinate amount of stress, much of it at toxic levels. Doubled-up arrangements may end abruptly; children may constantly fear that they will be forced to leave the places where they are staying. Mothers may tolerate abusive relationships, placing their children and themselves at risk, to avoid losing housing. Shelter environments can be vastly different depending on service providers, with some fostering caring environments and others offering less supportive settings. Even the physical structure of shelters varies widely, from more stressful large, congregate barracks-style settings, to communal living spaces shared with two or three families, to private rooms. Homeless children may also encounter the stress of short or medium time limits on how long they may stay in shelter. Shelters—and the hotels or motels that homeless families can afford—are usually in less desirable neighborhoods that offer few opportunities for children to safely relax and play. Furthermore, shelter staff often focus predominately on the needs of parents in order to resolve their homelessness and often lack the time and resources to address the needs of children (Nunez & Adams, 2014).

Homeless children experience three times the rate of emotional or behavioral problems of children not facing housing instability. As a reaction to the stressors associated with homelessness, children are often insecure, distrusting, irritable, lethargic, anxious, and depressed and frequently exhibit aggression or hostility, which can lead to developmental delays (Family Housing Fund, 1999). Research indicates that the multiple risk factors that homeless children experience have multiplicative rather than additive effects, regardless of whether they occur in isolation or accrue over time (Brooks, 2006; Masten, 2001). Children with two risk factors display four times as many behavioral problems as children with no risk factors or one risk factor (McFarlane et al., 2003; Rutter, 1979; Trentacosta et al., 2008).

Homeless children have twice the rate of learning disabilities (such as speech delays and below-grade reading or math achievement) of their housed peers (Family Housing Fund, 1999; Marchmont, 2010; My Child without Limits Advisory Committee, 2009; National Dissemination Center for Children with Disabilities, NICHCY, 2012). Despite these heightened vulnerabilities, studies indicate that homeless students with disabilities (broadly defined as five types of impairments: speech or language, cognitive, behavioral or emotional, sensory, or physical) are less likely than other students to receive assessments or special education services (Family Housing Fund, 1999; NICHCY, 2012; Zima et al., 1997). Because homeless students have higher rates of developmental delays and learning impairments, the rate at which they have disabilities would be expected to be much higher than that for the general student population. However, national rates are only 4% higher—17% versus 13%—for the 2013–2014 school year (NCES, 2014a, 2014b; NCHE, 2015).

Conditions commonly related to child homelessness, such as sleep deprivation, depression, and hunger, hinder learning and classroom performance. This can make it difficult for educators to distinguish between the harmful effects of homelessness and learning disabilities. A homeless student can be diagnosed as having a disability when none is present. At the same time, a homeless student's disability can also go unnoticed, if his or her poor classroom performance is attributed only to housing instability. Both errors can lead to children being placed in inappropriate classroom settings, impacting their educational attainment for the duration of their academic careers (Family Housing Fund, 1999; Homeless Children's Education Fund, Duquesne University School of Education, & Allegheny County Department of Human Services, 2009; NAEHCY, 2013; National Association of State Directors of Special Education, 2008; National Center for Children and Poverty, 2009; Smith, 2010).

The poor health of homeless students also hampers classroom performance; they suffer from chronic illnesses (such as neurological disorders and heart disease) and acute illnesses (including minor upper respiratory infections) at twice the rate of stably housed students (Wright & Weber, 1987). Homeless children are also seven times more likely to experience iron deficiencies that can lead to anemia (Family Housing Fund, 1999). One of the most prevalent nutritional issues is obesity; one in eight homeless preschoolers in a Los Angeles study was obese (Wood et al., 1990).

Even before birth, the health of children is inextricably linked to that of their mothers. Compared with 15% of women in the general population, half (50%) of homeless women had not had a prenatal visit in the first trimester of pregnancy. Lack of access to prenatal care, coupled with substance abuse, increases the risk of adverse birth outcomes such as low birth weight; one-fifth of homeless women report drug and alcohol abuse during pregnancy (Family Housing Fund, 1999). Even in the absence of substance abuse, the experience of homelessness alone is associated with low birth weight (Stein et al., 2007).

Poor housing conditions also influence the health of homeless children. Children born in low-income areas experience lower birth weights than those in neighborhoods with higher incomes. Many homeless families live in or have resided in old, overcrowded buildings with high exposure to tobacco smoke, air pollution, and other allergens. One-third (33%) of children in New York City shelters are affected by asthma when compared with 10% of children nationwide (Grant et al., 2007a; HHS, 2011).

Despite their health risks, homeless children have limited access to ongoing health care. As a result, homeless or highly mobile children are more likely than at-risk or poor but stably housed children to visit the emergency room (ICPH, 2012b). Furthermore, one-fifth (22%) of children in New York City shelters lack essential immunizations, while one-third (33%) of homeless children nationwide never visit a dentist (Grant et al., 2007b; Urban Institute, 1999).

Many risks associated with poor health are due to food insecurity. Homeless households are likely to experience higher levels of food insecurity—defined as limited or unstable availability of adequate amounts of nutritious and safe food for an active, healthy life—than their housed, low-income peers (Anderson, 1990; Gundersen et al., 2003; Lee & Greif, 2008; U.S. Department of Agriculture, 2016). While two in five (43%) poor families are food-insecure, the prevalence of food insecurity among homeless families is unknown (U.S. Department of Agriculture, 2016). In fact, little is known regarding differences between food-insecure homeless and other poor children.

Low-income children suffering from food insecurity experience worse physical and mental health, greater developmental delays, and lower academic achievement than their food-secure counterparts. Food-insecure infants and toddlers are two-thirds more likely to experience developmental delays, twice more likely to have fair or poor health, and one-third more likely to be hospitalized than those who are food-secure (Cook et al., 2004; Rose-Jacobs et al., 2008). Preschoolers facing food insecurity are almost two-thirds more likely to demonstrate behavior problems in the form of aggression, anxiety, depression, inattention, or hyperactivity (Whitaker, Phillips, & Orzol, 2006). Children with severe hunger experience roughly twice the risk for chronic health conditions and anxiety (Weinreb et al., 2002). Food insecurity is also associated with lower reading and mathematics scores among school-aged children (Jyoti, Frongillo, & Jones, 2005).

Due to the extremely high prevalence of violence experienced by homeless mothers, educators should be aware of its severe and long-lasting effects on child well-being. Children who grow up in households where domestic violence is prevalent are more likely to abuse drugs and alcohol, attempt suicide, and develop mental health issues when older. Domestic violence is also a multigenerational issue. Boys who witness and experience violence are almost four times more likely to perpetrate violence as men. Girls who experience physical or sexual abuse are three times more likely to be victimized as women (Desai et al., 2002; NNEDV, 2016).

While the focus of this chapter is on homeless children with parents present, educators should also be aware of the unique challenges faced by unaccompanied homeless youth. Due to a shortage of services and distrust of adult authority figures, the vast majority of the 1.6 to 1.7 million homeless minors are left to fend for themselves and are difficult to identify while on the streets or "couch surfing" (Burt, 2007; Zerger, Strehlow, & Gundlapalli, 2008). Physical and/or sexual abuse and neglect by family members are common reasons why youth leave home, while many others are thrown out following family conflict or financial hardship (Toro, Dworsky, & Fowler, 2007). Due to unstable childhoods and lack of safe alternatives, homeless youth are at greater risk of physical and sexual victimization, physical and mental health problems, and substance abuse than their housed peers (Zerger, Strehlow, & Gundlapalli, 2008). Educators should also be cognizant of the overrepresentation of those identifying as lesbian, gay, bisexual, transgender, or queer/questioning (LGBTQ) among homeless youth. Studies estimate that 15%–40% of homeless youth identify as LGBTQ, as opposed to 3%–10% of youth overall (NAEH, 2009; National Gay and Lesbian Task Force Policy Institute & National Coalition for the Homeless, 2006).[1]

How Well Do Homeless Students Perform in School?

Enrollment in high-quality child-care programs can help mitigate the negative effects of poverty and homelessness and help preschoolers become school-ready, with additional favorable long-term effects on graduation rates, grade repetition, and test scores (HHS, 1999b; National Forum on Early Childhood Policy and Programs, 2010; National Head Start Association, n.d.). However, homeless families are less likely to access these programs. Only one-quarter (24%) of urban homeless or highly mobile young children are enrolled in high-quality center-based care, roughly half the rate of poor but stably housed children (45%) and those at risk of homelessness (55%). Homeless parents are more likely to rely upon informal, relative care (46%) than at-risk (36%) and stably housed (22%) families (ICPH, 2012a).

Since 2007, when Head Start began prioritizing homeless children for enrollment, the proportion of homeless children in Head Start has increased (from 2.5% in 2007 to 4.5% in 2014; ICPH, 2015). Improved access benefits young homeless children, as participation in Head Start is associated with better cognitive, social, emotional, and educational outcomes than those for low-income children who do not participate (HHS, 1999b, 2010; National Forum on Early Childhood Policy and Programs, 2010; National Head Start Association, n.d.).

Toxic stress, trauma, and other factors such as poor health and hunger adversely impact homeless students' development and academic achievement. Whether there are differences between the classroom performances of homeless and other poor students is less clear. Some studies have observed no differences, while others suggest that homeless children have more negative academic outcomes, on average, than poor students. The circumstances of homelessness—in particular, high mobility—make homeless students challenging to study. Additionally, those living doubled-up or unsheltered are difficult to research, and most studies are limited to students residing in shelters (NCHE, 2012).

Research has shown that some homeless children are resilient despite the challenges that homelessness presents and meet or exceed the math and reading achievement scores of housed students. Nearly half (45%) of homeless students were resilient in a study of elementary school children in Minneapolis; the remainder performed substantially worse on assessments than other poor and stably housed students (Cutuli et al., 2013).

Many interpersonal and intrapersonal factors foster resiliency. High-quality parenting, for example, has been associated with higher levels of executive functioning among children, which can profoundly affect their capacity to develop positive social skills, build healthy interpersonal relationships, and eventually, parent their own children effectively (Herbers et al., 2011; Shaffer et al., 2009). Other factors include supportive relationships with other nurturing adults, positive bonds with caregivers, and supportive friends or romantic partners. Also important are interpersonal cognitive and self-regulation skills, positive self-perceptions and self-efficacy, and a sense of meaning in life. Neighborhoods with low levels of pollution and violence, cultures that provide positive standards, rituals, relationships, and supports, as well as bonds to positive sociocultural systems, including schools, also promote resilience (Masten, 2009; Wright, Masten, & Narayan, 2013).

All homeless children have the ability to be resilient. They can adapt and cope with trauma, as long as the balance between the positive and protective factors within themselves and their environment is reasonable (NCHE, 2013). However, the effects of homelessness can sometimes be too much for children. Homeless children are less resilient when they experience multiple risk factors, such as being separated from their families, having parents with substance-abuse or psychological disorders, or being exposed to violence or conflict. Engaging homeless children in cognitive tasks, even in such unfavorable circumstances, has been shown to decrease their stress levels (Cutuli et al., 2010).

The experiences of homeless children are both diverse and challenging. Schools can play a key role in supporting children's resilience by providing opportunities and settings in which children can form caring, positive relationships with adults. A school can provide a safe environment, where students are free to explore and learn. Fostering resilience among homeless students does not require extraordinary talents or resources; educators simply need to be aware of the characteristics of resilient children, understand the factors influencing students' capacity to cope, and support students in achieving positive outcomes (Masten, 2009).

Ten Teaching Tips

1 Show acceptance of the child and treat the child with respect. Respect the child's right to privacy. Some children do not want the class to know that they are homeless.
2 Work with the social worker to meet the needs of the child and provide support to the family.
3 Recognize that the parent may be a victim of abuse and watch for signs that the child may be abused.
4 Avoid any negative judgmental statements.
5 Be sensitive to any assignments that require a home, for example, doing a picture of your home or your room. Avoid homework assignments that require internet access.
6 Take care of the child's basic needs by making sure the child has water and healthy snacks.
7 Provide multiple opportunities for success through art.
8 Make the art room as stress-free as possible.
9 Be cognizant of the child's physical health and work closely with the school nurse when the child is exhibiting medical problems.
10 Watch for signs that the child may need to be evaluated for possible learning disabilities or other special needs.

Note

1 See Chapter 6, LGBTQ Trauma + Art Education.

References

Aidala, A., et al. (2007). Housing need, housing assistance, and connection to HIV medical care. *AIDS Behavior, 11*(6), 101–115.

Anderson, S. A. (1990). Core indicators of nutritional state for difficult-to-sample populations. *Journal of Nutrition, 120*(11S), 1555–1600.

Bassuk, E., et al. (1996). The characteristics and needs of sheltered homeless and low-income housed mothers. *Journal of the American Medical Association, 276*(8), 640–646.

Bassuk, E., et al. (1998). Prevalence of mental health and substance use disorders among homeless and low-income housed mothers. *American Journal of Psychiatry, 155*(11), 1561–1564.

Brooks, J. E. (2006). Strengthening resilience in children and youths: Maximizing opportunities through the schools. *Children and Schools, 28*(2), 69–76.

Buckner, J. C., et al. (1993). Mental health issues affecting homeless women: Implications for intervention. *American Journal of Orthopsychiatry, 63*(3), 385–399.

Burt, M. (2007). Understanding homeless youth: Numbers, characteristics, multi-system involvement, and intervention options. Testimony given before the U.S. House Committee on Ways and Means, Subcommittee on Income Security and Family Support. Washington, D.C.

Chicago Coalition for the Homeless (2014). 22,144 homeless students enrolled in Chicago public schools this past year.

Civic Enterprises (2006). The silent epidemic: Perspectives of high school dropouts.

Cook, J., et al. (2004). Food insecurity is associated with adverse health outcomes among human infants and toddlers. *Journal of Nutrition, 134*(6), 1432–1438.

Cutuli, J. J., et al. (2010). Cortisol function among early school-aged homeless children. *Psychoneuroendocrinology, 35*(6), 833–845.

Cutuli, J. J., et al. (2013). Academic achievement trajectories of homeless and highly mobile students: Resilience in the context of chronic and acute risk. *Child Development, 84*(3), 841–857.

Dallas Independent School District (2014). McKinney-Vento Homeless Children and Youth Education Program: 2013–2014.

Desai, S., et al. (2002). Childhood victimization and subsequent adult revictimization assessed in a nationally representative sample of women and men. *Violence and Victims, 17*(6), 639–663.

Every Student Succeeds Act (2015). 20 U.S. Code 6301.

Family Housing Fund (1999). Homelessness and its effects on children.

Gamache, G., et al. (2003). Overrepresentation of women veterans among homeless women. *American Journal of Public Health, 93*(7), 1132–1136.

Golding, J. (1999). Intimate partner violence as a risk factor for mental disorders: A meta-analysis. *Journal of Family Violence, 14*(2), 99–132.

Grant, R., et al. (2007a). Asthma among homeless children in New York City: An update. *American Journal of Public Health, 97*(3), 448–450.

Grant, R., et al. (2007b). The health of homeless children revisited. *Advances in Pediatrics, 54*(1), 173–187.

Gundersen, C., et al. (2003). Homelessness and food insecurity. *Journal of Housing Economics, 12*(3), 250–272.

Hall, I., et al. (2008). Estimation of HIV incidence in the United States. *Journal of the American Medical Association, 300*(5), 520–529.

Herbers, J. E., et al. (2011). Direct and indirect effects of parenting on the academic functioning of young homeless children. *Early Education and Development, 22*(1), 77–104.

Himmelstein, D., et al. (2009). Medical bankruptcy in the United States, 2007: Results of a national study. *American Journal of Medicine, 122*(8), 741–746.

Homeless Children's Education Fund, Duquesne University School of Education, and Allegheny County Department of Human Services (2009). Educating homeless children in Allegheny County: An evaluation of families, agencies, and services.

Homeless Emergency Assistance and Rapid Transition to Housing Act of 2009. P. L. 111–022. Enacted S. 896 (2009).

Institute for Children, Poverty, and Homelessness (2011). Profiles of Risk: Education.

Institute for Children, Poverty, and Homelessness (2012a). Profiles of Risk: Child Care.

Institute for Children, Poverty, and Homelessness (2012b). Profiles of Risk: Child Health.

Institute for Children, Poverty, and Homelessness (2013). *The American Almanac of Family Homelessness.*

Institute for Children, Poverty, and Homelessness (2015). *The American Almanac of Family Homelessness.*

Jyoti, D., Frongillo, E., & Jones, S. (2005). Food insecurity affects school children's academic performance, weight gain, and social skills. *Journal of Nutrition, 135*(12), 2831–2839.

Lee, B. A., & Greif, M. J. (2008). Homelessness and hunger. *Journal of Health and Social Behavior, 49*(1), 3–19.

Los Angeles Unified School District (2014). Homeless Education Program, 2013–2014.

Marchmont, S. (2010). If you're homeless, you're more likely to have a learning disability. *Medill Reports.* Retrieved from http://news.medill.northwestern.edu/chicago/news.aspx?id=158191

Masten, A. S. (2001). Ordinary magic: Resilience processes in development. *American Psychologist, 56*(3), 227–238.

Masten, A. S. (2009). Ordinary magic: Lessons from research on resilience in human development. *Education Canada, 49*(3), 28–32.

McFarlane, J. M., et al. (2003). Behaviors of children who are exposed and not exposed to intimate partner violence: An analysis of 330 black, white, and Hispanic children. *Pediatrics, 112*(3), 202–207.

McKinney-Vento Homeless Education Assistance Improvements Act of 2001. 42 U.S. Code 11431 (2010).

Metropolitan Policy Program at Brookings (2010). The Suburbanization of Poverty: Trends in Metropolitan America, 2000 to 2008.

My Child without Limits Advisory Committee (2009). Introduction to developmental delay.

National Alliance to End Homelessness (2009). Incidence and vulnerability of LGBTQ homeless youth.

National Alliance to End Homelessness (2010). Economy bytes: Doubled up in the United States.

National Association for the Education of Homeless Children and Youth (2013). Homeless education 101: Facts and resources. Retrieved from http://www.naehcy.org

National Association for the Education of Homeless Children and Youth and First Focus (2010). A Critical moment: Child and youth homelessness in our nation's schools.

National Association of Community Health Centers (2014). Access is the answer: Community health centers, primary care and the future of American health care.

National Association of State Directors of Special Education (2008). Homeless and special education.

National Center for Children and Poverty (2009). Homeless children and youth: Causes and consequences.

National Center for Education Statistics (2014a). Common Core of Data (CCD)— Local education agency (school district) universe survey, 2013–2014.

National Center for Education Statistics (2014b). Common Core of Data (CCD)— State nonfiscal public elementary/secondary education survey, 2007–2013.

National Center for Homeless Education (2010). Education for homeless children and youth program data collection summary.

National Center for Homeless Education (2012). Summary of the state of research on the relationship between homelessness and academic achievement among school-aged children and youth.

National Center for Homeless Education (2013). Research summary: Resilience and at-risk children and youth.

National Center for Homeless Education (2015). Federal data summary school years 2011–2012 to 2013–2014.

National Center on Homelessness among Veterans (2011). Prevalence and risk of homelessness among U.S. veterans: A multisite investigation.

National Coalition against Domestic Violence (n.d.). Domestic violence and substance abuse.

National Dissemination Center for Children with Disabilities (NICHCY2012). Categories of disability under IDEA.

National Forum on Early Childhood Policy and Programs (2010). Evaluation science brief: Understanding the Head Start impact study.

National Gay and Lesbian Task Force Policy Institute and National Coalition for the Homeless (2006). Lesbian, gay, bisexual and transgender youth.

National Head Start Association (n.d.). Benefits of Head Start and Early Head Start Programs.

National Health Care for the Homeless Council (2000). HIV/AIDS and homelessness: Recommendations for clinical practice and public policy.

National Health Care for the Homeless Council (2010). Homelessness and health: What's the connection?

National Health Care for the Homeless Council (2012). HIV/AIDS among persons experiencing homelessness.

National Network to End Domestic Violence (n.d.). omestic violence and sexual assault fact sheet.

National Network to End Domestic Violence (2016). Domestic violence counts 2015.

New York State Technical and Education Assistance Center for Homeless Students (2015). Data and statistics on homelessness, school year 2013–2014.

Nunez, R., & Adams, M. (2014). Primary stakeholders' perspectives on services for families without homes. In M. Haskett, S. Perlman, & B. Cowan (Eds.), *Supporting Families Experiencing Homelessness* (pp. 209–232). New York, NY: Springer.

Rose-Jacobs, R., et al. (2008). Household food insecurity: Associations with at-risk infant and toddler development. *Pediatrics, 121*(1), 65–72.

Rutter, M. (1979). Protective factors in children's responses to stress and disadvantage. In M. V. Kent & J. E. Rolf (Eds.), *Primary Prevention in Psychopathology, Vol. 8: Social Competence in Children* (pp. 49–74). Hanover, NH: University Press of New England.

Shaffer, A., et al. (2009). Intergenerational continuity in parenting quality: The mediating role of social competence. *Developmental Psychology, 45*(5), 1227–1240.

Shinn, M. (2013, June). Efficient targeting of homelessness prevention services. Paper presented at the International Homelessness Research Conference. Philadelphia, PA.

Shultz, J., et al. (1999). HIV seroprevalence and risk behaviors among clients attending a clinic for the homeless in Miami/Dade County, Florida, 1990–1996. *Population Research and Policy Review, 18*(4), 357–372.

Smith, C. (2010). School districts struggle to help homeless kids as number grows statewide. *InvestigateWest.* Retrieved from http://www.invw.org/taxonomy/term/2388.

Stein, J., et al. (2007). Applying the Gelberg–Anderson behavioral model for vulnerable populations to health services utilization in homeless women. *Journal of Health Psychology, 12*(5), 791–804.

Toro, P., Dworsky, A., & Fowler, P. (2007). Homeless youth in the United States: Recent research findings and intervention approaches. In D. Dennis, G. Locke, & J. Khadduri (Eds.), *Toward Understanding Homelessness: The 2007 National Symposium on Homelessness Research.* Washington, D.C.: U.S. Department of Health and Human Services, U.S. Department of Housing and Urban Development.

Trentacosta, C. J., et al. (2008). The relations among cumulative risk, parenting, and behavior problems during early childhood. *Journal of Child Psychology and Psychiatry and Allied Disciplines, 49*(11), 1211–1219.

U.S. Census Bureau (2014). *2014 American Community Survey 1-year Estimates.*

U.S. Census Bureau (2015). *2015 American Community Survey 1-year Estimates.*

U.S. Department of Agriculture (2016). *Household Food Security in the United States in 2015.*

U.S. Department of Education (2015a). *Consolidated State Performance Reports, School Year 2013–2014.*

U.S. Department of Education (2015b). *ED Data Express.* Available from http://www.eddataexpress.ed.gov

U.S. Department of Health and Human Services (1999a). *Blending Perspectives and Building Common Ground: A Report to Congress on Substance Abuse and Child Protection.*

U.S. Department of Health and Human Services (1999b). *Serving Homeless Families: Descriptions, Effective Practices, and Lessons Learned.*

U.S. Department of Health and Human Services (2007). *Characteristics and Dynamics of Homeless Families with Children.*

U.S. Department of Health and Human Services (2010). *Head Start Impact Study: Final Report.*

U.S. Department of Health and Human Services (2011). *Asthma Prevalence, Health Care Use, and Mortality: United States, 2005–2009.*

U.S. Department of Housing and Urban Development (2012). *HUD's 2011 CoC Application.*

U.S. Department of Housing and Urban Development (2015a). *2014 Annual Homeless Assessment Report to Congress: Part 2.*

U.S. Department of Housing and Urban Development (2015b). *2015 Annual Homeless Assessment Report to Congress: Part 1.*

U.S. Department of Housing and Urban Development and U.S. Department of Veterans' Affairs (2011). *Veteran Homelessness: A Supplemental Report to the 2010 Annual Homeless Assessment Report to Congress.*

U.S. Department of Justice (2000). *Full Report of the Prevalence, Incidence, and Consequences of Violence against Women: Findings from the National Violence against Women Survey.*

U.S. Department of Labor (2011). *Trauma-Informed Care for Women Veterans Experiencing Homelessness: A Guide for Service Providers.*

Urban Institute (1999). *Homelessness: Programs and the People They Serve, Findings of the National Survey of Homeless Assistance Providers and Clients—Technical Report.*

Vera Institute of Justice (2005). *Understanding Family Homelessness in New York City.* Washington, D., et al. (2010). Risk factors for homelessness among women veterans. *Journal of Health Care for the Poor and Underserved, 21*(1), 81–91.

Weinreb, L. (1990). Substance abuse: a growing problem among homeless families. *Family Community Health, 13*(1), 55–64.

Weinreb, L., et al. (2002). Hunger: Its impact on children's health and mental health. *Pediatrics, 110*(4), e41–e49.

Wenzel, S., et al. (2000). Antecedents of physical and sexual victimization among homeless women: A comparison to homeless men. *American Journal of Community Psychology, 28*(3), 367–390.

Whitaker, R., Phillips, S., & Orzol, S. (2006). Food insecurity and the risks of depression and anxiety in mothers and behavior problems in the preschool-aged children. *Pediatrics, 118*(3), e859–e868.

Wilder Research (2010). *2009 Homeless Adults and Children in Minnesota Statewide Survey: Physical and Sexual Abuse.*

Wood, D., et al. (1990). Health of homeless children and housed, poor children. *American Academy of Pediatrics, 86*(6), 858–866.

Wright, J., & Weber, E. (1987). *Homelessness and Health.* Washington, D.C.: McGraw-Hill.

Wright, M. O., Masten, A. S., & Narayan, A. J. (2013). Resilience processes in development: Four waves of research on positive adaptation in the context of adversity. In Goldstein, S., & Brooks, R. B. (Eds.), *Handbook of Resilience in Children* (pp. 15–37). New York, NY: Springer Science+Business Media.

Zerger, S., Strehlow, A. J., & Gundlapalli, A. V. (2008). Homeless young adults and behavioral health: An overview. *American Behavioral Scientist, 51*(6), 824–841.

Zima, B. T., et al. (1997). Sheltered homeless children: Their eligibility and unmet need for special education evaluations. *American Journal of Public Health, 87*(2), 236–240.

4   Child Abuse

Signs and Reporting Procedures— What the Art Educator Should Know

Oriana C. Hunter, Donalyn Heise, Beverley H. Johns, and Adrienne D. Hunter

A young lady at one of my alternative education high schools gave me a book she wanted me to read. It was *A Child Called It*, by David Pelzer. It was a Friday afternoon, and I was going out of town for the weekend, and took the book to read with me on the plane. As I read this true story of horrendous abuse, I suddenly thought, "Oh no! Is she trying to tell me something?" I worried myself sick, knowing that I was going to have to address this issue. Ultimately, it turned out that the reading class was having a pizza party for each student who could get ten people to read his or her assigned book, and I was her tenth person! But this was an incident that I, as her art teacher, absolutely had to follow up and report on as necessary.

Adrienne D. Hunter

A child wants his or her school setting to be a safe haven and wants his or her teacher to be a protector and supporter. This chapter explores the problem of child abuse, its impact on the education of children, the role of the art educator in detecting whether a child may be being abused, and in establishing a positive and supportive relationship with the student.

Overview of the Severity of the Problem

Child abuse and neglect, collectively termed child maltreatment, represent a health crisis at the national and international levels (Hoft et al., 2017). As many as one in eight children in the United States are victims of maltreatment before the age of 18 years (Leetch et al., 2015). For 2014 alone, the Child Welfare Information Gateway reported 3.2 million children who were the subject of at least one report to child protective services that year, of which 702,000 were substantiated as cases of child abuse or neglect—statistics that have varied little from year to year and are believed to grossly underestimate the actual incidence rate (Hoft et al., 2017; Berkowitz et al., 2017; Schilling et al., 2014; Kodner et al., 2013). Sadly, approximately 1500 cases of child abuse or neglect lead to death each year (Schilling et al., 2014). The United States is ranked third of 27 developed nations for annual deaths due to child maltreatment for children under the age of 15 years, and the annual financial cost of the initial evaluation of child abuse alone is $124 billion, reflecting child maltreatment as a pediatric public health crisis (Hoft et al., 2017).

There is an increasing body of evidence that the negative effects of abuse and neglect extend across multiple domains of functioning and developmental time points (Wilson, Samuelson, Staudenmeyer, & Widom, 2015). Children who are the subject of repeated episodes of child maltreatment are at risk for lasting physical impairment and decreased brain development, as well as increased incidence of attachment disorder, cognitive challenges impacting education, social difficulties, and mental health difficulties. As such, child maltreatment can be considered to be a toxic stressor with lifelong health impacts. Child abuse has been linked to increased lifetime incidence of major health conditions contributing to early morbidity and mortality, including cardiovascular disease, lung disease, cancer, hypertension, and liver disease (Hoft et al., 2017; Sugali, 2014).

Children involved in the child welfare system because of their experiences with abuse and neglect develop many social, emotional, and behavioral challenges that can have a long-lasting effect on their future well-being. These children are more likely to experience negative interactions with law enforcement and the judicial system later in life (Hoft et al., 2017). Studies have found support for the link between childhood maltreatment and future violent behavior and incidents of criminal violence. A relationship of cause and effect between childhood sexual abuse and violent behavior has been found in some studies. Individuals with a history of being abused as children were almost three times more likely than matched controls to become perpetrators of child abuse (Milaniak & Widom, 2015). The more frequently a child suffers maltreatment, the more likely he or she will commit delinquent offenses (Evans & Burton, 2013).

Defining the Problem

There are no clear definitions of child abuse or maltreatment, as the scope of the harm to the child may range from immediately accepted examples like hitting or sexual assault, to the more subtle injuries of neglect or emotional or psychological abuse. Actions that fall within the categories of child maltreatment continue to change, requiring that caregivers take an active role to re-educate themselves about these changing definitions. Generally speaking, child maltreatment is broadly defined by federal legislation and is specifically defined at and varies at the state level.

National legislation known as the Child Abuse Prevention and Treatment Act (CAPTA, 2010), initiated in 1974, came about as a result of the growing concern about harm being done to children across the United States and has been amended and reauthorized numerous times over the subsequent decades to reflect evolving awareness of the scope of the problem (Child Welfare Information Gateway, 2017a). CAPTA requires that states have procedures and agencies in place for reporting abuse and neglect. In order to receive these federal and community-based grants and funding to assist with these efforts, states and communities must adhere to specific policies developed at the federal level (McLeod & Nelson, 2013). Despite these national and state efforts to identify children who have been the victims of maltreatment and to provide the services necessary to protect them, it is often painfully clear to those who are directly involved with care of these vulnerable children, whether in medical, legal, or educational settings, that the resources available are often insufficient to address their immediate and long-term needs.

In general terms, CAPTA defines abuse as "any recent act or failure to act on the part of a parent or caretaker, which results in death, serious physical or emotional harm, sexual abuse, or exploitation, or an act or failure to act which presents an imminent risk of serious harm" (CAPTA Reauthorization Act, 2010). Child maltreatment is subcategorized by the Department of Health and Human Services into physical abuse, sexual abuse, emotional abuse, and neglect, although specifically included situations and the language describing them vary by state (Leetch et al., 2015; Wider, 2012). In general, physical abuse is considered to be non-accidental injury to a child, including hitting, kicking, biting, burning, choking, or any other damage that results in a physical injury or impairment. Some states expand this definition to include threats of harm and child trafficking.[1] Sexual abuse is typically described as physical contact by bodily intrusion or genital contact (molestation) or exposure of a child to a known sexual predator (Wider, 2012). Many states additionally expand these definitions to include sexual trafficking and sexual exploitation, such as prostitution or child pornography (Child Welfare Information Gateway, 2017b). Emotional abuse is defined as behaviors that result in psychological harm to the child, including close confinement or isolation of a child; verbal abuse including threats or demeaning language; terrorizing such as placing children in chaotic or dangerous situations; or denying emotional responsiveness (Wider, 2012). Neglect is considered to be the failure of a parent or caregiver to provide basic needs including food, shelter, supervision, or medical care such that a child's health or safety are endangered or are at risk. Many states include abandonment, which means failure to provide support for a reasonable period of time or when a child suffers serious harm due to absence of appropriate supervision; within their definition of neglect, however, some states define abandonment under separate language (Child Welfare Information Gateway, 2017b).

An individual episode of child maltreatment may fall within a single category or within several categories, and may occur as an isolated event or as a chronic pattern of behavior. Physical abuse is cited in 58%, sexual abuse in 24%, neglect in 61%, and emotional abuse in 27% of reported events of child maltreatment annually (Leetch et al., 2015). Due to the difficulty of identifying harm that does not leave physical evidence, psychological maltreatment or emotional abuse has the potential to be easily missed and is likely to be underreported. In a United States and United Kingdom study, 8% to 9% of women and 4% of men reported exposure to severe psychological abuse during their childhoods (Hibbard et al., 2012).

Given the multifaceted and life-long potential consequences of child maltreatment, there is an effort to further categorize ongoing, multi-category patterns of child maltreatment as child torture. Child torture is defined as a longitudinal experience characterized by at least two physical assaults or one extended assault; two or more types of psychological maltreatment; and neglect that results in long-term suffering or even death (Knox et al., 2014).

Given the degree of variability in the language and laws regarding child maltreatment by state, it is important as an art educator or health-care provider to be familiar with the child abuse laws and reporting practices in your state.

Demographics

Any child can be a victim of abuse or neglect. Child maltreatment can occur at any age, in any location, to children of any ethnicity, race, or socio-economic status. The perpetrator may be male or female, a parent, a stranger, or another caregiver. All children in a family may be victims, or only one child. As a potential reporter of child maltreatment, it is extremely important not to be blinded or biased by one's perceptions of what a victim of child abuse or neglect should look like, or conversely to assume that a child is not a victim of maltreatment based on appearance or the child's social situation.

The statistical prevalence of various populations among victims has been changing over time. While there is no specific gender variability among victims of physical abuse, victims of sexual abuse are more likely to be female. Historically, children between the ages of 6 to 8 years are most likely to be the victims of maltreatment. Teenagers are more likely to be the victims of physical or sexual abuse; however, infants and toddlers, due to their size and physical vulnerability, are more likely to suffer severe injuries or fatalities from abuse (Schilling et al., 2014; Leetch et al., 2015). In many cases, a child is at increased vulnerability to maltreatment and is exposed to situations that increase their risk of maltreatment, and multiple factors may exist concomitantly.

Many of the factors that put children at increased risk of maltreatment are factors that make a child more difficult to care for, including special needs or prematurity, or are due to a perceived inability of the child to meet parental expectations, whether behavioral, social, or physical. Such factors range from the presence of physical or developmental delays to children who express physical aggression, antisocial behavior, or are oppositional to parental guidance. Other factors put children at increased situational risk of abuse. Maltreatment is more likely to occur if parents have unrealistic expectations of developmental milestones, in families where parental discipline styles are punitive, in homes in which domestic violence occurs, or if a parent had been abused as a child (Schilling et al., 2014).

Factors in the home that increase a child's risk of maltreatment include low socio-economic status, unemployment, family isolation, multiple children below the age of 5 years, frequent changes to the household unit, parental substance abuse or mental health issues, or a single parent with live-in partner in the home. Biological parents account for 81% of physical abuse or neglect, but only 36% of sexual abuse. The perpetrators of physical abuse are more likely to be female, whereas the perpetrators of sexual abuse are more likely to be male (Schilling et al., 2014; Leetch et al., 2015; Moles et al., 2014). Further complicating matters, in up to 80% of cases, the perpetrator views his or her actions as an appropriate form of discipline (Wider, 2012), leading to a large variation in the law from state to state and even internationally regarding where appropriate parental discipline ends and child abuse begins (Child Welfare Information Gateway, 2017b).

As such, the factors that contribute to child abuse and risk are very complex, representing a significant challenge to identifying victims of child abuse. There remains, as of yet, no clear consensus for a single, best screening method to identify children who are victims of or who are at risk for maltreatment (Hoft et al., 2017). Due to the unique opportunity that a school offers for evaluation of and monitoring of a child's behavior and emotional health by numerous adult contacts, as well as opportunities to form relationships of trust, the educator, particularly the art educator, is in a unique position to identify victims of child maltreatment. Identification and reporting are essential in addressing the needs of children who are abused or neglected.

Additionally, it is important to be aware that children in the classroom may already be in the process of evaluation by child protective services. Other children may be in the process of seeking emancipation status because of abuse, as more states have laws that establish procedures for this status. When these children come to school, they too can exhibit a great deal of fear and anxiety because they are unsure whether the school environment will be a safe haven for them.

Identification of Child Maltreatment

Identifying children who are victims of abuse and neglect is difficult. When thinking about physical abuse, the idea of a child being hit or burned or locked in a closet often comes to mind. When thinking about neglect, one might think of children who are not fed or clothed properly. As has been discussed previously, the breadth of actions that are within the definition of child abuse is far more extensive than one might be aware exists, or that one might easily imagine. However, for the children who are victims, such hurtful behavior represents the reality of their lives.

Physical signs of abuse are myriad, and within the medical venue, certain patterns of injury can have strong predictive power for identifying abuse.

Such detailed medical assessment is outside of the scope of an educator; however, many more subtle clues to the presence of abuse are identifiable to an observer with a keen eye for details and a patient ear for listening.

When assessing a child for possible physical signs of abuse, an injury may be obvious— a cast or a black eye—or may not be outwardly visible, or may be hidden by the child. The information on the list below is included as a resource and is not intended to be used by the teacher to make a diagnosis. Many of these injuries are not easily seen. If the teacher notes any possible indications of the following, he or she should have the school nurse evaluate the child. Red flag injuries that warrant further questioning include, but are not limited to:

- head injuries, particularly those that involve bleeding within the skull, bleeding of the retina, or skull fractures in young children;
- rib fractures in young children;
- certain types of fractures of the arms or legs in young children;
- multiple injuries at the same time;
- bite marks larger than 1 inch in width;
- bruising around the mouth, especially in young children;
- healing bruises or new injuries after an absence from school;
- any trauma to the genitals or anus. It is not up to the teacher to investigate, but to send the child to the nurse;
- cigarette burns;
- circumferential burns that would indicate submersion in hot water;
- circumferential bruising to the neck that might indicate choking;
- bruises or burns in the shape of objects (i.e. electrical cord, electric stove burner, hand, shoe);
- bruises to the chest, back, neck, or buttocks, especially in young children;
- child is not appropriately clothed for the weather;
- child has not received medical treatment for serious injuries or illnesses; and
- numerous dental cavities.

(Leetch et al., 2015; Wider, 2012)

When speaking to a child or parents, it is important to pay close attention not only to what is said, but also to body language. Avoid questions that lead the interviewee towards a specific answer. Ask open-ended questions—"How did you hurt your hand?" rather than "Did someone burn you?" Recognize that a child may not recognize an act of harm as wrong, or may developmentally lack the understanding of what is happening to them needed to clearly explain what has happened. Provide a safe, private environment to ask questions. Give them time to answer and be attentive to what they say. If a child is explaining an injury, does the story make sense for the severity of injury? Is the activity described appropriate to the child's level of development? Is the child or parent unable to provide an explanation of the injury, or does the story change frequently? Concerning interview findings include:

- story of injury does not make sense of developmental stage or severity of injury;
- story of injury changes;
- description of episodes of prior child abuse, domestic abuse, or animal abuse by child or caregiver;
- age-inappropriate knowledge of sexual activities or substance use;
- aloof or unreliable caregivers; and
- caregiver frustration with age-appropriate behavior or development.

(Kodner et al., 2013; Leetch et al., 2012; Wider, 2012)

There is evidence that children are more likely to exhibit indirect signs of needing help when they have been abused or neglected rather than directly asking for help (Daniel et al., 2014). Art educators must look for those indirect signs to establish a positive relationship with students. School is a critical environment for children's development, healthy or not (Gallagher-Mackay, 2014).

A child's behavior or patterns of behavior may additionally signal a need for closer investigation, including the following:

- frequent absences from school or skipping school, especially if representing a change from usual attendance;
- feigned illness;
- frequently hungry;
- appears frightened of parents or other adults;
- cries or acts out to avoid going home;
- poor school performance, especially if representing a change;
- increased promiscuity;
- fear, phobias, guilt;
- isolation or withdrawal from classmates; and
- acting out.

(Wider, 2012)

If your conversation with or observation of a child causes you to suspect that the child needs further physical examination than what is clearly visible in the execution of your usual duties as a teacher, a school health care provider should be consulted for further evaluation.

The Role of the Art Educator

Teachers are likely to be professionals to whom a child will turn for help, but teachers also have to be proactive in looking for signs that the child needs help (Daniel et al., 2014). Art educators, together with their other colleagues within the school, should look for signs of abuse and neglect as described previously.

If an art teacher notices any of these signs or other changes in behavior, they should report it immediately. Unexplained absences should be thoroughly investigated because the child may be being abused while not in school. Sometimes a child isolates him- or herself because he or she is afraid of getting too close to someone. The child may act out for no apparent reason. Sometimes, after the child has acted out and has calmed down, the child may disclose that he or she has been abused.

One of the authors remembers that one of her students had a two-hour temper tantrum. Knowing that the child should never be left alone, the teacher patiently waited with the child during the tantrum, preventing the child from self-harm. After the tantrum was over and the child calmed down, it was disclosed that he was being sexually abused by his father. A report was immediately made to the child welfare authorities, the report was found to be true, and the student was removed from the abusive home. After an incident such as the one described above, and once the child is calm, the child is vulnerable but may feel safe because an individual cared enough to stay with him or her; the child may then disclose personal information because he or she has developed a sense of trust with that person.

Sometimes, even when a child shows visible signs of abuse, there has been verbal confirmation of the abuse, and the events are reported to authorities, the student may come to feel fear and regret for disclosing the abuse to the teacher. For the victim, there may be ongoing fear of further abuse, retaliation against other family members or pets, or fear of angering or disappointing his or her parents. For the victim, the psychological impact of trauma and reporting is ongoing and creates uncertainties for the victim regarding the future. One time a student came to school with multiple bruises and cuts. When asked how that happened, the student shared tearfully that his mother had done it. The tears in his eyes were also of concern. After the incident was reported to the principal, the student was called in to speak to the school counselor and the principal. The student returned to the art room angry and yelling at the art teacher, saying his mother did not hurt him. The student may have been protecting himself from further abuse if his mother found out he told someone; he may have been protecting his mother or was afraid of what would happen if the truth were revealed.

Children are not equipped to deal with abuse and the consequences of revealing some secrets. Therefore, it is paramount that skilled professionals are notified who can assist in the child's emotional well-being. Often this first step is the school counselor or psychologist. An important consideration is letting the child know that you are a mandated reporter and that you are going to seek help for the child.

Art teachers are in a unique position to look for indirect signs of abuse. The child may reveal those signs through their art work. They may be drawing or painting what they are unable or don't want to say. If an image seems alarming, first ask the student to tell you about the image. Notice how the child responds. Listen to the verbal description and notice if their body language seems uncomfortable. Sometimes, violent or disturbing images are simply depictions of things they saw on television and are not signs of abuse. If the image is indeed communicating abuse that is uncomfortable to say orally, the child may want to conceal the truth to protect him- or herself or to protect their parent(s). If you notice the child fidgeting while describing the picture, report that to the school counselor so they can use their expertise to investigate further. Be aware of zero-tolerance policies, in place at many schools, where drawing a violent image dictates that the child will likely be expelled or suspended. Recognize that such images may be a cry for help and consult with the student and see/hear his or her explanation of the image before reporting to the professionals as dictated in your faculty manual, in case the child requires further evaluation for possible child maltreatment.

Teachers are required to report any signs of abuse as mandatory reporters. As such, most schools have policies in place that instruct teachers about the correct procedures for reporting. Some require teachers to notify the school counselor or school administration. Check with your administration to clarify your legal and ethical responsibilities. In addition to immediately reporting any signs of abuse, teachers can establish positive communication networks with child protective agencies and work in partnership with them. Child protective services may be able to connect families with interventional resources. Some early family intervention strategies have been shown to help prevent child maltreatment and assist parents (Pecora et al., 2014). It is critical that we, as art educators, keep up with current practices and network with other agencies to do our part to protect children.

There are other aspects of professionalism that may become important during the process of reporting suspected child maltreatment. Even if a claim of child abuse is substantiated, continue to show courtesy, compassion, respect, and, very importantly, tact. If a claim of abuse is substantiated, remember that it is not the role of educators to judge or "convict" the parents. Extreme family stressors may be present, such as domestic abuse, substance abuse, poverty, or mental health issues. A parent may fail to recognize their actions as neglect or abuse, whether because they themselves were the victims of abuse, or through lack of adequate parenting education, young age, or intellectual disability.

Maintain the same privacy that one would expect of a doctor's office and avoid gossip or discussion of the case beyond what is necessary to perform the job of reporting. Confidentiality is paramount and has the potential to impact legal proceedings. Sometimes the media may contact a teacher for a statement after child abuse is reported. Do not speak to the media without permission from the school district. Many districts have policies and procedures that must be followed. For instance, some schools designate a communication specialist to speak to the media, someone who is skilled at protecting the child throughout the investigation.

The priority is to protect the child from harm, whether from the initial trauma, or from the resulting investigation. Be compassionate to the dramatic stresses and life changes that the child is experiencing. Some forms of abuse, such as emotional and psychological maltreatment, that can harm a child cause emotional distress, or unintentional maladaptive behavior (Hibbard et al., 2012), as were described previously.

Therefore, the teacher must maintain professionalism and strive to provide safety and support for the child as the investigational and legal process proceeds.

Reporting, Barriers to Reporting, and Complexity in Reporting

After police, educators are the main group who report suspected maltreatment of children most frequently in the United States and in Canada. At the same time, studies over the last 20 years have shown that teachers often do not report suspected abuse or neglect (Gallagher-Mackay, 2014). Teachers, like health-care providers, form a partnership of trust with parents in the care or education of a child—a partnership that must still be maintained during and after a report has been filed, an added emotional burden for the reporter (Sterling, 2014). All jurisdictions within the United States have legislation that requires that school district personnel are mandated reporters of child abuse and must share information with child welfare authorities in the local area.

That said, there are many factors that impact a mandatory provider's decision to file or not file a report of suspected child maltreatment. Studies of emergency department providers suggest that these factors range from the influence of personal biases to perception of having not enough time to further pursue a red flag observation due to professional obligations (Tiyyagura et al., 2015). Parallels to the classroom are not difficult to imagine as class sizes and complexity of educational needs of students increases, or where the ability to privately interview a student may be difficult within the structure of the school schedule or without drawing attention to a student. Biases might include a desire to trust that caregivers are truthful in describing an injury, or fear of falsely judging them by reporting one's suspicion. Biases might include those guided by the affluent socio-economic status, profession, appearance or dress, "niceness," family structure, neighborhood, or respected status within the community, of the child or caregivers. Other barriers to reporting might include hesitation over lengthy reporting practices that remove reporters from their professional obligations, fear of becoming involved as a witness in a lengthy investigation, or fear of disrupting a family's peace and privacy if an investigation were to prove unsubstantiated (Tiyyagura et al., 2015).

Ultimately, if a reporter is undecided as to whether to file a report with child protective services, it may be helpful to think of the consequences of not reporting. The temptation may be that if it happens again, he or she would file a report at that time. Within the medical community, the first episode of an injury suspicious for child maltreatment is known as a sentinel injury. Such injuries are usually mild, such as bruising, and often have a poor explanation for how the injury occurred. There is strong evidence within the medical literature that sentinel events are observed in a high proportion of fatal and serious non-accidental traumas resulting from child maltreatment. In one study of child abuse fatalities, 19% had been evaluated by a physician within the month prior to their death, usually as ER visits for complaints like fussiness or poor feeding and many had sentinel injuries, which in hindsight were highly suspicious for trauma. Another study showed that one-fifth of children with fractures secondary to abuse had also been seen by a physician prior to their fracture (Leetch et al., 2015). Each of these prior visits represented a potential opportunity when earlier recognition may have spared the victims from worse harm, had their symptoms been recognized as child maltreatment at that time. Similarly, educators have the opportunity for close interaction with and observation of the children in their care, an opportunity to monitor changes in their care, and an opportunity to identify alarming findings whether due to a child's appearance, actions, or words. Educators have tremendous opportunity to make a difference in children's lives, and even to save lives, through their role as mandatory reporters of child maltreatment.

While the specific details of what happens after a report is filed vary from state to state, it is usual that a child protective services representative will be assigned to investigate whether maltreatment has occurred and to determine what future actions will be required to ensure the safety of the affected children. Further medical testing or home visits may occur. The resulting investigation may demonstrate that no harm occurred; may demonstrate the need for assistive services for the family or for the children; may demonstrate the need for removal of the child from the care of a caregiver during further investigation; or if substantiated, may result in criminal investigation. Filing a report does not necessarily lead to removal of children from their home and may in fact identify modifiable behaviors and connect families with community resources which may help to protect them (Wider, 2012; Sterling, 2014).

Drawing parallels from health care, a number of strategies have been identified which may help to improve the reporting process and reduce hesitation in reporting (Sterling, 2014). Many of these strategies may be adapted to the educational setting, including:

- opportunity for prompt case discussion with peers, including social workers, psychologists, or health-care providers;
- consistent and frequent education of reporters about the importance of reporting suspicion of child maltreatment;

- accurate education of reporters regarding the role of child protective services in an investigation; and
- case-based education for reporters and modeling of intervention strategies.

(Tiyyagura et al., 2015)

Such strategies could empower educators in the reporting of suspected child maltreatment with ready resources, skills for intervention, a supportive reporting environment, and accurate education.

Compliance with the law requires a number of skills, which should be considered prior to the time of need in order to be able to exercise them well when an instance of child abuse is suspected. In our experience, an educator must be able to:

1   Identify signs of abuse and neglect and write them down with details and dates. Try to be objective and focus on things you have seen, or have heard, rather than assumptions or inferences. Include direct quotes when possible. If describing an injury, describe not only the injury, but also the description of how, when, and where the injury occurred. Given the fact that there may only be indirect signs that the child is in desperate need of help, this is not always easy.

2   Assess whether there are grounds for a report. This is as much an art as it is a science, and requires both knowledge of signs of possible maltreatment, as well as an element of judgment. Often educators use their intuition to determine whether the child may be abused or neglected. In general, most states require prompt reporting in the event of reasonable suspicion of child maltreatment. It is important to remember that the job of an educator is to report suspicion; not make the decision about whether the child was actually abused or neglected. The child welfare agency will make that judgment.

3   Recognize that once a report is made, the actions taken will be beyond the control of the reporter. The goal of filing a report, if abuse is present, is to help the child and family to receive the support services they need. The reporter may fear bringing the wrath of the family down upon the reporter for perceived judgment of their parenting, or perceived lack of compassion. The educator prides him- or herself on establishing a positive relationship with the child and the family and is then torn about risking a breach of that relationship if a report of abuse or neglect is made.

4   Be aware of the school's protocols for reporting suspected child maltreatment, as well as resources within the school to support the child, the teacher, and possibly the family. Although the law clearly defines the legal reporting obligation of a teacher, administrators and fellow faculty may not always be supportive of a mandated call.

It is important as a reporter to identify a support structure and coping strategies to help you during the reporting process and subsequent investigation.

5   Be aware of the process for reporting suspected child maltreatment, whether by phone or online. Remember that your role as a reporter is to provide factual information and to identify a suspicion of maltreatment. In addition to documenting the details, time, and dates of interactions with the child and other involved parties, it is a good idea to document in writing the times and dates of filing reporting documentation, the names of any hotline personnel with whom you spoke, as well as any notifications to your school administration.

6   Educate yourself regarding the local process of how an investigation proceeds after a report is filed. Good resources for information include school social workers or psychologists and the local child protective services branch. Students or family may ask "What happens next?" or may have preconceived perceptions or misapprehensions regarding the role of child protective services that may need to be addressed early on in order to preserve communication and partnership between family, student, and educators.

7   Maintain compassionate, respectful, objective communication with the family of a suspected victim of child maltreatment. It may be helpful to reiterate the legal obligation of educators as mandatory reporters. It is often helpful to reiterate the shared goal of parents and educators to ensure the child's safety and to prevent future harm. You may be able to utilize school social workers or administrators to assist with these conversations.

Final Thoughts

Educators, particularly art educators, are in a unique position to identify and report child maltreatment at any age, through their unique knowledge of child development, their close interactions with children, and the role of trust and guidance that they establish with their students. While the reporting process may strain the relationship between the family and the school, it offers the opportunity, when child maltreatment is identified, to make a lifelong impact on the victim's physical and psychological health, and to help them to find safety. Early identification of child maltreatment also helps victims to access support resources in the community and to begin the process of healing. While there is no perfect blueprint for identifying child maltreatment, constant awareness and careful observation leading to early reporting when strong suspicion of child maltreatment exists, are among the most important skills that an educator can provide in the battle against this social crisis.

Ten Teaching Tips

1 Teachers should look for obvious warning signs of abuse or neglect; bruises, burns, hunger, lack of sufficient clothing, or lack of adequate health care;

2 Look for changes in the child's artistic creations, such as seemingly violent or disturbing imagery. Ask the child to tell you about the image and be aware of their body language as they speak. Document and report any concerns immediately;

3 Design art lessons that allow all students to visually communicate emotions, allowing for artistic expression, functioning as an art teacher and not an art therapist;

4 When a history of abuse is known, design art lessons that avoid any reminders of the abuse/neglect that the child has experienced;

5 Art teachers should also look for those indirect "cries for help" that children may be giving through their art work, abnormal behavior, or their isolation from others;

6 Remain with a child during any outburst, meltdown, or tantrum to ensure their safety and to build respect and a trusting relationship;

7 Teachers must remember that they are mandated reporters and are not to decide for themselves whether they should report abuse; leave that job to the child welfare agency;

8 Teachers should work together with the social worker, psychologist, and administrator to share observations about a child's behavior;

9 Teachers must be attuned to the needs of the children and parents in their classrooms and have the ability to connect parents with support services available to families who are struggling or who may be at risk for abusing or neglecting their children; and

10 Teachers should examine their own biases and monitor their own behavior to ensure that they are not treating certain children in a negative way because of personal biases, or allowing their biases to blind them to evidence of child maltreatment.

Note

1 More information can be found in Chapter 7, The Role of the Art Educator in Meeting the Needs of Students Who Are Victims of Human Trafficking.

References

American Academy of Pediatrics (2012). Psychological maltreatment. *Journal of Pediatrics*, 130(2), Published online July 30, 2012.

Berkowitz, et al. (2017). Physical abuse of children. *The New England Journal of Medicine, 376(17)*, 1659–1666.

Cataldo, M. (2014). Safe haven: Granting support to victims of child abuse who have been judicially emancipated. *Family Court Review, 52(3)*, 592–609.

Child Abuse Prevention and Treatment Act (amended and reauthorized December 20, 2010). 42 U.S.C. secs. 5101 et seq.; 42 U.S.C. secs. 5116 et seq.

Child Welfare Information Gateway (2017a). About CAPTA: A legislative history. Washington D.C.: U.S. Department of Health and Human Services, Children's Bureau. Retrieved September 10, 2017 from www.childwelfare.gov/pubPDFs/about/pdf#page=2&view=Summary of legislative history.

Child Welfare Information Gateway (2017b). Definitions of child abuse and neglect. Washington D.C.: U.S. Department of Health and Human Services, Children's Bureau. Retrieved September 10, 2017 from www.childwelfare.gov/pubPDFs/define.pdf#page=1&view=Introduction

Daniel, B., Burgess, C., Whitfield, E., Derbyshire, D., & Taylor, J. (2014). Noticing and helping neglected children: Messages from action on neglect. *Child Abuse Review, 23*, 274–285.

Evans, C., & Burton, D. (2013). Five types of child maltreatment and subsequent delinquency: Physical neglect as the most significant predictor. *Journal of Child and Adolescent Trauma, 6*, 231–245.

Gallagher-Mackay, K. (2014). Teachers' duty to report child abuse and neglect and the paradox of noncompliance: Relational theory and "compliance" in the human services. *Law and Policy, 36(3)*, 256–289.

Hartley, D., Mullings, J., & Marquart, J. (2013). Factors impacting prosecution of child sexual abuse, physical abuse, and neglect cases processed through a children's advocacy center. *Journal of Child and Adolescent Trauma, 6*, 260–273.

Hibbard, R., Barlow, J., MacMillan, H., & Committee on Child Abuse and Neglect and American Academy of Child and Adolescent Psychiatry, Child Maltreatment and Violence Committee (2012). Clinical report: Psychological maltreatment. *Pediatrics, 130(2)*, 372–378.

Hoft, M., & Haddad, L. (2017). Screening children for abuse and neglect: A review of the literature. *Journal of Forensic Nursing, 13(1)*, 26–33.

Knox, B., Starling, S., Feldman, K., Kellogg, N., Frasier, L., & Tiapula, S. (2014). Child torture as a form of child abuse. *Journal of Child and Adolescent Trauma, 7*, 37–49.

Kodner, C., & Wetherton, A. (2013). Diagnosis and management of physical abuse in children. *American Family Physician, 88(10)*, 669–675.

Leetch, A., Leipsic, J., & Woolridge, D. P. (2015). Evaluation of child maltreatment in the emergency department setting: An overview for behavioral health providers. *Child and Adolescent Psychiatric Clinics of North America, 24*, 41–64.

McCleod, B., & Nelson, R. (2013). An incremental approach to fully funding the Child Abuse Prevention and Treatment Act. *Social Policy, Fall*.

Milaniak, I., & Widom, C. (2015). Does childhood abuse and neglect increase risk for perpetration of violence inside and outside the home? *Psychology of Violence, 5(3)*, 246–255.

Moles, R. L., & Asnes, A. G. (2014). Has this child been abused? Exploring uncertainty in the diagnosis of maltreatment. *Pediatric Clinics of North America, 61(5)*, 1023–1036.

Pecora, P., Sanders, D., Wilson, D., English, D., Puckett, A., & Rudlang-Perman, K. (2014). Addressing common forms of child maltreatment: Evidence-informed interventions and gaps in current knowledge. *Child and Family Social Work, 19*, 321–332.

Schilling, S., & Christian, C. W. (2014). Child physical abuse and neglect. *Child and Adolescent Psychiatric Clinics of North America, 23,* 309–318.

Sterling, J. (2014). The conversation: Interacting with parents when child abuse is suspected. *Pediatric Clinics of North America, 61(5),* 979–994.

Suglia, S., Clark, C., Boynton-Jarrett, R., Kressin, N., & Koenen, K. (2014). Child maltreatment and hypertension in young adulthood. *BMC Public Health, 14,* 1149.

Tiyyagura, G., Gawel, M., Koziel, J. R., Asnes, A., & Bechtel, K. (2015). Barriers and facilitators in detecting child abuse and neglect in general emergency departments. *Annals of Emergency Medicine, 66(5),* 447–454.

Wider, L. C. (2012). Identifying and responding to child abuse in the home. *Home Healthcare Nurse, 30(2),* 75–81.

Wilson, H., Samuelson, S., Staudenmeyer, A., & Widom, A. (2015). Trajectories of psychopathology and risky behaviors associated with childhood abuse and neglect in low-income urban African American girls. *Child Abuse and Neglect, 45,* 108–121.

5 Behavioral Characteristics of Children Living in Crisis and the Impact on Learning

Beverley H. Johns

It is indeed hard to concentrate on learning when children are worried about whether they will be abused when they get home, where they will be sleeping that night, or whether they will have any food to eat. Children who are living in crisis or who have suffered trauma are emotionally fragile and exhibit a variety of behaviors depicting the turmoil within their lives.

Art educators can play a significant role in meeting the needs of the most vulnerable children. This chapter provides an overview of the many challenges the children face and provides specific strategies that can be utilized to build positive relationships with these children in need.

Schools are now dealing with the issues of child hunger, well-being, and the negative effects of poverty (Varlas, 2013). Childhood trauma at an early age is hypothesized to play a significant role in anxiety disorders such as post-traumatic stress disorder and social anxiety disorder (Bishop, Rosenstein, Bakelaar, & Seedat, 2014). Studies have found that approximately 50% of sheltered homeless children in Boston suffered from at least one developmental delay or required further psychiatric evaluation for depression or anxiety (Zima, Wells, & Freeman, 2004).

The more adversity a child copes with, the greater the chances of long-term developmental consequences. Significant adversity in childhood is associated with impaired cognitive and physical development (Walkley & Cox, 2014).

A study conducted in Los Angeles County found that sheltered homeless children were almost 20 times more likely to have depressive symptoms than prepubescent children in the general population. They were 1.5 times more likely to have symptoms of a behavioral disorder, and they were four times more likely to score at or below the 10th percentile in receptive vocabulary and reading than other children of the same age. At the same time, few homeless children receive treatment (Zima, Wells, & Freeman, 2004).

Some research has shown that as many as 38% of children of homeless families have behavioral and emotional disorders of clinical significance (Harpaz-Rotem, Rosenheck, & Desai, 2006).

Almost half of all children who enter the child welfare system do so between the ages of birth to 5, and more than 25% of these young children exhibit symptoms of trauma (Fusco & Cahalane, 2014). These children need early intervention services to meet their needs.

In a study conducted with formerly homeless mothers and their children, aged kindergarten to second grade, who were now living in a supportive housing community, it was found that the children were at risk for externalizing behavior problems, internalizing behavior problems, and experiencing school problems. There is a relationship between adversity in the family and conduct problems (Lee, August, Gewirtz, Klimes-Dougan, Bloomquist, & Realmuto, 2010).

Because of their frustration or fear, or both, children may act out. Their behavior may be communicating that they are lacking structure and routine in their lives, may need additional attention, or have basic needs that are not being met. They may be bullied and consequently they engage in bullying behavior. The United States Department of Education Office for Civil Rights reports that bullying persists in our schools today (Dear colleague letter, October 21, 2014). The children may show high levels of fear, anxiety, or externalizing behaviors that clearly will impact their learning.

It will be important that the adults working with these children understand the function of their behavior, engage in active listening, try to understand the children's feelings, and try to make life better for them.

Behavioral Characteristics and Impact on Learning

Fear and Anxiety

These children may be coming to school feeling the weight of the world on their shoulders. They are afraid of what is going to happen to them. If they are being abused, they are worried about when the abuse will happen again. They may also be worried that someone will find out about it and they will be punished. They are worried about where they are going to sleep that night. They are afraid they may be taken away from mom and/or dad. They may be afraid of getting hurt. This fear and anxiety may show itself in either withdrawal of the student or acting-out behaviors. Children who are worried may have difficulty completing tasks and bring a great deal of emotional baggage to academic tasks that are given to them. They are unsure of themselves and fear that they will fail. At times, it may be easier for them to give up or not to even begin because of the fears they face.

Fear may result in the students becoming overly upset when the classroom structure and routine is upset or when the teacher is out sick. The student may be fearful of trying new things and become anxious during a test or when called on in front of other students (Craig, 2008).

Lack of Concentration and Attention

Children suffering trauma or children of homeless families may have difficulty focusing and attending to tasks because they have multiple worries on their minds. They may be hyper-vigilant to danger and are so focused on survival and potential threats that this behavior interferes with the development of attention to task at school (Craig, 2008). Their minds are on a myriad of other things, and they may find it very difficult to pay attention to tasks. They may also be tired because of lack of sleep and have difficulty paying attention because they are exhausted.

The teacher must be very careful not to become angry or nag at the student who is having difficulty paying attention. The student may not be able to control this lack of attention and concentration.

Withdrawal

Children may withdraw because they have learned this as a coping strategy to remove themselves from what may be the horror or trauma in their lives. They are afraid to trust anyone and therefore stay to themselves and may be unresponsive to the teacher's efforts to establish a positive relationship. Often, adults then back down and do not try to establish a relationship. That, however, is not productive. The teacher needs to provide support but at the same time be careful to not be intrusive. The teacher shows that he or she is there for the student and provides positive and nurturing comments that are accepting of the student.

Students may withdraw because they are afraid of failure and are unsure of themselves. Their academic skills may be delayed because they have missed school. They may withdraw because they are suffering from untreated physical illness. They may be withdrawn because there is a delay in their receptive vocabulary (Zima, Wells, & Freeman, 1994). Complex trauma from exposure to significant stressors can create an almost continual state of anxiety and the feeling that the world is not safe (Lawson & Quinn, 2013).

Internalizing Behaviors such as Depression

Children who have suffered trauma and children in homeless families may have a sense of hopelessness. Children who are depressed can be pessimistic about their ability to succeed and may lack motivation or may lack the persistence to master skills. They may feel powerless and helpless. There has been some documentation of the relationship between hopelessness and suicide (Guetzloe & Rockwell, 2003). School personnel must give students a sense of hope as a factor in resilience. It is critical to build in success-oriented instruction. It requires the teacher to nurture and protect the children within the classroom. The teacher should model optimistic behavior and use a language of hope that includes literature, songs, and pictures that depict a message of optimism (Guetzloe & Rockwell, 2003).

Externalizing Behaviors

While some children who have experienced trauma or are in homeless families may show signs of withdrawal and remove themselves from difficult situations, other children will exhibit externalizing behaviors such as acting-out tantrums, bullying behaviors, or inappropriate and derogatory verbal comments. These children often react by behaving aggressively toward adults in the school and their peers. Anger, accompanied by physical aggression, may be a common emotion (Walkley & Cox, 2013).

They may be looking for control and therefore they become defiant toward adults in authority and other children. They don't want to comply with rules. They may engage in bullying. The U.S. Department of Education has stressed that there is an increase in the number of complaints that are being received concerning the bullying of students with disabilities (Dear colleague letter, October 21, 2014).

Because of their internal conflicts, students who experienced trauma may act out because they don't know how to control their own behavior. Their internal feelings exhibit themselves with externalizing behaviors. Educators must teach children that bullying cannot be tolerated and must teach them appropriate alternatives to deal with their anger.

Educators have to understand the emotional turmoil that these children are experiencing and provide clear rules and expectations for them. Educators must avoid power struggles with these students and provide opportunities where they can be given power and control. Choice, peer tutoring, and reasonable responsibilities can provide these children power and control in an appropriate manner.

The above are just some of the characteristics that may be exhibited by children who have experienced trauma or are from homeless families. The question is what we can do to help and nurture them.

Understanding the Function of Their Behavior

These children may exhibit externalizing behaviors that may include acting out or refusing to work. It will be important to know what the child's behavior is communicating and what the function of the behavior is. The student may be acting out to receive positive attention from adults. The student may engage in negative externalizing behaviors when unable to keep up with the academic work that is expected because of missing school or because of so many other things on his or her mind: Will there be someplace to sleep or something to eat? Will he or she be abused again? Is the child acting out because of worry that is exhibiting itself in the only way the child knows to communicate the behavior—by acting out?

These children may also possess a whole array of withdrawing behaviors because of sadness or depression they are feeling. They may also withdraw because they are afraid of getting too close to people or to places for fear that they will be taken away from those individuals and places.

The educator must be an understanding individual and has to explore the possible functions of the behavior. Good teachers are detectives who work to figure out what the behavior of the student is telling. Students' needs cannot be met until they are understood. If a student is acting out because he or she needs attention, it will be critical that adults provide attention for positive behaviors. If a student is acting out when expected to do academic work, the educator must look at the work. Is it too difficult for the student, is there too much work given to the student at one time, can the student read the assignment? Whatever the reason may be, the educator will need to adapt instruction to meet the needs of the student.

Adults may believe that these children can control their behavior. This may not be the case, and it is important for the adult to understand this. Misbehavior may not be within the child's control. Their behavior may be a result of traumatic events they have faced and they have little, if any, control over their behavior (Craig, 2008).

What Can Educators Do?

Meeting Their Basic Needs

In the hierarchy of basic needs, students must have their primitive needs met. A child cannot learn if he or she is hungry or tired or believes that their clothing isn't like the other students. The child may be acting out because they cannot concentrate because of hunger. He or she may be self-conscious because their clothes are worn or dirty, or may be worried that their appearance and hygiene are not as good as other students.

Many of today's schools provide breakfast and lunch for students. Clothing and opportunities for those students who do not have other options to take a shower may be offered at school. For those students who are coming from homeless families, meeting those needs in a discreet manner can reduce embarrassment.

For children who have suffered trauma, they are living in fear and need to know that, while they are at school, they are safe from harm.

Creating Positive Personal Relationships

Little (2000) discusses the need for connection. Adults within the school should create a connection with their students. Adults will need to create a one-on-one relationship with students: that relationship should focus on the child's interests and strengths, will not be judgmental about the situation of the child but will be supportive instead, and will not allow other students to judge the student negatively. The adults will protect the child from hurt within the school setting and will build the student up, giving the student hope and promise of what he or she can be.

Creating a Sense of Security with Structure and Routine

Because these children's lives may be chaotic, it is important that the classroom provide stability for the student. In order to do that, the student must understand the rules of the classroom and will need frequent, positive reminders of those rules. If there will be a change in routine, the students will need to be prepared for the change in routine. Manno, Bantz, and Kauffman (2000) provide these ways in which the school can create an environment of structure and routine: communicating clear behavioral expectations, offering instruction geared to the appropriate level and interest of the student, and decreasing the portrayal of violence within the school and the media.

Expectations and tasks should be developmentally appropriate for the student so that the student is able to feel a sense of security.

Focusing on the Positive

These students have probably met with a great number of negative comments. Their parent(s) have so many stressors in their lives that it is difficult for them to recognize the positive behavior that the children exhibit. Educators will need to look for every positive behavior that the student exhibits and should sincerely recognize the student for those behaviors.

We also must teach students the importance of improving their attitude and coping with difficulty. Research has shown that positive affect can be self-induced (Bryan, 1998). A simple strategy to build those coping skills is as follows: For one minute prior to doing a task, the child closes his or her eyes and thinks of something that makes them happy.

Effective and caring educators build confidence in their students through accomplishments. They accent the skills and talents of their students (Johns, 2000).

Ten Teaching Tips

1 Understand the function of children's behavior: Is the student's behavior for access to attention, power, and control; is it to escape a task; or is it to meet a sensory need? Once the function(s) of the behavior have been determined, develop a plan to meet the needs of the student.
2 Engage in active non-judgmental listening.
3 Provide supportive assistance to the student.
4 Provide frequent positive reinforcement to the student.
5 Provide success-oriented instruction.
6 Avoid power struggles.
7 Build in choice in assignments.
8 Assure that the student's basic needs of food, proper hygiene, safety, and clothing are met in a discreet manner.
9 Utilize interest-based interventions.
10 Provide structure, routine, and clear expectations.

References

Bassuk, E., & Rosenberg, L. (1988). Why does family homelessness occur? A case-control study. *American Journal of Public Health, 78(7)*, 783–788.

Bryan, T. (1998). Social competence of students with learning disabilities. In B. Wong (Ed.), *Learning about Learning Disabilities* (pp. 237–307). San Diego, CA: Academic Press.

Craig, S. (2008). *Reaching and Teaching Children Who Hurt.* Baltimore, MD: Brookes Publishing.

Fusco, R., & Cahalane, H. (2014). Young children in the child welfare system: What factors contribute to trauma symptomology? *Child Welfare, 92(5)*, 37–58.

Guetzloe, E., & Rockwell, S. (2003). Preventing hopelessness in children and adolescents. *Beyond Behavior, 12(3)*, 20–24.

Harpaz-Rotem, I., Rosenheck, R., & Desai, R. (2006). The mental health of children exposed to maternal mental illness and homelessness. *Community Mental Health Journal, 42(5)*, 437–448.

Johns, B. (1997). Making school a place to call home. *Reaching Today's Youth, 2(1)*, 34–36.

Johns, B. (2000). The peace-filled classroom. *Reaching Today's Youth, 4(2)*, 27–31.

Lawson, D., & Quinn, J. (2013). Complex trauma in children and adolescents: Evidence-based practice in clinical settings. *Journal of Clinical Psychology: In Session, 69*, 497–509.

Lee, S., August, G., Gewirtz, A., Klimes-Dougan, B., Bloomquist, M., & Realmuto, G. (2010). Identifying unmet mental health needs in children of formerly homeless mothers living in a supportive housing community sector of care. *Abnormal Child Psychology, 38*, 421–432.

Little, M. (2000). Reframing challenging behaviors by meeting basic needs. *Reaching Today's Youth: The Community Circle of Caring Journal, 4(2)*, 21–26.

Manno, C., Bantz, J., & Kauffman, J. (2000). Cultural causes of rage and violence in children and youth. *Reaching Today's Youth, 4(2)*, 54–59.

U.S. Department of Education, Office for Civil Rights (2014). Dear colleague letter. Letter re: Bullying of students with disabilities. Washington, D.C: United States Department of Education.

Varlas, L. (Ed.) (2013). Aligning health and education in today's economic context. *ASCD Education Update, 55(7)*, 1, 4.

Walkley, M., & Cox, T. (2013). Building trauma-informed schools and communities. *Children and Schools, 35(2)*, 123–126.

Zima, B., Wells, K., & Freeman, H. (1994). Emotional and behavioral problems and severe academic delays among sheltered homeless children in Los Angeles County. *American Journal of Public Health, 84(2)*, 260–264.

6 LGBTQ Trauma + Art Education

Mindi Rhoades

The past decade, and specifically the past few years, have been truly momentous for the lesbian, gay, bisexual, transgender, and queer/questioning (LGBTQ) community and its efforts for equality, often called the gay rights movement. Here are brief definitions of relevant terms:

Lesbian—a female-identified person attracted (romantically, physically, and emotionally) to other females.

Gay—a male-identified person attracted to other males; can be used generically to include lesbians.

Bisexual—a person attracted to males and females.

Trans—a transgender person who does not identify with the gender corresponding to their anatomical sex.

Queer—an umbrella term encompassing a range of non-heterosexual and transgressive identities.

Questioning—a person undecided and questioning their sexual orientation.

More recently, there is increasing pressure to expand the acronym to include other gender/sexuality orientations:

Intersex—a person whose reproductive or sexual anatomy is not exclusively male or female.

Asexual—a person who does not experience and/or act upon sexual attraction.

Ally—a person who supports and advocates for LGBTQ people and their rights.

In 2003, Massachusetts became the first state to legalize same-sex marriage, setting off a flurry of anti-gay sentiment resulting in many state laws specifically banning such unions. It also triggered the federal *Defense of Marriage Act*

(DOMA, 1 U.S.C. sec. 7; 28 U.S.C. sec. 1738C, 1996) defining legal marriage as between one man and one woman.

On June 26, 2013, the Supreme Court ruled in *United States v. Windsor* that a same-sex couple, married in Canada but living in New York when one of the spouses died, could not be denied the federal estate tax exemption for surviving spouses as violating the Due Process and Equal Protection clauses of the Fifth Amendment. The Court ruled that DOMA was unconstitutional. On June 26, 2015, in *Obergefell v. Hodges* the United States Supreme Court ruled that under the Due Process and Equal Protection clauses of the Fourteenth Amendment, same-sex couples who had married in states recognizing these unions but living in states that had enacted legislation defining marriage as a union between one man and one woman, could not be denied their constitutional right of having their marriage recognized. Thus the *Obergefell* decision guaranteed same-sex couples the right to marry in all states, making gay marriage the law of the land and eliminating a longstanding justification for and result of unequal treatment based on homophobia and bigotry.

This legal progress follows larger trends of cultural progress toward acceptance of lesbian, gay, bisexual, transgender, and queer/questioning (LGBTQ) people in the United States and Western world. Television shows like *Modern Family* and *Orange is the New Black* and even Disney's *Good Luck Charlie* have introduced and embedded LGBTQ characters in realistic, sympathetic, normalizing, and meaningful ways. Professional and college athletes are "coming out," often to the open arms and hearts of their teammates, fans, and family. Casual cultural use of terms like "Woman Crush Wednesdays" (where female users of Facebook, Twitter, and other sites recognize and offer tribute to other females they love/respect), "Man Crush Mondays" (where men do the same), and the "Bromance" (where men demonstrate a notable public fondness for other men) emphasize a shift toward less rigid and more fluid expressions of connections, intimacy, and attractions.

But these achievements do not erase longstanding and deeply entrenched homophobia, bigotry, and the disparate treatment and hostility still faced by many LGBTQ people. The constant stress of such marginalization and mistreatment, or even the fear of it, can be as damaging and long-lasting as any single traumatic event, though many LGBTQ people encounter those, too. In particular, families, schools, and churches—the very institutions we expect to offer people support—can be minefields for LGBTQ youth.

The progress in schools for LGBTQ youth, alongside these legal and cultural gains, has been less dramatic. While acknowledging that many things have improved for many LGBTQ youth in many places, there is still much room for growth. In 1999, what became the Gay, Lesbian and Straight Education Network (GLSEN) conducted their first *National School Climate Survey* to gather data about the treatment and experiences of lesbian, gay, bisexual, and transgender (LGBT) students, a survey they have conducted every two years since, the most recent in 2013 (Kosciw, Greytak, Palmer, & Boesen, 2014).[1]

Specific trends toward improvement include lower rates of verbal and physical harassment and assault, based on real or perceived sexual orientation and gender expression. In slightly over a decade, students report a 20% drop in hearing homophobic remarks frequently or often, including a steady decline since 2001 in the use of the most common anti-LGBT epithet, "that's so gay," and the lowest level of negative gender remarks reported (p. 10).[2]

While such positive trends are heartening, they do not erase or compensate for the hostile school environment and trauma many LGBT students still inhabit and experience. According to GLSEN's *2013 National School Climate Survey*:

- Over 70% hear the word "gay" used negatively at school often or regularly.
- Almost 65% report other homophobic language use (dyke, fag).
- Over 30% heard negative remarks about transgender people.
- Over 50% of students report homophobic, trans-phobic, and gender-negative comments from teachers and other school staff.
- Many LGBT students face more direct forms of harassment.

Again, according to GLSEN's *2013 National School Climate Survey*:

- Almost 75% of LGBT and over 50% of trans* students were verbally harassed.
- Over 30% were physically harassed.
- 16% were physically assaulted for (real or perceived) sexual orientation.
- 11% were physically assaulted for (real or perceived) gender non-conformity.
- Almost 50% experienced cyberbullying.
- Over 50% of LGBT students harassed or assaulted don't report the incidents.
- Over 60% of students who report harassment get no official response/action from school faculty, staff, or administration. Worse, at times LGBT students are told they caused their own harassment or assault through their dress, demeanor, or behavior.

Trans* students report additional harassment:

- Over 40% are not allowed to use their preferred name.
- Almost 60% are required to use the rest room corresponding with their sex at birth.
- Over 30% are prevented from wearing "inappropriate" clothing according to their sex at birth.

(GLSEN, 2013)

Even though the U.S. Department of Education issued a policy letter in May of 2016, explaining that trans students deserve equal rights and protections, and instructing schools to respect them, many schools and districts still resist. By July 2016, approximately half of all states filed lawsuits challenging the application of Title IX's civil rights protections to trans students. Several states created anti-transgender laws around bathroom use, most notably North Carolina's House Bill 2, insisting that in state facilities, people use the rest room aligned with the sex on their birth certificates (Emma, 2016). In response to this wave of anti-trans legislation, many major corporations, such as Target, fought back by issuing statements about their inclusive policies for employees and shoppers (Mclean, 2016). Other corporations, including Bank of America and Paypal, have terminated plans to locate or expand in North Carolina. Events, like the NCAA basketball tournament and multiple concerts and performances, have also been canceled in North Carolina.

Such hostility, or even the constant threat of it, can create and sustain a sense of trauma that continually negatively impacts LGBT students in their school experiences and lives:

- Over 50% of LGBT and almost 40% of trans* students felt unsafe in school.
- Over 30% report discomfort in gender-segregated spaces.
- Over 30% skipped a day in the past month because of feeling unsafe.

The GLSEN *National School Climate Survey* (2013) reports that LGBT students who experience high levels of trauma miss school three times as often as non-LGBT peers, have higher rates of depression and lower self-esteem, have lower GPAs, and are only half as likely to pursue post-secondary education.

Trauma and LGBTQ Students

Across the board, LGBTQ students need teacher and adult support. For many minorities, home and family serve as a place of comfort, acceptance, and solidarity. For many LGBTQ students, these traditional support networks may not exist, or may even be disapproving or hostile (Dragowski et al., 2011). Top concerns for LGBTQ youth are family acceptance, school problems/bullying, and the fear of being "out," while non-LGBTQ youth worry about college/career plans and financial concerns related to college/career goals. While many students are planning and preparing for their futures, many LGBTQ youth are focused on surviving their present situation. This concern is not unfounded. In a 2012 survey, *Growing Up LGBT in America*, conducted by the Human Rights Campaign (HRC), 33% of LGBT youth say their family is not accepting of LGBT people, with 46% reporting their family is where they regularly hear anti-LGBT messages (HRC, 2012, p. 15).

These constant pressures have a cumulative negative impact on LGBT youth. In the HRC survey, a student states, "[I]t's really hard on me.

I deal with so much ignorance on a daily basis" (HRC, 2012, p. 6). Another offers, "The people in my community and family aren't really accepting of the LGBT community and it's hard for me to lie about who I am" (HRC, 2012, p. 20). Even more demoralizing, one youth admits, "It's very easy to look at me and tell I'm gay and it makes me feel afraid to walk around knowing there are people here in my hometown who hate me and people like me, enough to attack me" (HRC, 2012, p. 15). LGBT youth need love, support, and acceptance. When they have these, they thrive; when they don't, on average, they face harsher consequences than their non-LGBT peers.

These harsh consequences can often involve homelessness. Statistics show that LGBTQ youth make up a much larger percentage of the homeless population than non-LGBTQ youth. Although estimates calculate the proportion of LGBTQ people in the general population to be between 2% and 10%, in places like New York, LGBTQ youth comprise 15% to 40% of the homeless population (Ream & Forge, 2014). The dominant narrative about homeless LGBTQ youth is that they were "kicked out" specifically because of their sexuality or gender expression, which accounts for between 14% and 39%, but Ream and Forge (2014) argue that it is often a contributing cause, given societal and parent/guardian prejudices and expectations. Also, most homeless LGBTQ youth go through the child welfare system on their way to homelessness. Within this system, they often face the same, or even greater, mistreatment and abuse. Almost all LGBTQ youth in foster care are verbally harassed, with many experiencing emotional and physical abuse as well (Ream & Forge, 2014). Even a system set up to help youth in crisis can be punitive for these particular youth and their crises.

LGBTQ students who do thrive may face similar societal pressures and trauma, without suffering the same level of injury or harm from it, demonstrating "resilience," or the ability to adapt and cope successfully with stress, adversity, and challenges (Heise, 2014; Mustanski, Newcomb, & Garafalo, 2011; St. Athatos, Watson, & Sulkowski, 2016). Given that trauma and constant disapproval can destabilize a student's sense of safety, stability, security, and self, Heise (2014) asserts that all educators should attend to these factors and help students establish "healthy, lifelong strategies for dealing with pain and tragedy" (p. 27). While addressing such issues and teaching such skills may seem outside the purview of traditional educational approaches, these skills support students in a holistic manner. Students who feel safe, supported, and secure are more prepared to learn and excel than those consumed by concern about how their sexuality and/or gender expression impact their physical and emotional health and well-being. With this support, students who succeed develop what Rutter (2012) calls "the steeling effect," or the accumulation of positive adaptation and coping strategies to stress, that results in resistance to or inoculation toward future stresses (Heise, 2014, p. 28).

Art education can play a positive role in helping address and hopefully ameliorate some of the trauma LGBTQ students experience. Heise believes that art educators, in general, can "play an important role in preventing devastating effects of trauma by fostering resilience through art" (2014, p. 27). The following sections explore the potential of art educators in fostering LGBTQ youth resilience followed by more general suggestions.

The remaining sections present the general steps all educators can take to better support LGBTQ students followed by those more specific to art educators. The following are resources and recommendations.

What Can Educators Do?

There are many successful strategies for improving education and support for LGBTQ students. One is implementing district-level, comprehensive bullying and violence prevention programs and policies that explicitly include "sexual orientation, gender identity, and gender expression . . . with clear and effective systems for reporting and addressing [negative] incidents" (GLSEN, 2013, p. 14; see also Aragon et al., 2014; Iverson & Seher, 2014, p. 43). Another strategy is ensuring that "school policies and practices, such as those related to dress codes and school dances, do not discriminate against LGBT students" (GLSEN, 2013, p. 14). Districts and schools can also accommodate LGBTQ students by making changes to available facilities, like gender-neutral bathrooms and changing areas, bearing in mind that although some adults depict trans and gender non-conforming people as predators, they are in fact much more vulnerable in these spaces and much more likely to be victimized.[3]

At the school level, there are also opportunities for supporting LGBTQ students. Gay–Straight Alliance (GSA) groups send a clear message that there are people who support LGBTQ students, want to find ways to help them connect, and can help students access additional resources. In the GLSEN (2013) survey, although approximately 18% of students were "restricted from forming or promoting a GSA," and although only half of the students reported having a GSA (or similar club) at their school, this was higher than ever before (GLSEN, 2013, p. 5). GSAs provide many benefits, especially for LGBT students. In schools with GSAs, students are less likely to hear homophobic remarks or slurs, less likely to hear negative remarks about gender expression, less likely to feel unsafe, about 50% less likely to be victimized, and more likely to report homophobic remarks. Overall, they help LGBT students feel more "connected to their school community" (GLSEN, 2013, p. 7).

Individual teachers can also take steps to be supportive and inclusive of LGBTQ students. Teachers can make their acceptance and support of LGBTQ students explicit and clear through signage and symbols, such as rainbow flag, ally, or Safe Space stickers. Teachers can enforce a policy of not allowing homophobic or anti-LGBTQ remarks in their classrooms (Check & Ballard, 2014, p. 11). In a more proactive manner, teachers can "examine their curriculum for inclusiveness" (Aragon et al., 2014, p. 12), making sure to "[incorporate] LGBTQ social issues and [people] in their curricula" (Check & Ballard, 2014, p. 11), and "provid[e] appropriate and accurate information regarding LGBTQ people, history, and events" (p. 14). Additionally, all teachers can create assignments allowing student choice around topic/subject matter, including LGBTQ-related ones. Teachers can also provide resources or access to resources that provide additional information and support for LGBTQ students.

What Can Art Educators Do?

While all educators are responsible for teaching and protecting all students, art educators are generally characterized as being more supportive of marginalized student populations, of individual expression, of challenging the status quo, and of finding value, beauty, and strength in diversity. In some schools, art classes serve as a safe haven for outcasts, misfits, and "weird" kids. LGBTQ students often migrate to these spaces and the teachers who create and manage them. Art educators can capitalize on this reputation and art's special affordances, flexibility, and individualization.

Like all educators, art educators can often customize their specific materials and curricula in service of achieving student learning objectives. Art educators can start by "examin[ing] their curriculum for inclusiveness" (Aragon et al., 2014, p. 12), and then deliberately and explicitly include LGBTQ art, artists, and issues in teaching art and visual culture education (Check & Akins, 2004; Check & Lampela, 1999; Lampela, 2005, 2007, 2010; Lampela & Check, 2003; Sanders, 2007). Check and Ballard claim systematic "omission and misrepresentation of [LGBTQ] art content and material [amounts to] intellectual violence" (2014, p. 7). When information about artists' relationships and partners is appropriate, pertinent, and usually mentioned, LGBTQ biographic information should be included. Including positive representations of LGBTQ people in art, history, current events, and popular culture examples can yield positive results. Robinson and Espelage (2011) note that pop culture (e.g., Lady Gaga, *Glee*) may be effective in helping LGBTQ and non-LGBTQ middle and high school youth become more aware, informed, and respecting of LGBTQ people and concerns (Aragon et al., 2014, p. 12). These examples help normalize the presence of LGBTQ people and show their embedded-ness in families, communities, workplaces, politics, religious institutions, etc.

Art educators can also provide multiple ways for students to explore LGBTQ issues productively. Check and Ballard note the "value and importance of 'inviting student lives' into our classrooms" to create "opportunities to connect to students, their lives, and art" (2014, p. 10). Art educators can create assignments and projects that provide spaces for all students to explore identity issues—their own and those of other people. Art educators' general strategies for supporting marginalized and traumatized students fall into several key categories: art as therapy (self-expression, resilience); art as a framework for meaning-making (engaging big ideas); and art as communication and connection/interaction (multimedia literacies). Art educators can ensure, whenever possible, students have options for inserting their lives, investigating their concerns, and developing the skills and knowledge they desire. This gives LGBTQ students opportunities to conduct research, find ideas and inspiration, and use arts-based processes and practices to explore issues related to marginalized identities, sexualities, and forms of gender expression.

Art education can also help LGBTQ students deal with stress and trauma through its more therapeutic and introspective aspects. While most art educators are not certified therapists, they are still able to present art and art-making as valuable tools for personal development. Reflective art-making projects "can help students struggling with identity" (Pelton-Sweet & Sherry, 2008, p. 173). In particular, LGBTQ students value the processes of self-expression—textually, materially, and virtually—in their process of identity exploration and formation (Pelton-Sweet & Sherry, 2008). Without attempting to provide students with official therapy or a substitute for it, Heise believes art educators can "[listen, affirm, and utilize] the therapeutic qualities of art education to create an environment that allow[s] students' creative expression and opportunity to engage in the aesthetic process," using their own lives and experiences as the basis for their art-making (2014, p. 29). Heise, admitting her own "tendency to give sympathy, to advise, or to counsel students," encourages restraint, emphasizing the need to provide students with "a safe, nurturing environment . . . to help them sort through their feelings in a non-judgmental atmosphere" (p. 29). Check and Ballard (2014) note that art educators can adapt and adjust classroom practices and assessments to deal with students' concerns and interests openly or more privately, according to student wishes and educational context. Through these openings, art educators may gain more personal and direct insight into their students' lives, and must enter this exchange responsibly, creating and maintaining safe spaces for students to do this work.

Art-making is also a helpful process, a set of tools that enables active participants to engage their bodies and minds to grapple with the events and issues and concerns of their own lives as well as those of others (Roeck, 2008, p. 55). In this way, not only does the personal become political, the personal and political become artistic; students experience aesthetic engagements with representations and processes of meaning-making "that respon[d] to cultural and social situations" (p. 55). This is an assets-based approach to working with marginalized and traumatized populations (Heise, 2014; see also Craig, McInroy, McCready, & Alaggia, 2016; Mustanski et al., 2011). Art-making can provide a mechanism through which traumatic events and personal challenges become the sources of rich imagery, strong metaphors, and deep significance (Heise, 2014, p. 29), providing students with space to process these things more abstractly and obliquely.

Art-making can also serve as a framework or model that "develops creative problem solving, flexibility, and resourcefulness," "addresses a variety of perspectives," "requires persistence and vision," promotes a "sense of purpose," and fosters "social competence" (Heise, 2014, p. 28). Further, art is a "meaning-making endeavor" that addresses universal themes like "humor, identity, life cycles, patterns, and transformation" (p. 28). Art-making requires framing and reframing ideas and challenges, then playfully experimenting with materials and these ideas in ways that provide students with hope, possibility, strength, stamina, grit, and resilience (Heise, 2014; see also Wolin & Wolin, 1993). There are also many examples of artists "who overcame great obstacles in their lives" (Heise, 2014, p. 28), sometimes directly and explicitly related to their sexuality and gender expression. Art-making can "provoke a safe haven for people in times of stress," and foster the development of "insight, independence, relationships, initiative, humor, and morality" (p. 28). These creative factors all form a set of "strong coping skills," including resourcefulness and an orientation toward participating in and learning from new experiences (p. 29).

Art-Making as Activism: "Artivism"

While not the first to explore the more social justice-oriented aspects of art-making, Sandoval and Latorre's (2008) term "artivism" helpfully fuses "art" and "activism" to create a framework for collective, creative, community-based projects that challenge sociocultural and political inequities. Sandoval and Latorre's research focused on primarily Latino communities in Los Angeles using new media and public space to tell their histories as part of the larger story of the area, to make them and their contributions visible and valued. Artivism holds potential as an approach for any marginalized people or populations, including members of the LGBTQ community. This collective, critical, creative approach can provide marginalized youth with the ability to speak to larger audiences more directly, using their own voices to tell their own stories, stories that sometimes "contradict and complicate dominant ones" (Rhoades, 2012, p. 317).

One of the best examples of artivism is *20 Straws: Growing Up Gay in the Midwest* (Rhoades, 2007), a 30-minute documentary short that was created, filmed, screened, distributed, and used as a teaching and training tool around LGBTQ youth's identities and their experiences in schools, outside of schools, in workplaces, and online. Video artist Liv Gjestvang started Youth Video OUTreach as a project to empower LGBTQ youth to use video as a way to tell their own stories themselves. Over the course of a year and a half, Liv worked with a group of other teaching artists and facilitators to support youth through this process.[4] Liv broke film-making into small, manageable steps, with exercises around interviewing, photographing, and visual poetry which then provided valuable source material once the youth were ready to compile their film. The process also included workshops and trainings around big ideas the film needed to address: gender, sexual identity, oppression, and empowerment.

As the youth worked on creating the film, they also worked to create a vision for using the film. After their proposal was accepted for *The Right to*

Be Different (2010), the largest LGBT Human Rights Conference on record (coinciding with the *Gay Games* in Montreal, Canada), the group devised a fundraising plan so they could attend. They were the youngest presenters at the international conference. They also submitted the film to different LGBT film festivals, securing showings at the *San Francisco Gay and Lesbian Film Festival, Sacramento Film Festival,* and winning Best Documentary Short at the *Indianapolis GLBT Film Festival.*

Additionally, Youth Video OUTreach began using the film as an informational and educational resource. Liv and the participants formed a speakers' bureau and contacted potentially interested parties, offering to screen the film on-site and then host a Q&A or more formal informational/training sessions afterwards. Screenings/outreaches were conducted at schools, for community groups, at churches, and for businesses. The DVD was also available online for individual or organizational purchase.

These youth telling their own stories in their own words is activism. They address the problems that can accompany being LGBTQ, but they also insist on sharing the benefits and joys. They want to tell a more complex tale, but one with hope, one where they have agency. As part of this, they wanted audiences to leave with a fuller understanding of their issues, and also with a way to translate their greater awareness into meaningful practices. As a result, the film ends with the following list, each line appearing and disappearing, one by one:

Things individuals can do:

- Learn about LGBTQ issues.
  - Educate others.
- Ask about LGBTQ books at your library.
  - Read them.
- Don't use hateful language.
  - Say something to those who do.
- Don't be a bully.
  - Stand up to people who are bullied.
- When someone comes out, listen.
  - Remember, it is their story to tell.
- Join your school's Gay–Straight Alliance (GSA).
  - If there's not one, start one.
- Be aware of political issues.
  - Vote.

(Gjestvang, 2007)

While documentaries about LGBTQ youth were not numerous or popular when Liv started this project, the ones that existed were made by adults reflecting on their own experiences or telling youths' stories for them. This one was made by the youth themselves, assisted and supported by adults, and assigning positive steps for everyone to take after seeing their stories.

There are also other pop culture examples of this kind of artivism that are more crowd-sourced and allow more open-ended participation. A prime example of a publicly collaborative arts-based response to the trauma of being LGBTQ is Dan Savage's online video project. In response to a string of publicized suicides of (presumably) LGBTQ youth, Savage and his husband, Terry Miller, launched *It Gets Better*, a website offering video testimonies encouraging LGBTQ youth not to commit suicide, instead to hold on because "it gets better" and "love and happiness can be a reality in their future" (Savage, 2010, para. 3). Videos are from celebrities, politicians, organizations, and businesses—anyone can participate by leaving a positive public message. While it has not saved all LGBTQ youth, it has certainly saved some. It is too traumatic to believe you are alone, that you don't deserve to be happy, that something is wrong with you, that things will always be so painful, or that it might get even worse. Savage created a space for LGBTQ youth (and adults) to see they have supporters, that there are people who survived, and that being LGBTQ can be a wonderful gift, not a terrible curse.

This kind of artivism helps youth "reframe adversity to see possibility instead of despair," "transform their thinking from victim to survivor," and "shifts the focus from the trauma to their sources of joy and strength" (Heise, 2014, p. 29). The *20 Straws* film and the *It Gets Better* project exemplify art-making as artivism, as something that helps students become "empowered as change agents in their own lives," and as "change agents in their world" (p. 29).

Conclusions

Not every LGBTQ youth is a direct victim of violence, but they all face the still-present societal prejudices that exist against LGBTQ people. As Heise (2014) notes, "Violence—direct or indirect—can be traumatic, with immediate and long-term consequences" (p. 27). The constant stress of being marginalized and the worry of what being LGBTQ might provoke in others—from slight displeasure to physical harm, from biased treatment to bruised bones—take an incredible toll. Schools are often the site of much of the stress LGBTQ youth encounter. Therefore, educators and administrators must play an active role in addressing these issues. Educators can help by addressing LGBTQ bias and bullying directly, by making schools and classrooms safe spaces for LGBTQ youth, by providing them with caring adults to listen and support them. Teachers can help by including LGBTQ information, people, work, and issues into their curriculum in deliberate and meaningful ways. Teacher education and preparation programs need to address the specific challenges, needs, and ways to support LGBTQ youth. In particular, art educators can extend a welcoming environment to LGBTQ students, include LGBTQ art and artists, and provide students with options to address LGBTQ topics in assignments. Art educators can also teach LGBTQ youth—all youth, really—that art is a tool for self-reflection, but artivism (Sandoval & Latorre, 2008) can also be a tool for change. We can use art in the service of social messages and progress. We can use it for good.

Ten Teaching Tips

1 Create and maintain a safe learning environment for *all* students.
2 Prevent hate speech and derogatory terms around gender and sexuality.
3 Educate yourself about LGBTQ issues so you can educate others.
4 Position yourself explicitly as an ally (verbally, stickers, posters, and clothing).
5 Avoid assuming all LGBTQ students experience trauma around gender and sexuality.
6 Include LGBTQ art, artists, and pop culture examples in curriculum.
7 Name artists as LGBTQ when relevant and/or in common with other artists.
8 Allow students to choose topics, art, and artists that allow them to investigate and insert their lives and concerns into the curriculum.
9 Invite students to use art-making as a medium for coping with and expressing trauma and other negative experiences, feelings, and events.
10 Find ways to embed artistic skill development within larger projects that question and challenge the injustices students see and encounter.

Additional Resources

Online LGBTQ resources have profoundly changed coming out and being LGBTQ, and continue to proliferate. The resources below are current as of this printing.

American Civil Liberties Union (ACLU)

The ACLU works to defend and preserve the individual rights and liberties guaranteed to everyone in this country, including lesbians, gays, bisexuals and transgender people.

www.aclu.org

www.aclu.org/library-lgbt-youth-schools-resources-and-links

www.aclu.org/know-your-rights/lgbt-high-school-students

American Psychological Association (APA) and Just the Facts Coalition

Offering resources for principals, educators, and school personnel dealing with sexual orientation and gender identity issues.

http://www.apa.org/helpcenter/sexual-orientation.aspx

Gay, Lesbian and Straight Education Network (GLSEN)

Every day GLSEN works to ensure that LGBT students are able to learn and grow in a school environment free from bullying and harassment.

www.glsen.org

https://www.glsen.org/educate/resources/guides

Gay–Straight Alliance Network (GSA Network)

An LGBTQ racial and gender justice organization that empowers and trains LGBTQ youth leaders and allies in an intersectional effort for safer schools and healthier communities.

http://www.gsanetwork.org/about-us

Human Rights Campaign (HRC)

The largest civil rights organization for lesbian, gay, bisexual and transgender equality.

http://www.hrc.org/

http://www.hrc.org/topics/children-youth

It Gets Better

Convincing LGBTQ youth that "it gets better," and creating the changes needed to make it so.

http://www.itgetsbetter.org

National Art Education Association's (NAEA) Lesbian, Gay, Bisexual, Transgendered Issues Caucus (LGBTIC)

Providing visibility, support, and advocacy for lesbian, gay, bisexual, and transgender issues and people within the field of art education, in the arts, and throughout culture more broadly.

> https://www.arteducators.org/community/articles/69-lesbian-gay-bisexual-transgendered-issues-caucus-lgbtic

Safe Schools Coalition: A Public–Private Partnership in Support of GLBTQ Youth

Helping schools become safe places where all families belong, all educators can teach, and all children can learn, regardless of gender, gender identity, or sexual orientation.

> http://www.safeschoolscoalition.org/index.html

Teaching Tolerance: A Project of the Southern Poverty Law Center

Helping educators who care about diversity, equity, and justice to find news, suggestions, conversation, and support.

> www.tolerance.org

The Trevor Project

The leading national organization providing crisis intervention and suicide prevention services to lesbian, gay, bisexual, transgender, and questioning (LGBTQ) young people ages 13-24.

> www.thetrevorproject.org

Welcoming Schools (part of HRC)

HRC's efforts to make schools safe and equitable for LGBTQ students.

> www.welcomingschools.org

YouthResource

A website created by and for LGBTQ youth.

> http://www.youthresource.com/

Notes

1 Statistics in the following paragraphs are from the GLSEN 2013 *National School Climate Survey* Executive Summary unless otherwise noted.
2 GLSEN hypothesizes that increasing availability of LGBT-related school and social resources contributes to this positive shift.
3 Many transgender students do not want to use gender-neutral bathrooms, but rather the bathroom of the sex with which they identify. See NBC Out website, where there's an account of a transgender boy who sued successfully to use the boys' bathroom, and Behrman (2017), where three women students successfully settled a lawsuit with a school district to rescind a policy restricting them to use either unisex bathrooms or bathrooms matching their biological gender.
4 The author of this chapter primarily served as Liv's project assistant and sometimes teaching artist.

References

Aragon, S. R., Poteat, V. P., Espelage, D., & Koenig, B. W. (2014). The influence of peer victimization on educational outcomes for LGBTQ and non-LGBTQ high school students. *Journal of LGBT Youth, 11*, 1–19.

Behrman, E. (August 4, 2017). Court settlement finalized with Pine-Richland regarding transgender bathrooms. *Pittsburgh Post-Gazette.*

Check, E., & Akins, F. (2004). Queer lessons in the art classroom. *Democracy and Education, 15(3–4)*, 66–71.

Check, E., & Ballard, K. (2014). Emotional, intellectual, and physical violence directed toward LGBTQ students and educators. *Art Education, 67(3)*, 6–11.

Check, E., & Lampela, L. (Summer, 1999). *Teaching More of the Story: Sexual and Cultural Diversity in Art and the Classroom.* Advisory. Reston, VA: National Art Education Association.

Craig, S. L., McInroy, L., McCready, L. T., & Alaggia, R. (2016). Connecting without fear: Clinical implications of the consumption of information and communication technologies by sexual minority youth and young adults. *Journal of LGBT Youth, 12(3)*, 254–275.

Defense of Marriage Act (1996). 1 U.S.C. sec. 7; 28 U.S.C. sec. 1738C.

Dragowski, E. A., Halkitis, P. N., Grossman, A. H., & D'Augelli, A. R. (2011). Sexual orientation, victimization, and posttraumatic stress symptoms among lesbian, gay, and bisexual youth. *Journal of Gay and Lesbian Social Services, 23(2)*, 226–249.

Emma, C. (July 8, 2016). Ten more states sue Obama administration over transgender bathroom directive, *Politico.* Retrieved from http://www.politico.com/story/2016/07/obama-transgender-bathrooms-states-sue-225303

Gjestvang, L. (Producer), & Youth Video Outreach Collective (Directors) (2007). *20 Straws: Growing Up Gay in the Midwest* [motion picture].

Heise, D. (2014). Steeling and resilience. *Art Education, 67(3)*, 26–30.

Human Rights Campaign. (2012). *Growing Up LGBT in America.* Retrieved from hrc-assets.s3-website-us-east-1.amazonaws.com//files/assets/resources/Growing-Up-LGBT-in-America_Report.pdf.

Iverson, S., & Seher, C. (2014). Using theatre to change attitudes toward lesbian, gay, and bisexual students. *Journal of LGBT Youth, 11*, 40–61.

Kosciw, J. G., Greytak, E. A., Palmer, N. A., & Boesen, M. J. (2014). *The 2013 National School Climate Survey: The Experiences of Lesbian, Gay, Bisexual and Transgender Youth in Our Nation's Schools.* New York: GLSEN.

Lampela, L. (2010). Expressing lesbian and queer identity in the works of three contemporary artists of New Mexico. Instructional Resources, *Art Education, 63(1),* 25–32.

Lampela, L. (2007). Including lesbians and gays in art curricula: The art of Jeanne Mammen. *Visual Arts Research, 33(1),* Issue *64,* 34–43.

Lampela, L. (2005). Writing effective lesson plans while utilizing the work of lesbian and gay artists. *Art Education, 58(2),* 33–39.

Lampela, L. & Check, E. (Eds.) (2003). *From Our Voices: Art Educators and Artists Speak Out about Lesbian, Gay, Bisexual and Transgendered Issues.* Dubuque, IA: Kendall/Hunt.

Mclean, R. (April 20, 2016). Target takes stand on transgender bathroom controversy. CNN Money. Retrieved from http://money.cnn.com/2016/04/20/news/companies/target-transgender-bathroom-lgbt/.

Mustanski, B., Newcomb, M. E., & Garofalo, R. (2011). Mental health of lesbian, gay, and bisexual youths: A developmental resiliency perspective. *Journal of Gay and Lesbian Social Services, 23(2),* 204–225.

NBC Out (May 30, 2017). Transgender Wisconsin student can use boys' bathroom, federal court says. Retrieved from http://www.nbcnews.com/feature/nbc-out/transgender-wisconsin-student-can-use-boys-bathroom-federal-court-says-n766436.

Obergelfell v. Hodges, 576 U.S. ____ (2015).

Pelton-Sweet, L. M., & Sherry, A. (2008). Coming out through art: A review of art therapy with LGBT clients. *Art Therapy: Journal of the American Art Therapy Association, 25(4),* 170–176.

Ream, G. L., & Forge, N. (2014). Homeless lesbian, gay, bisexual and transgender (LGBT) youth in New York City: Insights from the field. *Child Welfare, 93(2),* 7–22.

Rhoades, M. (2012). LGBTQ youth + video artivism: Arts-based critical civic praxis. *Studies in Art Education, 53(4),* 317–329.

Robinson, J. P., & Espelage, D. L. (2011). Inequities in educational and psychological outcomes between LGBTQ and straight students in middle and high school. *Educational Researcher, 40(7),* 315–330.

Roeck, K. (2008). Exploring how to change stereotypical attitudes toward students who are LGBT. *Democracy and Education, 18(1),* 53–56.

Rutter, M. (2012). Resilience as a dynamic concept. *Development and Psychopathology, 24(2),* 335–344.

Sandoval, C., & Latorre, G. (2008). Chicana/o artivism: Judy Baca's digital work with youth of color. In A. Everett (Ed.), *Learning Race and Ethnicity: Youth and Digital Media* (pp. 81–108). The John D. and Catherine T. MacArthur Foundation Series on Digital Media and Learning. Cambridge, MA: The MIT Press.

Savage, D. (September, 2010). What Is the It Gets Better Project? It Gets Better Project. Retrieved from http://www.itgetsbetter.org/pages/about-it-gets-better-project/.

St. Athatos, M. E., Watson, R., & Sulkowski, M. L. (2016). Peer victimization and resilience among LGBTQ youth. *Communique, 45(2),* 1–33.

U.S. v. Windsor, 576 U.S. ____ (2013).

Wolin, S. J., & Wolin, S. (1993). *The Resilient Self: How Survivors of Troubled Families Rise above Adversity.* New York, NY: Vallard Books.

7 The Role of the Art Educator in Meeting the Needs of Students Who Are Victims of Human Trafficking

Beverley H. Johns and Adrienne D. Hunter

It is estimated that nearly 30 million people worldwide are being exploited. They are being forced to work or provide sex for their captors. The trade in humans is big business and it is highly profitable (Luscombe, 2014). In fact, it is one of the most lucrative criminal activities, with estimated profits of $32 billion dollars annually (Rafferty, 2013).

Some may think that this horrific practice is occurring only within other countries, but not in the United States. However, the United States is one of the top three destinations for human sex trafficking. The United States government has estimated that approximately 50,000 women and children are trafficked into this country each year to work as prostitutes. The average age of victims is between 12 and 14. Sex trafficking victims are getting younger, and it is not uncommon to find them in every major city in the United States (Tomes, 2014). Among children in schools in the United States are those who are slaves.

Children who have run away from home because of possible abuse or neglect and are living on the streets or in out-of-home placements are at greater risk of trafficking. It is suggested that there is a link between child maltreatment and maladaptive physical and psychological outcomes, including emotional problems, aggressive behavior, substance abuse, and suicide (Rafferty, 2013).

Turner (2014) argues that while inter-country adoption seems to offer a chance for a happier life for some children, those children may be victims of human trafficking schemes. The United States is the leading country for adoptions, and inter-country adoptions account for about 15% of all United States adoptions. A number of children are offered for adoption illegally or are adopted by those who should not be permitted to adopt children. Parents in other countries are coerced into selling their children into orphanages; others are tricked into signing papers when they are told the signature is needed to get their children medical treatment but they are really relinquishing their rights. In other instances, Americans tricked parents into releasing their rights as parents so the children could get an education in the United States, saying the children would be returned to them, but then of course they were not.

The act of moving a child from one country to another does not constitute human trafficking. The question is the purpose of moving the child. The action must occur with the specific purpose of exploiting the child through sexual exploitation, slavery, or the removal of organs (Alexander, 2014).

Children who are victims of sexual trafficking face many challenges. They may have sexual diseases, they may have their own children, and they have physical and psychological scars. Children who are victims of sexual trafficking are vulnerable to arrest. In some states, law-enforcement officials may arrest children believed to be prostitutes and incarcerate them in juvenile centers. These children should be seen as victims, not criminals. Victims do not want to report abuse because they are afraid of the police and what the police may do to them. Some may have developed the Stockholm Syndrome (Tomes, 2014). According to the Rape, Abuse and Incest National Network (2014), the Stockholm Syndrome describes a victim's emotional bonding with their abuser as a survival strategy. It is subconsciously utilized as a survival instinct in a threatening and controlling environment.

At least two different populations of children emerge among those who are victims of trafficking within the United States: They are children from other countries, and those who are from the United States (Tomes, 2014).

Howard (2013) studied how Benin is promoting healthy childhoods and anti-trafficking. He discusses the importance of village vigilance committees. He also stresses the importance of sensitization to children's needs. It is critical to get the children into school and keep them there.

What can art educators do for students who face the potential of this trauma or who are living this trauma?

Being Informed

Art educators need to read and learn as much as possible about the human trafficking crisis and what is happening within the local area in which they work. They may not think that this is a problem where they live, but it certainly could be. Art teachers cannot ignore the fact that victims of trafficking may be within their classrooms, because it is possible that they are, and it is essential to have the knowledge and tools to help.[1]

Prevention

In terms of prevention, art educators can look for signs in their students that they may be distressed. Students will often communicate their frustrations about what is happening at home within their art work. When art educators notice that students' art work shows signs of problems, they can network with the school social worker, the guidance counselor, or school psychologist to alert them about potential problems. Schools need to create school vigilance committees. The art educator plays a critical role in this vigilance because he or she may see signs that a student may be in distress.

The art teacher is able to offer creative opportunities for the students to work individually and/or as a group in creative endeavors. A variety of materials and techniques could be offered, such as clay, paint, collage, print-making, sculpture, and fiber arts. The lessons should always be open-ended to encourage maximum individuality and creativity.

It may not be appropriate within the normal class setting to have students face their problems publicly, but rather to provide them with an opportunity for self-expression and to allow them to find solace and strength through the successes experienced in creating art. Due to the open nature of the art room, clues will often surface in the course of ordinary conversations. These clues may come in the form of questions that one student asks another, or just general conversational comments. Sometimes, it is not what the student says, but rather, what the student does not say. The attention of the art teacher is essential, and at times might be critical for the safety of the students.

Super Hero Theme

One of the authors shared this project:

The Super Hero theme was chosen because it was very open-ended. It offered infinite possibilities to safely and non-judgmentally express emotions and challenge the imagination while creating art. Giving the Super Heroes fantastic powers gave the students a sense of empowerment.

For this project, I explained to the students that they would be making life-sized Super Heroes and that they could give their Super Hero special super powers. We had a lively, often silly discussion about super powers. I asked each student to lie on a long sheet of white craft paper, while I very loosely traced around her or him. The students were permitted to choose how they wanted to pose: hands up, arms out, legs bent. The student then had the framework to create a Super Hero. Realizing that some students would not be comfortable being traced, I always gave them the option of selecting one of my extra pre-drawn bodies. (These were always prepared ahead of time.) The students then were able to create their own Super Heroes using a large variety of materials. I had available for them materials such as: pencils, paint, specialty fabrics like felt, velvet, lace and netting, glitter, feathers, plastic gems. Some students asked to work together in a pair, and this was permitted, but I did not suggest that the class pair up. Not only does "pairing up" often leave someone out, but most of my student artists preferred to work alone. While the materials were available to all students, I never recommend having students share their paint trays. They usually don't like to share their colors, and will often get upset when their colors get "dirty." The students were permitted to choose where they worked on their Super Heroes: Some students hung their Super Hero on the wall to be worked on, some chose to spread them out on the floor, either sitting or lying on their Super Hero or sprawled out beside it as they worked, and still others felt more comfortable remaining in their seats at their tables, draping their Super Hero over the edge of the table. The students were instructed to move around the room carefully as they got their own materials, and to speak quietly as they "checked out" each other's Super Heroes.

Size: Using life-size sheets of paper, the students were free to express themselves in a "big" way. Many had never worked so large, and it was a freeing experience. It also eliminated a common art problem for students who are not prepared to take risks in the classroom: They had a designated area to fill up, and therefore did not create a tiny little picture floating in the middle of the paper.

The outline: The outline was important because it presented a departure point. Where do I start? For some of the students, it was difficult to work so large, and these students generally sectioned off areas until the whole outline was filled in. Others found it necessary to fill in the background to set the stage for their Super Heroes. For students who wanted to preserve their backgrounds, we did not cut out these Super Heroes, but rather hung them as they were created.

The plethora of materials: Having a wide variety of materials from which to choose eliminated the "I can't draw" factor. It also served to spark their creativity and challenge them to have fun with their Super Heroes.

Classroom management expectations: My expectations for classroom behavior were clear—I expected them to get their own materials, to move around the room carefully, to see what their peers were working on, to talk quietly, and to relax and enjoy themselves. The atmosphere of the classroom was conducive to safely and successfully creating art while having fun with their peers.

Display: Creating a display for the Super Heroes validates the students' feelings and artistic endeavors. It builds self-esteem, promotes pride, and encourages the students to take risks in learning. It is important to note that I always give the students a choice as to whether their name is visible on the front of their Super Heroes or safely hidden on the back. Some Super Heroes were cut out while others were hung with their backgrounds, and they were displayed throughout the school for everyone to enjoy. The students were given the choice of writing a story about their Super Hero and its super powers, and some students chose to have their stories displayed along with their art work.

Art teacher reflections: The students enjoyed explaining the super powers that they had "given" to their Super Heroes. Some were fashion statements, some cartoon-like, and all had some combination of super powers. While none of the Super Heroes looked at all like their creators, the students' personalities shined through.

When art educators notice problems in school attendance, they can alert others within the school who can then determine why the student is not attending school on a regular basis. One of our authors shares this experience:

> While working in an alternative education high school, I had a principal tell me that I had to rescind the A that I had given to my star art student, because she had not completed the necessary attendance requirements.

Upon reviewing my attendance book, we realized that this student had perfect attendance in my art class. In comparing my attendance book with the school attendance record, we found that this student only came to school on the two days a week that I was teaching art at that school. In the end, I did not rescind the A grade, but I did sit down with the student and talk to her. As a trusted teacher, I was able to suggest to her that she attend her other classes if she wanted to graduate. Unfortunately, the pressures of her home life became overwhelming and she dropped out of school.

Monitoring Attitudes

Teachers must ensure that their attitude toward trafficked students is that they are victims. They are not the ones who are responsible for what they are doing. They have been coerced into this way of life. It is critical that we understand that these children need help; they do not need criticism about their values. They are trying to survive and need our support. A model that punishes them is counterproductive to their needs for support.

Here is an experience shared by one of the authors:

> While teaching teen-aged girls in a shelter program, I presented a lesson on counted cross-stitch. The lesson was very well accepted, and the girls asked for materials to continue working on their own. I was happy to be able to oblige. During the course of the lesson, the girls talked freely to one another, working on their projects, as I moved around to work individually with each student. I overheard a conversation, spoken very openly and very matter-of-factly, between two young ladies, which stopped me in my tracks. I was astounded when I heard one young lady say to the other, "We can work on this when we are waiting in the motel room." The other young lady said, "Yeah, it gets so boring just waiting." It was said so casually and with such acceptance. I didn't say anything to them at that time, but after class, I reported the conversation to one of the counselors. I was told that they were aware of the situation, and that the young ladies were in the shelter for protective custody from their pimps. The important part of this story is that I did not express any moral judgment, I provided the young ladies with a creative outlet that they enjoyed, but I did make sure that the appropriate counselors were notified.

Providing Support and Positive Relationships

These students are living in fear and have a difficult time trusting any adult. Positive relationships take time. The adult must remain non-judgmental and supportive. The art educator can build the student's esteem and confidence by praising the student for his or her creativity. The art educator can reinforce the student for school attendance and provide encouragement for the student to come to school. The art educator can and should listen attentively to what the student is saying.

Rehabilitation

Art educators may find themselves working with children who are in a rehabilitation and reintegration program. These are children who have been located and are now being provided a positive program to assist them. These children can benefit from art education as a necessary support and service. According to Fallot (2011), research on trauma-informed care has shown positive results in helping victims of violence to cope with their experiences and to avoid being victimized again. Art is an excellent way of teaching students to cope with their experiences. Art can provide a safe space for children to express themselves, and can help them say what cannot be said with words. The creative process can help foster resilience by helping children articulate individual strengths and personal attributes that help them survive traumatic events (Heise, 2013).

Conclusion

The art educator is a key player in a vigilance team within the school. Through art work, students can express their fears and their hopes for a better life. Art provides a positive outlet for students who are victims of such trauma. We must focus on protective factors that are believed to foster resilience such as safe and nurturing environments, high expectations, and ongoing opportunities for meaningful participation (Heise, 2013). Having at least one person who cares can facilitate resilience in youth. The art educator can be that person who cares and who builds on the strengths of the student.

Ten Teaching Tips

1 Educate yourself about human trafficking.
2 Build a positive and supportive relationship with the student.
3 View the student as a victim, not a criminal.
4 Pay close attention to the student's art work to see if there are messages of concern.
5 Watch for changes in the student's behavior and be alert to school attendance problems.
6 Network with pupil personnel staff and administrators in your school to discuss warning signs the student may be showing.
7 Provide choices in materials and techniques used in art projects.
8 Build success into each art experience and respond positively to the students' work.
9 Listen closely to conversations the student has with others and with you. Decode the message being given.
10 Exhibit the student's art and stress what each student has accomplished.

Note

1 See Chapter 4, Child Abuse: Signs and Reporting Procedures—What the Art Educator Should Know.

References

Alexander, J. (2014). Why the United States should define illegal adoption practices as human trafficking. *Houston Journal of International Law, 36(3)*, 716–748.

Fallot, R. (2011). Trauma-informed care: A values-based context for psychosocial empowerment. *Preventing Violence against Women and Children: Workshop Summary*. Washington, D.C.: The National Academies Press.

Heise, D. (2013). Fostering resilience through art. In K. Tavin & C. B. Ballengee-Morris (Eds.), *Stand Up for a Change: Voices of Arts Educators* (pp. 112–120). Reston, VA: National Art Education Association.

Howard, N. (2013). Promoting "healthy childhoods" and keeping children "at home": Beninese anti-trafficking policy in times of neoliberalism. *International Migration, 51(4)*, 87–102.

Luscombe, B. (2014). Bring back all girls. *Time Magazine*, May 26, 31–34.

Rafferty, Y. (2013). Child trafficking and commercial sexual exploitation: A review of promising prevention policies and programs. *American Journal of Orthopsychiatry, 83(4)*, 559–575.

Rape, Abuse and Incest National Network. Retrieved October 21, 2014, from https://rainn.org/get-information.

Tomes, M. (2014). A child is not a commodity: Stopping domestic child sex trafficking. *University of Florida Journal of Law and Public Policy, 24*, 213–234.

Turner, C. (2014). Sometimes it is better not to be unique: The U.S. Department of *State* view on intercountry adoption and child trafficking and why it should change. *Duke Forum for Law and Social Change, 6*, 91–112.

8 Alternative Educational Services for Students Who Have Experienced Psychological Trauma

Athena Petrolias, Beverley H. Johns, and Adrienne D. Hunter

The United States has various types of alternative school programs across the country. Alternative programs refer to services that are offered to students off the grounds of the elementary, middle, or high school that the student would ordinarily attend. Alternative school options for students are different across the 50 states and may include, but not be limited to, schools for students with disruptive behavior, charter schools, cyber schools, voucher schools, residential schools, home-schooling options, general learning centers, blended college/high school programs, career-themed schools, and special education alternative schools. The list of alternative school options continues to grow. The leadership of the education departments of each state may or may not dictate rules or regulations on how alternative schools are structured, operated, and monitored. Some states may not have any requirements or guidelines for operating alternative schools, while others may have clearly articulated rules and regulations for students identified for alternative education.

According to a 2014 survey of the United States done by the Institute of Education Sciences, there are 43 states and the District of Columbia who have formal definitions of alternative education. These programs primarily serve students with behavioral problems (Porowski, O'Conner, & Luo, 2014). Many of those behavioral problems may be the result of psychological trauma. The most common alternative services include regular academic instruction, counseling, social/life skills, behavioral services, and job readiness. The study did not mention the role of art in these programs. It is hoped that art is seen as an integral therapeutic part of the behavioral services and the academic instruction as well.

One of the authors shared her perspective on teaching art in alternative education programs and the impact of art on the students:

> When I was hired to teach art in 1974, the phrase "alternative education" had not yet been coined. I was hired to teach art to "institutionalized children." Over the course of many years, the label may have changed, but I was still teaching students who couldn't attend their home schools

for a variety of reasons: they were homeless, they were disruptive, they were truant, they had been expelled, and they were students who had experienced psychological trauma.

Teaching art in an alternative education program can be like teaching in a state of limbo. You aren't teaching "regular education students," and yet you aren't teaching what other people considered "special education students," despite your classes being inclusive. Many art teachers say it was like teaching art in isolation. There was and continues to be a dearth of professional development and professional teaching organizations that support teaching art in alternative education. It wasn't until I started making presentations on teaching art in alternative education programs for the National Art Education Association that I began to meet other art teachers in similar situations. These art teachers invariably said, "Finally! I have felt so alone teaching my students!"

Why? While there are a variety of school programs or programs within schools under the category of "alternative education," very few of these programs announce or promote their educational art programs, if offered. Occasionally someone will publish or present about a special art project or program that was offered for a limited time, but there is very little information available about permanent educational art programs within alternative education programs.

My journey by trial and error in teaching myself how to work with my alternative education art students has been a journey of lifelong learning for me as a teacher. I wish I had kept a journal documenting the progress of my students and myself, as a teacher. It is my firm belief that art opens the door for other learning. I have watched my students go from being reluctant to do any art work at all to refusing to leave the art room because they "have to finish this!" Students, who claimed to hate art, claimed they had no artistic ability whatsoever, suggested ideas for new, exciting projects that our whole school could participate in. I have seen very angry students enter my classroom and leave with smiles on their faces as they headed to their next class. I have seen the pride that students who generally set themselves up for failure display when they have successfully completed a project. I have witnessed how the lessons learned in art were generalized into other parts of their lives. Critical thinking skills such as making plans in sequential order, considering the cause and effect of actions, looking for alternatives and options when something doesn't work, looking at the big picture, and keeping track of details became a part of their survival tool kit. You really know you are making an impact when an "institutionalized" student asks you if he can return to your school after he is "out of the system." You know that art is making an impact when your classroom becomes a safe haven in a life of turbulence.

As Beth Kreinin, a retired alternative education teacher, said:

> Working with "at-risk" kids in an academic environment can present a number of challenges. Kids without self-esteem, unable or unwilling to engage with others, have a difficult time recognizing and/or verbalizing their academic deficits and needs. Art in the alternative education environment is an incredible way to bring students together. Many kids who aren't comfortable with "straight" academic subjects, like math and science, can get on board with an art project where they are using math to help devise the size of a mural, making papier-mache buildings for a history project, or creating clay vessels and painting them to hold science experiments. Art fills the void for interaction; it provides hands-on therapy without the traditional setting, allowing for self-expression, peer collaboration, and a comfortable way to reconnect with those academic subjects. Art attracts these kids because it's theirs to share. Projects have a beginning, middle, and end, with immediate gratification of having completed something they can hold and call their own, or share with others. What better way to link cognitive learning, socialization, and self-esteem.
>
> (2017)

In an early study, it was found that students who attended alternative schools showed improved positive peer relationships, commitment to school, and improved school performance (Lehr, 2004). In another study, students perceived a higher rate of support at the alternative school than in the traditional school (Edgar-Smith & Palmer, 2015). Critical also was the school staff modeling of empathy and non-retaliation. Staff were trained to show unconditional acceptance, and they were trained in instructional and behavioral management strategies. Strong achievement goals established by the teachers played a critical role in how engaged the students were in their school.

The National Dropout Prevention Center at Clemson University (2017) found these characteristics of effective alternative school programs: small teacher/student ratio of one to ten, a small student base, clear mission and discipline code, caring faculty, continual staff development, staff with high expectations for student achievement, an individualized learning program, a flexible school schedule, and a total commitment to ensure each student meets success.

Portland, Oregon, has built what is known as a strong, comprehensive, and innovative educational alternative system that re-engages out-of-school youth in addition to serving other vulnerable students (U.S. Department of Education, National Center for Education Evaluation and Regional Assistance, 2014). They work to reconnect with those students who may have mental health problems or who have experienced trauma. Their focus is on the engagement of students.

In strong alternative schools, there is considerable time devoted to cultivating connections between teachers and students (Raywid, 1994). An example of one such model follows.

A Model of Alternative Education in Pennsylvania

This section describes one model for providing a relevant education to a group of students whose needs were not met in a traditional setting. Alternative education in Pennsylvania is one model of providing non-traditional education to students that also offers art for credit. Policy and practice supports effective education for youth who have been temporarily excluded from public education. The hope is to provide readers with realistic ideas as they design innovative programs to effectively meet the needs of youth whose needs have not been met within traditional settings.

The current alternative education statute under which the Pennsylvania Public School Code, Department of Education Act is formally known as Alternative Education for Disruptive Youth (AEDY, 1997). Pennsylvania superintendents from the 501 different school districts asked for help in addressing negative behaviors in their respective districts. The lawmakers in Pennsylvania listened, and created state rules that specifically addressed youth with disruptive behavior.

AEDY provides six reasons that may allow a school district to place a student (grades six to twelve) into an alternative education setting:

1   Disregard for school authority, including persistent violation of school policy and rules.
2   Display of or use of controlled substances on school property or during school-affiliated activities.
3   Violent or threatening behavior on school property or during school-related activities.
4   Possession of a weapon on school property, as defined by Pennsylvania Crimes Code (1980), relating to possession of weapons on school property.
5   Commission of a criminal act on school property.
6   Misconduct that would merit suspension or expulsion under school policy.

The objective of a Pennsylvania state-approved Alternative Education Program (AEP) is to ultimately change the behavior of the student referred, and to return the student to the originating school system. Behavioral goals are established at intake, and periodic reviews on behavioral improvements are scheduled at least twice in a school year.

The referring school entity is required to complete a comprehensive referral form that outlines all the interventions that have been attempted to assist the student with negative behaviors. Extensive data is collected by Pennsylvania's Department of Education at the end of each year on the students referred to the AEDY program.

Students who do not meet any of the six requirements for referral to an AEDY program are not permitted to attend an approved alternative school. An AEDY program is required to emphasize changing negative behaviors and does not encourage students or school systems to have students remain in the alternative settings despite successes in the alternative setting. The goal, according to the state of Pennsylvania, is to return the student to the referring school program. The alternative setting is temporary, even if the student is succeeding in the alternative setting. Students with minor behavioral or academic issues, school phobia, or home issues impeding their learning are not candidates for the AEDY placements.

Before the state's AEDY statutes became law, alternative programs in Pennsylvania served students without any "entry criteria" to a program. School phobia, family issues, teen pregnancy or teen parenthood, parent/ child conflicts, and minor student/school conflicts were all examples of reasons for considering an alternative program in Pennsylvania. Students with issues that now do not meet Pennsylvania's definition of AEDY are required to seek alternatives in other types of educational programming.

An AEP—the "Right Stuff"

Southwestern Pennsylvania's Allegheny County boasts an AEP with a 57-year history of serving at-risk students. The program is currently run by the Allegheny Intermediate Unit, a state educational service agency. The program's strength is the quality and stability of the staff. There is little change in staff from year to year, and hiring practices emphasize a "missionary mentality" to help support students with a multitude of family and personal issues that may impede their educational experiences. Many of these students have suffered psychological trauma. The culture of the program has had almost 60 years of fostering the "advocacy" element of the program's mission: "The Allegheny Intermediate Unit's AEP is an educational system providing instruction, school counseling, and advocacy for students (grades 7 to 12) who have been temporarily excluded from a traditional school setting for a variety of circumstances" (Mission Statement from Alternative Education Program Allegheny Intermediate Unit, 2017).

The AEP currently operates three free-standing state-approved alternative schools, and three school programs, one in a juvenile detention facility, another in the county jail, and the third is a shelter program. The six sites are connected through a centralized record system that allows for an efficient accessing of records for a transient population of students. An at-risk student in a typical school year may move from a short stay at the detention facility to an alternative school and then back to the detention facility.

The centralized record system allows the program guidance counselors to work together to address the academic needs of students moving through court and schools systems to support credit and graduation requirements.

The professional development of the program has emphasized a better understanding of the culture of the students and families served by providing staff with diversity training. A few years ago, the state of Pennsylvania began to emphasize fostering protective factors that enhance the resiliency of at-risk youth, and the program worked to incorporate Nan Henderson's "Resiliency in Schools" concepts (Henderson & Milstein, 1996).

Mental Health 101, an Allegheny County-sponsored training for educators, was shared with the staff to better understand these students and some of the aspects of mental health at-risk youth may bring to the classroom. For the two most current school years, the AEP has had an in-depth focus on psychological trauma. The AEP addresses the impact of trauma on students, with strategies to address trauma in a learning environment based on trainings offered by the University of Pittsburgh and regional experts on trauma.

Recently teachers and counselors have taken greater ownership of their professional development, suggesting more effective ways for the organization to increase capacity for serving students. The "one and done" in-service is enhanced with smaller more collaborative learning groups to gain effective training in topics to improve student achievement in alternative education. Peer collaboration and action research have been introduced to the staff and are now formal options for a differentiated supervision/evaluation opportunity. Teachers and guidance counselors have also begun structuring small group discussions on topics first presented at large in-service presentations to process information presented.

Aspects of the brain and the adolescent were emphasized this school year at the local detention center, with six lunchtime sessions with University of Pittsburgh's Dr. Judy Cameron, a neuroscientist, and the center's teaching/counseling staff. These sessions allowed the educators an opportunity to dialogue with a noted expert on brain development about their work at the detention center and to discuss best strategies to interact with students for optimal enhancement of student brain circuits. These varied efforts demonstrate a future trend in more individualized professional development approach for educators.[1]

The alternative education teachers and counselors work with both academic deficiencies and behavioral challenges every day. Understanding trauma and its impact on students in the classroom better prepares staff for their daily interactions in delivering instruction. Strategies for working with at-risk students may include providing consistent daily classroom routines, creating calm learning environments, and predictable transitions. A safe, structured classroom, and awareness of the issues the students bring to the daily classroom, will help improve the learning opportunities of at-risk youth (Henderson & Milstein, 1996).

The AEP has approximately 70 certificated professionals who work with youth from various school systems and court placements at six different locations. It is the professionals of the program that bring the "right stuff" to the front-line interactions with our students and foster the successes of the clients served. The "right stuff" is defined by the former director of the AEP, Ronald Covato (2017), as "the ability to love the least lovable of society's children." Since the program's inception in 1959, advocacy for students has been the consistent thread woven through the years of changes in locations and service delivery. The most important factor in the success of the AEP is demonstrating the "right stuff"—students intuitively know when teachers or counselors truly care about them, often just from the tone of voice and an educator's disposition in daily interactions with students. It is in the small, nurturing environments with caring adults that our alternative education students succeed.

In addition, the educators with the "right stuff" have the ability to love the least lovable of society's children and work together to foster a positive school culture and climate. The delivery of instruction and learning opportunities to "at-promise" young people in the diverse settings of alternative schools flourishes with a positive school culture and climate. A quality, well-trained staff with compassion and the "right stuff" will provide the foundation for a successful alternative education program.

Art education in the program is offered for credit at the alternative schools. Students have many ideas and the schools offer a positive way to explore their creativity and problem-solving skills in a community school setting. Students are presented with a wide variety of mediums in a supportive and nurturing environment. Art teacher Sarah McGinnis offers a structured, choice-based model where students have the freedom to select a variety of options of projects. They can explore a variety of mediums and have license to create their own independent works with individualized instruction. Student ideas are fostered by the teacher, who allows them to problem-solve and make choices along the way. Skills are taught and the projects are facilitated with frequent conferences. Self-assessment is encouraged. Final works are celebrated with displays in the school and at community art shows.

Other Examples of Alternative Programs that Promote Art as a Means to Reach Students

In the Baltimore County Schools, Maryland, the Inverness Center was established in 1993 as a middle-school-level alternative program. In this program, teachers utilized art, technology, health, and physical education in order to teach content material (Lloyd, 1997). The center is known as a show place of student work where their artistic endeavors are always displayed.

In an alternative program in Boston, students worked on project-based problems that required the use of basic literacy and numeracy skills. The program was a practicum that was developed as part of an art education class at the School for the Visual Arts at Boston University. The University students taught art for five weeks of their semester. Students at the alternative school chose a social concern, researched it, wrote about it, and created a visual work that reflected the concern. The university students taught artistic processes to the students at the alternative school, and working side by side, shared problems and solutions while making art (Simpson, 2007).

Another program in the Midwest had a kiln and students created ceramic pieces. Students took great satisfaction in creating gifts that they could give family members.

In the state of Oklahoma, there is a program known as Arts in Alternative Education whereby alternative schools can apply for grants for eligible arts education programs. This program was designed by the Oklahoma State Department of Education where arts education programming such as dance, literary arts, media arts, and more are eligible. Any program, which must raise a 5% matching fund, may receive a grant for up to $2,500 per school year, but is also required to assess student learning to determine the effectiveness of the grant. The Oklahoma Arts Council also has a program known as "Find a Teaching Artist" which is a resource list of artists in Oklahoma who have been vetted by the Oklahoma Arts Council. The list is available to schools for their art education program (Oklahoma Arts Council, 2017).

Dr. Joseph Lagana, Executive Director Emeritus, Allegheny Intermediate Unit, stresses the vital role that the therapeutic value of art education plays for students in alternative education programs:

> The arts are essential for the full development of all children and youth. Therapy through the arts is particularly powerful in counseling troubled youth including those who are incarcerated. Therefore, the arts should be a key component in the development and delivery of alternative education programs. Preceding "cognitive" activities with a focus on the "affective" is a wise and effective means to reach troubled youth.
>
> The arts tap into and draw out all aspects of youth talent and have the potential to assist them to do well in their academic subjects by informing their teachers or counselors of their deeper thoughts, concerns, and interests. In addition, the therapeutic value of art is a critical ingredient for the alternative education curriculum. A trained art educator who understands that youth may express themselves in a variety of ways other than direct dialogue can be an invaluable member of the education team. Using the "power" of art is an invaluable approach to reach, unlock, and address the challenges associated with distracted youth. The basic understanding of the importance of art education in teacher training is vitally important in fostering insights and commitment to help guide youth to a healthy, productive, meaningful, and self-sustaining path in life (2017).[2]

Ten Teaching Tips

1 Incorporate art with academics to enhance relevant instruction.
2 Model empathy and non-retaliation.
3 Focus on the strengths of the students.
4 Utilize art to promote social and emotional well-being, stressing strengths of students.
5 Provide support to students by building a positive relationship with them.
6 Know your students' strengths, weaknesses, and interests.
7 Provide predictable transitions by preparing students for those transitions and utilizing picture cues that guide students on what is expected of them.
8 Provide a calm environment in the art setting.
9 Provide step-by-step directions with picture cues on what to do in any art project.
10 Provide frequent, positive recognition to students.

Notes

1 See Chapter 10, Neurobiological Impact of Trauma, for more information on the workings of the brain.
2 While this chapter discusses alternative education programs and Chapter 16, Non-Traditional Educational Settings, Center Schools, and Students with Behavioral Disorders, focuses on non-traditional settings, both present art education practices that can and should be generalized to traditional inclusive schools. Integrating art with academics and problem-solving needs to be an important part of all school curriculums. See Chapter 13, Integrating Art and Academics: A Collaborative Approach.

References

Barr, R. D., & Parrett, W. H. (2016). Alternative schooling—Types of alternative schools, alternative school models, international alternative schools, conclusion. Retrieved September, 2016, from http://education.stateuniversity.com/pages/1746/Alternative-Schooling.html.

Covato, R. (2017). Personal interview between Covato and Hunter.

Edgar-Smith, S., & Palmer, R. (2015). Building supportive school environments for alternative education youth. *Preventing School Failure, 59(3)*, 134–141.

Flower, A., McDaniel, S., & Jolivette, K. (2011). A literature review of research quality and effective practices in alternative education. *Education and Treatment of Children, 4*, 1–22.

Henderson, N., & Milstein, M. M. (1996). *Resiliency in Schools: Making It Happen for Students and Educators.* Thousand Oaks, CA: Corwin Press.

Kreinin, B. (2017). Personal interview between Kreinin and Hunter.

Lagana, J. (2017). Personal interview between Lagana and Hunter.

Lehr, C. (2004). *Alternative schools and students with disabilities: Identifying and understanding the issues.* Information Brief 3. Minneapolis, MN: University of Minnesota, Institute of Community Integration.

Lloyd, D. (1997). From high school to middle school: An alternative program for both. *Education Digest, 62(7)*, 1–4.

Maryland Department of Health and Mental Hygiene, Missouri Department of Mental Health, and National Council for Community Behavioral Healthcare (2012). *Youth Mental Health First Aid USA: For Adults Assisting Young People* (2nd edition). Baltimore, MD: Mental Health Association of Maryland.

National Alternative Education Association (2014). Exemplary practices 2.0: Standards of quality and program evaluation. Retrieved on April 10, 2017 from the-naea.org/NAEA/wp-content/uploads/2014/03/NAEA-Exemplary-Practices-2.0-2014.pdf.

National Dropout Prevention Center/Network at Clemson University (2017). Key elements of successful programs. Retrieved August 4, 2017 from http://dropoutprevention.org/effective-strategies/alternative-schooling.

Oklahoma (2017). Retrieved August, 4, 2017 inhttp://www.arts.ok.gov/Arts_in_Schools/Arts_in_Alternative_Education.html.

Pennsylvania Crimes Code (1980). 18 Pa.C.S. sec. 912.

Pennsylvania Public School Code of 1949, 24 P.S. sec. 19-1901-1906C, as amended, Act of June 25, 1997, P.L. 297, No. 30.

Porowski, A., O'Conner, R., & Luo, J. L. (2014). How do states define alternative education? U.S. Department of Education: Institute of Education, Sciences; National Center for Education Evaluation and Regional Assistance; Regional Educational Laboratory Mid-Atlantic. Retrieved on April 10, 2017 from https://ies.ed.gov/ncee/edlabs/regions/midatlantic/pdf/REL_2014038.pdf.

Raywid, M. (1994). Synthesis of research/alternative schools: The state of the art. *Educational Leadership, 52(1)*, 26–31.

Simpson, J. (2007). Connections to the world: Visual art in urban schools. *The Journal of Education, 188(1)*, 41–53.

Slaten, C., Irby, D., Tate, K., & Rivera, R. (2015). Towards a critically conscious approach to social and emotional learning in urban alternative education: School staff members' perspectives. *Journal for Social Action in Counseling and Psychology, 7(1)*, 41–62.

Swarts, L. (2004). Alternative education accountability: Kentucky's approach. In V. Gaylord, D. R. Johnson, C. A. Lehr, C. A. Bremer, & S. Hasazi (Eds.), *Impact: Feature Issue on Achieving Secondary Education and Transition Results for Students with Disabilities, 16(3)*. Minneapolis, MN: University of Minnesota, Institute on Community Integration.

Wilkerson, K., Yan, M., Perzigian, A., & Cakiroglu, O. (2016). Supplementary reading instruction in alternative high schools: A statewide survey of educator reported practices and barriers. *The High School Journal, Winter*, 166–178.

9 Mental Health Issues and the Art Classroom

Steven Kelly and Darla Dawn Absher

While teaching in a juvenile detention center, I was approached by the school counselor, who was quite agitated. She showed me a drawing of a figure with elongated limbs supported by crutches, and asked me what I thought of it. I immediately recognized the drawing as a reproduction of a Salvador Dali painting, and opened one of our art reference books to the plate. I told her I thought it was a good attempt at reproducing a master-piece. She was extremely relieved, and said, "Phew! I thought I was going to have to do some heavy duty counseling!" I asked her if she had spoken to the student about it, and she said, "No." I suggested that she ask the student why he chose that particular picture to replicate. She returned to me later and said that the student just thought it was "an interesting picture, and wanted to see if he could draw it." Sometimes we read too much into children's art work.

Adrienne D. Hunter

The goal of this chapter is to help art teachers, or any teacher, to meet the needs of all students, including those who may suffer from mental illness. We are also providing information to teachers that will assist in the early recognition of the signs of mental illness, and thus perhaps a better outcome for these students.

The art classroom of today is eclectic and each child is unique, bringing his or her own individuality to the table. Teachers need to appreciate this: The challenge is how to understand these children and to try to understand what is truly taking place in their minds.

Today's art room may look like this. On the first day of school, a teacher may look around and see several eager students in a sea of differing overt personalities and behaviors, first noticing the students in the back who pain-fully try not to be noticed, flanked by students who act out to be noticed, but hope to not get caught. There are other students who nervously bounce their legs, maintaining a perpetual motion in their seats, or trim their pencil like a beaver fashioning a log for a dam. There may be a fair representation of races, religions, and cultures. A teacher must quickly assimilate all of the small details and begin to form opinions of the participators, cooperators, collaborators, and trouble-makers, while attempting to suspend all preconceived notions, keep an open mind, and hope for the skills to learn something new from the individuals in the classroom.

Over the next few weeks, a teacher will begin to notice "that" boy or "that" girl who, for some reason not totally understood, is unique. Are they the "trouble-makers"? They do act up; however, they are also likeable. Why are their behaviors challenging behaviors? These are the kids who cannot sit still; who appear unable to follow directions. They may blurt out nonsense during instruction. They submit incomplete work or work with doodles, incomplete sentences, or anything else that may not pertain to the assignment. When redirected, they explode like a F5 tornado, not only redirecting the teacher's attention, but also perhaps requiring administrative support. The current framework of society would support an attention deficit/hyperactivity disorder (ADHD) evaluation, which if diagnosed, would likely lead to medications. Yet children are faced with many challenges in the home and in the school. The reason behind their behavior could be simple; however, many times this is a multifaceted problem, and it will take attention, support, and patience to assist and guide this child throughout the school year, understanding that this child can be as successful as all the other students.

There may also be a child who stares blankly or looks off to the right or left. They may smile or laugh at something that is not funny. Why are they smiling; What are they laughing at? When questioned, they may look slightly confused and be unable to provide an explanation of why they smiled or laughed. Another child may appear to be fearful of "something," yet they cannot label the cause of the fear they are experiencing. Sometimes the same child may appear to be talking to themselves in a room full of other students, but when prompted they are unable to tell you who they are talking to. Sometimes this can be fearful or comforting, depending on the child and the voice. These children need to be spoken to in a low voice and not startled. They may be responding to internal or external stimuli. This looks a little different than the imaginary friend that some children, usually of preschool age, report experiencing. None of these children want to be different; they do not truly understand what is taking place in their brains.

Some of the children in an art room may have difficulty with sensory issues. A simple example of this for some children is sensitivity to sound. They can yell or scream; however, let someone else yell or scream, or any other loud noises occur in the environment, and they are not able to handle this noise. This child may be observed sticking their fingers in their ears and starting to rock. This child may also shake his or her head as if saying "no." They appear fearful and scared or angry. A simple solution in this situation is to remain calm, speak in a low and slow voice, and offer reassurance to the child as you attempt to get the classroom quiet again.

Middle school appears to be a difficult time for many. Some challenging behaviors may include increased risk-taking behavior, increased aggression, or even moodiness. It is often thought that this is "normal" adolescent behavior. According to the *Merriam-Webster Online Dictionary* (2017), the definition of normal is "according with, constituting, or not deviating from a norm, rule, or principle." Can any human being ever be described as "normal"? The best way to truly describe "normal" is a setting on a washer. An adolescent who seems happy-go-lucky, who comes from a family that appears stable and great, may then all of sudden one day punch a peer in the face. He or she may then begin to exhibit increased anger, agitation, and annoyance. This child can be experiencing many different difficulties, and it is important to get a clear understanding of what is occurring in his or her life. No one, including the above child, fits into just one box: A clear understanding of the whole child is needed to explain why the child is exhibiting these behaviors. When a teacher understands the uniqueness of a child, the teacher is then able to assess the needs of the child and have a better understanding of where the child is coming from. When the teacher understands the dynamics, this will assist in designing effective ways to teach, as well as presenting the students with effective ways to learn.

In some of the higher grades, students may exhibit totally different behaviors not congruent with the rest of their classmates. There may be a student who just does not seem present. He or she always appears unkempt and maybe even has a little body odor. This child may have at one time been involved with school activities, and then slowly stopped; earned decent grades, but now does not; ceases interaction with adults or peers; or now exhibits an entire lack of affect or is apathetic toward school in general. It is of greatest concern when children give up activities but do not replace them with something else.

There also may be a student with a fantastic imagination, accompanied with the most creative art work, who whispers in the corner. He or she may share that "they" frequently talk about him or her on the radio, making demeaning statements; but the student's artistic talent is linked to an unexplainable event that has something to do with the unidentified voice.

Some of the mental health problems that begin in high school may look very different from the onset of mental illness later in life or adulthood. A young person may have a lot of things to say; however, they may have a very difficult time expressing themselves. This is where expression through art may speak volumes.

It is not uncommon for adolescents to report experimentation with drugs during this time. Upon interviewing and working with youth, we found that many also report drug use as a direct attempt to self-medicate. Drug use may allow them to feel not sad for a short time, it may alleviate the voices they do not understand, or they are for a time able to escape the abuse or traumatic pain they are experiencing.

These examples may appear to be a little extreme, but will be present in many schools. They are examples of ways mental illness may manifest itself in schools and communities. The National Alliance on Mental Illness (NAMI, 2017) defines mental illness as a condition that impacts a person's thinking, feeling, or mood and may affect his or her ability to relate to others and function on a daily basis. They emphasize that each person will have different experiences, even those with the same diagnosis.

What does the average person know about mental illness? A few people will have become informed enough by either doing research or actually experiencing events related to someone suffering from mental illness. Just as people with diabetes can be brilliant, so can those suffering from these emotional illnesses be brilliant. Unfortunately, the majority of the population most often relies on the preformed schemata developed by the media. Historically, the media has portrayed mental illness in a poor light, biased toward entertaining without educating. Thus, from a young age, the general population subconsciously draws opinions from books, cartoons, periodicals, movies, and broadcast news.

What do the media teach about mental illness? Watching *Halloween*, *Psycho*, or *Friday the 13*th may lead to the formulation of an opinion that all persons who are mentally ill are psychopathic killers. Follow that up with the evening news on television which may suggest that all people suffering from schizophrenia are violent, or watch the series *Wonderland*. When reading newspapers about the latest murder or arson, the perpetrator is often described as being depressed. Watching *One Flew over the Cuckoo's Nest* or *Dream Team* might lead to a generalization that the mentally ill are "crazy," incompetent, and having over-the-top fun in their delusions and lunacy.

However, it is not all bad. Some individuals can be wrongly portrayed as having a mental illness and yet are seen as geniuses who can become rich with their savant abilities to count things, as in *Rain Man*. In *Good Will Hunting*, Will was able to overcome depression by conversations with a therapist and was able to move beyond his problems in just a semester (although this is not necessarily a realistic time frame). John Nash, a brilliant mathematician, was portrayed enduring brutal electroconvulsive therapy treatments in the movie *A Beautiful Mind*. While the films above are certainly better portrayals of mental illness by the media, they make light of the illnesses they portray or exaggerate the treatments that could be effective for the disorder. Would anyone elect to have electroconvulsive therapy after watching *A Beautiful Mind*? Most people would not. However, having seen the gentle procedure as it is performed today, most would consider it in certain situations. It can be a very effective treatment for depression that has been non-responsive to medications.

As defined in the *Open Education Sociology Dictionary* (2017), a "stigma is a severe social disapproval [of] a person on the grounds of a particular characteristic which distinguishes them from others in society, e.g., mental illness or physical disability." Link and Phelan (2001) defined stigma in terms of the convergence of four interrelated components: people distinguish human differences; the dominant cultural group labels these differences and links them to undesirable characteristics; negatively labeled groups or individuals are placed in separate categories from the non-stigmatized; and as a result of the first three components, labeled individuals lose status. Is it fair to say that what is presented by the media has created a set of negative and often unfair beliefs which stigmatize mental illness? *Merriam-Webster* defines stigma as "a mark of shame or discredit" (2017). Should it be shameful or discrediting to be diagnosed with an illness? Should people feel shame when taking a blood pressure pill, injecting insulin, or having been diagnosed with heart disease? There is enormous family support for those who suffer from cancer or have a heart attack. Why do people become so uncomfortable when talking about mental illness? After all, it is a medical problem too.

The Centers for Disease Control and Prevention (CDC) Statistics Report for 2017 reports that in 2015, 30.3 million people had diabetes in the United States. That is about one in every 11 people. The CDC (2016) also reports that about 75 million adults had high blood pressure. That is about 1 in every 3 adults. According to the National Institute of Mental Health (NIMH, 2016), approximately 43.8 million adults experience a mental illness each year. That is about one in every five adults in the United States. To put this in perspective, for every 20 readers of this chapter, two should watch their diet because of diabetes, six have struggled with high blood pressure, and finally, four readers are struggling with a mental health problem. By bringing this ignored statistic to the forefront, enlightenment can be achieved. Knowledge opens the door to understanding; a little bit of understanding leads to empathy; and empathy gives art teachers the power to accept and use these tools to teach.

There are ways for art teachers to go about expanding their knowledge of mental illness. For example, there are many free and or fee-based continuing education units offered in communities across the country. They can be found by contacting local NAMI offices; boards of social work and counseling; and local mental health facilities. It is not necessary to be a mental health professional to attend. When considering professional educational development, art teachers often do not consider going outside of the usual educational offerings.

According to the NIMH (2016), by the age of 14, half of lifetime mental illnesses begin. Research shows that a human's body will exhibit signs of mental illness before symptoms appear. The child may report somatic complaints, such as headaches and stomachaches, with no medical reason for them. This is a new insight into mental illness, as well as potentially offering ways to help children and adolescents in their formative years. In order for children to be diagnosed with a mental illness, they will have to see a doctor or mental health specialist. Providers gather a detailed history regarding the child and attempt to determine how long the child has been exhibiting the signs the parents or teachers are observing. The provider tries to determine the root of the cause. Diagnosing young children is difficult at times due to them not being able to fully explain what they are experiencing. A diagnosis should be used to guide treatment and provide understanding regarding what a child is experiencing. Mental illness can be treated; however, nearly two-thirds of children who need help will receive little if any help (NAMI, 2017). Early identification and treatment is imperative for children, highlighting the important role art teachers can play in early identification. This will allow these children to reach their full potential with the proper support and treatment.

Thanks to great research at the NIMH (2016), we know that 20% of our children currently, or at some point during their lives, have had a seriously debilitating mental disorder. The U.S. Department of Education (2016) estimates the current average classroom size to be 25 students. That could lead a teacher to infer that, at any given time, five of these students are or will be suffering from a mental illness.

When children have an untreated mental health problem, it can affect their functioning at home as well as the classroom and their community. Once it is known that some students are struggling with a mental illness, it is an art teacher's duty to gain some insight into what that may look like in an art room. According to *Mental Health America* (NIMH, 2016), the following signs may indicate the need for professional help.

- decline in school performance;
- poor grades despite strong efforts;
- constant worry or anxiety;
- repeated refusal to go to school or to take part in normal activities;
- hyperactivity or fidgeting;
- persistent nightmares;
- persistent disobedience or aggression;
- frequent temper tantrums; and
- depression, sadness, or irritability.

Knowledge opens the door to understanding—the most essential task in dealing with mental health issues in the classroom for teachers is to educate themselves.

Some of the signs and symptoms of mental illness in children and adolescents that we as clinicians have observed:

- increased conflict in relationships at home and at school;
- increased irritability, anger, or hostility;
- fighting, verbal aggression, and conduct problems;
- extreme sensitivity to rejection or failure;

- psycho–motor agitation;
- intense worrying or fear that interferes with participation in class or school;
- low self-esteem;
- social isolation and poor communication;
- extreme low energy or signs of always being fatigued;
- decreased interest in activities or enjoyment (anhedonia);
- frequent complaints of physical illness such as headaches and stomachaches;
- poor school performance;
- major change in sleeping or eating habits;
- struggles with parental divorce/situation;
- increased sadness, tearfulness, and crying;
- hopelessness;
- cutting or carving on one's skin; and
- thoughts or expressions of suicide.

These are just a small representation of some of the warning signs of mental illness in our youth. If any of these symptoms appear, it warrants a discussion with the school counselor, mental health team member, or professional present within the school. It is important to take note of the symptom(s) or behavior(s) and track frequency and severity, as this would be important information to share with any treating professional who could use it to make a diagnosis or first impression. This will also make it much easier to communicate with parents and students from a "just the facts"-based perspective which can help decrease defensiveness. No one wants to hear that their child has a problem, certainly not a problem they don't understand. Remember, just as a teacher may have formed opinions from the media, so have parents.

One topic that many are uncomfortable to talk about is suicide. According to the American Association of Suicidology (2011), suicide is the second leading cause of death for 15- to 24-year-olds and the sixth leading cause of death for 5- to 14-year-olds. Attempted suicides are even more common. Girls are more likely to attempt suicide, but boys are 4.34 times more likely to die by suicide than girls; 90% of these suicides have an underlying mental illness. Suicide affects nearly 20% of those with bipolar disorder and 15% of those with schizophrenia (2011).

Discussing suicide has been a taboo topic for some time. Many have believed if you speak of it, it will happen. This, however, is not the case. Asking the question or talking about suicide does not put the thought or idea into someone's mind. Research has shown that asking the question could and will save a life (NAMI, 2017). There are risk factors associated with suicide: A diagnosis of mental or addictive disorders, often co-occurring, are the greatest risk factors for suicide, with bipolar disorder and schizophrenia having the strongest association with suicidal behavior. Depression is also a factor. The loss of many things may make one feel helpless and hopeless, with no reason for living, especially in young children or adolescents. "Copy-cat" suicides have also occurred.

It is important to note if a student exhibits dramatic mood changes (high or low), anxiety, or agitation. Youth are resilient. They possess many protective factors that act as a safety net. The role of art teachers and social workers is to assist students in reaching their coping skills when needed.

Sher (2004) reports that there is no single factor that can determine if someone will commit suicide: It is a combination of a genetic predisposition; a psychiatric disorder or conflicting disorders, diagnosed or not; and sociological factors such as poor social relationships or support. Of note is that most psychiatric patients never attempt suicide, although it is suggested that a variety of risk factors may increase the likelihood that someone experiences suicidal ideation or a suicide attempt (Sher, 2004). While talking about suicide is considered to be taboo, it is one of the most preventable deaths. It is difficult scientifically to prevent childhood cancer; however, educating and discussing suicide and suicide prevention is the best form of intervention to prevent suicide.

There is an average of ten years between the onset of the symptoms of mental illness and receiving an intervention (Sher, 2004). The long-entrenched stigma obviously plays a role in the length of time it takes for someone to seek help, but that is not the only factor in play. The children in the busy art room who were discussed at the beginning of this chapter displayed all sorts of overt behaviors. Every teacher can name three children off the top of their head who misbehave regularly. What about those children who do not misbehave? What about those children who have withdrawn to the back of the classroom because they are not engaged in the instruction? Many educators may not have time to notice. This is one of the most frightening things about teaching children in crisis—the unknown "why" of the behavior of the children. Not drugs, teen violence, or gang activities cause death as frequently as suicide; statistically, suicide is the second leading cause of death in youth aged 15 to 24. This is alarming. We urge all teachers to learn about mental illness in adolescents.

According to NAMI (2017), some children in all schools will be suffering from the following disorders: ADHD, mood disorders, and anxiety. Various research articles state that there can be anywhere from 5% to 11% of children and adolescents with ADHD. This disorder is characterized by symptoms of inattention, hyperactivity, and impulsivity. The ADHD made famous by the media, stigmatization, and drug advertisements on television tends to be more hyperactive in nature. One important point to remember is that ADHD is not an emotional illness that occurs only in school. These behaviors will be present at home as well. It is important to get a clear diagnosis from a professional, as ADHD can be mistaken for symptoms of other disorders such as anxiety.

Everything changes. The *American Psychiatric Association's Diagnostic and Statistical Manual of Mental Disorders* (5th edition; DSM-5) revised and expanded certain diagnoses, and now guides clinicians to provide more accurate diagnoses. The road to mental health begins with an accurate diagnosis, and this improvement should prevent many children from slipping through the cracks.

For example, an 11-year-old boy was diagnosed with bipolar disorder at age 4. First, is it ethical to diagnose a child this young? How does mania look in a 4-year-old? This child was never successfully treated for his extreme, explosive rages. Too many children with significant impairments like this have suffered from a disorder that had not yet been defined. A new diagnosis in the DSM-5 aims to give these children a diagnostic home and ensure they get the care they need.

A clearer diagnosis for the above child might be a disorder called disruptive mood dysregulation disorder (DMDD), and its symptoms go beyond describing temperamental children to those with a severe impairment that requires clinical attention. Far beyond temper tantrums, DMDD is characterized by severe and recurrent temper outbursts that are grossly out of proportion in intensity or duration to the situation. These occur, on average, three or more times each week for one year or more. Between outbursts, children with DMDD display a persistently irritable or angry mood, most of the day and nearly every day, that is observable by parents, teachers, and peers. A diagnosis requires the above symptoms to be present in at least two settings (at home, at school, or with peers) for 12 or more months, and symptoms must be severe in at least one of these settings. During this period, the child must not have gone three or more consecutive months without symptoms. The onset of symptoms must be before age 10, and a DMDD diagnosis should not be made for the first time before age 6 or after age 18.

Mental illness should not be stigmatized, and it is the job of educators to cross that barrier when dealing with today's students. Observe students with an open mind. Recognize those that may be struggling emotionally. Approach them as individuals in a non-judgmental manner. Most important, listen to what they have to say. By listening, more information is conveyed. By allowing for more moments of silence than questioning, more information is forthcoming. Last, involving the families as part of the school is just a small part of the larger ecosystem that the student resides in.

Rather than focusing on each diagnosis, this chapter is an overview of what teachers may encounter in the art room. These topics reflect what we have seen the most often in recent years, although there are others. Teachers of children in crisis are providing great services to children, but their services are often unnoticed or unappreciated. We hope that they know that they are appreciated even though the words are rarely, if ever, spoken.

Ten Teaching Tips

First, a bonus tip, and the most important tip: The art room can be a dangerous place with scissors, toxic materials such as paints, and pencils. Know the students, especially if any of them have violent tendencies, and plan accordingly. Tearing up colored paper to create art is always a possibility.

1 Modify the standard teaching approach by providing more interactive instruction and building on the interests and strengths of the students.
2 Design lessons so students may get up and move around.
3 Each learning task is introduced, one step at a time.
4 Utilize visual aids.
5 Provide immediate feedback.
6 Provide one-on-one instruction.
7 Teach and practice organization skills, utilizing art.
8 Challenge but don't overwhelm.
9 Provide supports to promote on-task behavior.
10 Listen to what the students have to say.

References

American Association of Suicidology (2013). Youth suicide fact sheet. Retrieved May 24, 2017 from www.suicidology.org/14/docs/Resources/FactSheets/Youth2012.pdf.

American Psychiatric Association (2013). *Diagnostic and Statistical Manual of Mental Disorders* (5th edition).

Centers for Disease Control and Prevention (June 17, 2017). *National Diabetes Statistics Report, 2017*, 2. Retrieved July 20, 2017 from www.cdc.gov/diabetes/data/index.html.

Centers for Disease Control and Prevention (June 16, 2017). *Heart Disease Facts and Statistics*, 1. Retrieved July 20, 2017 from https://www.cdc.gov/dhdsp/data_statistics/fact_sheets/fs_bloodpressure.htm.

Link, B., & Phelan, J. (2011). Conceptualizing stigma. *Annual Review of Sociology* 27(3), 363–385.

Merriam-Webster Online Dictionary (2017). "Normal," *para.* 2.a. Retrieved on June 6, 2017 from https://merriam-webster.com/dictionary/normal.

Merriam-Webster Online Dictionary (2017). "Stigma," *para.* 1.b. Retrieved on June 6, 2017 from https://merriam-webster.com/dictionary/stigma.

National Alliance on Mental Illness (2017). *NAMI: National Alliance on Mental Illness*. Retrieved on May 24, 2017 from www.nami.org/Learn-More-Mental-Health-Condition

Open Education Sociology Dictionary (2017). "Stigma." Retrieved September 4, 2017 from sociologydictionary.org.

Sher, L. (2004). Weather, climate and suicidality. *Letter to the editor, ACTA Psychiatrica Scandinavica, 109*, 319.

U.S. Department of Education (2016). *National Center for Educational Statistics.* Retrieved May 2017 from www.nces.ed.gov/surveys/sass/tables/sass1112_2013314_tls_007.asp.

U.S. Department of Health and Human Services, National Institutes of Health, National Institute of Mental Health (2016). *NIMH strategic plan for research. NIH Publication No. 02- 2650).* Retrieved on May 24, 2017 from http://www.nimh.nih.gov/about/strategic-planning-reports/index.shtml.

10 Neurobiological Impact of Trauma

Carlomagno Panlilio, Elizabeth Hlavek, and Amanda Ferrara

On the third day of school, Matthew's teacher assigned him an essay about a challenge he has overcome. He began diligently writing as asked, but soon became distracted, staring listlessly out of the window. When his teacher approached him, asking why he was not writing, he burst out in tears. He explained that his cousin was shot and killed over the summer and this essay topic triggered a troubling memory from this traumatic event. His teacher allowed him to take a few minutes in the hallway to calm down as well as choose an alternative essay assignment. This psychologically traumatic event caused cognitive, behavioral, and emotional difficulties for Matthew as he began his writing assignment at the beginning of the year, and in many other situations as the school year went on. He volunteered this information to a caring adult, which allowed his teacher to be cognizant of his traumatic experience throughout the school year and react in a trauma-sensitive manner.

Unfortunately, many educators may work with students with traumatic histories and not even realize it. The prevalence for experiencing two or more traumatic events is very high for children from birth to 17 (Saunders & Adams, 2014). This means that, at some point, art educators may have a student in their class who has experienced some form of traumatic event. Knowing the impact of psychological trauma on a child's developing brain and related learning processes becomes that much more important. As art educators recognize the developmental impact of trauma, the next step is to recognize the potential benefits of art education and how to employ teaching strategies that can help these vulnerable students.

What Is Trauma?

According to the National Child Traumatic Stress Network (2017), trauma occurs when a child witnesses or experiences an event or a series of events that pose a real or perceived threat that overwhelms their capacity to cope. These traumatic experiences can be understood as occurring under two different sets of circumstances: acute trauma or chronic trauma. Examples of acute traumatic events include school violence, natural disasters, and sudden or violent loss of a loved one. Chronic traumatic situations include complex trauma, intimate partner violence, and wars or other political violence. Complex trauma within the chronic scenario describes exposure to multiple or prolonged traumatic events that negatively impact children's developmental trajectories. Complex trauma typically involves child maltreatment that is chronic, begins in early childhood, and occurs with the child's primary caregiver. These experiences often lead to negatively cascading effects that lead to vulnerabilities in functioning later in life. Given the serious nature of childhood trauma, it is important to understand how traumatic events impact brain development in children.

Trauma and the Brain

Brain development proceeds at an astounding rate from birth until the age of 5. The regions of the brain responsible for visual and auditory processing as well as body movement develop first. Brain regions that control higher-order processes such as conscious thought, decision-making, memory, reasoning, problem-solving, and self-regulation continue to develop from early childhood into adolescence.

Brain architecture is comprised of a network of 100 to 200 billion neurons that store and transmit information across different areas of the brain. The strength and complexity of these neural connections depend upon the child's interaction with his or her environment, particularly around sensitive periods of development. During these sensitive periods, children's interactions with caring adults, especially with their parents early in life, affect the development and organization of their brain architecture through what is known as experience-expectant brain stimulation. As infants continue to develop, experience-dependent stimulation of brain regions proceed as a result of specific learning experiences that vary widely based on individual differences and contextual influences.

During these important moments of development, it is important for caregivers and educators to be sensitive and responsive to children's signaling behaviors that provide a rich adult–child relationship, which promotes positive development. Unfortunately, when children experience adverse events in their environment, particularly complex trauma such as abuse and neglect, changes at the neurobiological level become quite evident.

The Biological Stress Response System

Children across different developmental stages may experience traumatic stress when exposed to acute and chronic traumatic events. Their bodies' major biological stress systems, such as the hypothalamic-pituitary-adrenal (HPA) axis, activate to produce a range of physiological reactions to deal with the real or perceived environmental threat (De Bellis & Zisk, 2014).

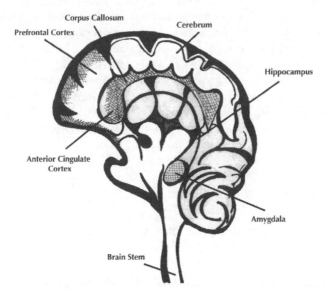

Figure 10.1 "Brain Illustration" drawn by Elizabeth Hlavek

Typical functioning of the HPA axis is usually assessed by measuring different levels of the hormone cortisol. During stressful events, cortisol levels become elevated but then return to baseline due to the negative feedback loop within the HPA axis (Trickett et al., 2014).

This short-term increase in cortisol levels is necessary to ensure survival. However, when stress responses remain active at high levels for an extended period of time in the absence of supportive relationships, organ systems and brain architecture may become damaged, leading to negative effects on learning, behavior, and health for these children. The excessive or prolonged activation of the stress response systems is known as "toxic stress," which can have damaging effects on the development of neural connections, brain structures, and brain functions, especially those dedicated to higher-order skills (Shonkoff et al., 2012).

Structural, Functional, and Connectivity Issues Related to Trauma

Alterations in brain structures that are typically associated with trauma, particularly as a result of toxic stress, include the hippocampus, corpus callosum, the anterior cingulate cortex (ACC), the amygdala, and the prefrontal cortex (PFC). The hippocampus is a brain area that is rich in corticosterone receptors (Trickett et al., 2014) and plays an important role in the process of information encoding and recall. It is also particularly important in the consolidating of short-term memory or sensory and perceptual information into long-term storage. Given the number of corticosterone receptors in the hippocampus, it becomes particularly susceptible to the increased cortisol levels as a result of toxic stress. This, in turn, is associated with reductions in hippocampal volume, which may not emerge until after puberty (Teicher et al., 2016). Decreased hippocampal volume may then be related to problems with encoding, retention, and recall of information learned in the classroom.

The corpus callosum is a band of myelinated neural fibers that connects the left and right cerebral hemispheres and aids in the lateralization process. The left hemisphere is often implicated in processing verbal abilities, positive emotions, and sequential, analytic processing. The right hemisphere is often implicated in processing spatial abilities (e.g., judging distance, reading maps), negative emotions, and holistic, integrative processing. It is important to note that despite this lateralization or specialization of functioning, the corpus callosum ensures that both hemispheres communicate and work together, which becomes more effective and efficient over time.

Unfortunately, traumatic experiences, particularly complex trauma such as maltreatment, are often associated with reduced integrity of the corpus callosum. Decreased thickness of the corpus callosum has been related with decreased IQ scores in maltreated children. It has been hypothesized that communication problems between the two cerebral hemispheres may play an important role in problem-solving, leading to lower IQ scores (Teicher et al., 2016). Additionally, sex differences in decreased corpus callosum integrity were evident, in that boys showed greater reduction than girls. Finally, when hemispheric balance is altered (e.g., using electroencephalogram-asymmetry studies), there is a resulting shift in how approach-avoidance decisions are made, particularly around anger and aggression, where the left hemisphere is specialized for approach responses and the right hemisphere is for avoidance responses.

The region of the brain that is collectively known as the ACC is usually associated with the processing of emotional information, as well as the monitoring of cognitive and motor responses during conflict situations (Shackman, Wismer Fries, & Pollak, 2008). In non-traumatized children, enhanced activation in the ACC region was observed when participants were presented with threat-related facial expressions as distractors. However, individuals with high levels of anxiety were shown to exhibit lower activation of the ACC region (Bishop, Duncan, Brett, & Lawrence, 2004). Experiencing toxic stress and the resulting dysregulation in the HPA axis may decrease metabolism in the ACC. Indeed, individuals with prior experiences of trauma and resulting post-traumatic stress disorder (PTSD) often show decreased ACC activation (Shackman et al., 2008). Decrease in activation levels for this particular brain region may indicate problems with emotional processing for children with traumatic experiences. This, in turn, may impact social interactions of children in the classroom.

The amygdala is an important structure for encoding information with emotional significance and is part of the limbic system. It has reciprocal connections to cortical sensory areas such as visual and auditory areas. As part of the attentional network, the amygdala is responsible for orienting attention in the presence of salient emotional stimuli in the environment. It exerts a "bottom-up," or sensory-driven, influence over cortical areas that will be used in the attentional network when emotional information is present. The amygdala helps with the assessment of emotionally expressive information in order to learn about environmental events that may pose a threat or provide a reward. Thus, emotional signals are used to enhance vigilance and to prepare the brain's learning networks in order to acquire new information from the environment. The orienting function of the amygdala has been shown to amplify attention to threat or bias attention toward anger-eliciting or sadness-eliciting information in the child's environment (Briggs-Gowan et al., 2015; Romens & Pollak, 2012; Shackman, Shackman, & Pollak, 2007), which may lead to an increase in anxiety, depressive symptoms, or aggressive behaviors. These, in turn, may lead to socio-emotional difficulties related to children's educational well-being.

The prefrontal cortex is a structure responsible for thought, consciousness, inhibition of impulses, integration of information, and use of memory, reasoning, planning, and problem-solving strategies. Production of moderate levels of cortisol by the HPA axis stimulates neural activity within the PFC, which underlies these executive attention and executive function abilities (Blair & Raver, 2015). It exerts a "top-down" influence on the amygdala when processing emotionally salient stimuli. Sufficient development of the PFC indicates children's readiness to begin formal schooling around 5 to 6 years of age. Maturation proceeds at later ages as children continue to learn self-regulatory capacities to promote sustained engagement in the learning process. For children with traumatic histories, however, experiencing toxic stress and the "flooding" of cortisol decreases activity in the PFC. There is also an associated reduction in the interconnectedness of the hippocampus with the PFC and the ACC, which is associated with a decrease in the top-down regulation of the amygdala by the PFC (Teicher et al., 2016). As PFC activity is reduced, there is an associated increase in brain regions associated with reactive emotional and behavioral responses to emotion-eliciting stimuli. This decrease in inhibitory control may then lead to poor judgment and more impulsive behaviors, particularly for children who experience complex traumatic events.

Many of these brain structures function in an interconnected manner that allows for the effective and efficient activation of the attentional networks. At home and in the classroom, children are constantly bombarded with incoming information from the environment. Children must somehow be able to engage in selective attention, given the brain's limited capacity to simultaneously process all of the incoming stimuli. During normal social development, children learn to modulate their attention to selectively attend to the most relevant internal and external information, while at the same time inhibiting or minimizing attention to irrelevant cues. This is important in the context of learning as children are required to attend to the lesson at hand, encode the information, and recall this at a later time during assessment. As highlighted above, these perceptual and attentional processes become altered due to early adversity, which may then influence the regulation of cognition, emotion, and behavior that places children at an increased risk for developing emotional and behavioral problems that can impact their educational well-being.

Trauma and Art Education

Traumatic experiences are encoded as a nonverbal sensation; while dialogue may not bring up psychologically traumatic memories, sensorimotor and visually based activities, such as art, can (Van der Kolk, 2006, 2014). In this regard, art can be extremely helpful in mitigating PTSD in children and adults by helping them to reconstruct the memory in their brain. The nonverbal traumatic memories stored in the right hemisphere can integrate with the verbal functions of the left hemisphere, providing an increased understanding of the trauma. When explored safely through simultaneous art-making and conversation, this integration can be extremely healing. Additionally, the act of art-making is affirming, and can promote an increased sense of self-esteem and mastery, both important for the healthy development of traumatized children. Imagination and imagery have the capacity to promote resilience and problem-solving (Malchiodi, 2002), which can serve to benefit all children, particularly those with traumatic backgrounds. In that regard, art is a crucial modality in trauma-informed education.

Art-making can also aid in sublimation, the act of transforming an undesirable, often primitive behavior into a socially acceptable act (Kramer, 2000). The gratification a traumatized child gets from aggressive behavior could be sublimated through splattering paint on a canvas.

However, the art educator needs to be sensitive to the nuances of the art process, which can have an adverse effect on a child making art. Since engagement in the art process is able to arouse traumatic memories, a child who has experienced traumatic events may be triggered while creating art. The properties of different artistic mediums can contribute to the trauma reaction a child may experience. For example, a simple pencil drawing tends be highly structured and engages more cognitive thinking. Fluid materials, such as watercolors, finger paints, and clay, engage the child on a kinesthetic-sensory level, and are likely to trigger right hemisphere memories, including traumatic ones. So, a child drawing a simple image that he or she is copying from a source may not induce traumatic memories, but a non-structured experimentation with acrylic paints could be over-stimulating and evoke traumatic memories, resulting in emotional regression.

The Expressive Therapies Continuum (ETC) (Kagin & Lusebrink, 1978; Lusebrink, 1990; Lusebrink & Hinz, 2016) provides a framework for artistic engagement as it relates to brain functions. It consists of three levels, each as a continuum of variations in visual expression (Lusebrink & Hinz, 2016). Starting from the bottom, the levels are: Kinesthetic-Sensory, Perceptive-Affective, and Cognitive-Symbolic. The ETC is compatible with Fuster's (2003) classifications of the brain.

The Kinesthetic-Sensory level is the most simplistic, and is characterized by an exploration of materials, textures, and surfaces. It corresponds to the brain stem, the area responsible for bodily movement. Examples of the Kinesthetic-Sensory level include scribbling, finger painting, and any other tactile but unstructured art activity. For traumatized children, engagement on this level can be grounding, but also regressive. The emphasis on movement could stimulate preverbal bodily memories (Elbrecht, 2013).

The Perceptual-Affective level relates to forms, boundaries, and emotion regulation. Perceptual components can be found in color boundaries and horizon lines, as well as differentiation between forms in an image. Affect is determined by line quality, color intensity, and other components of an image that infer emotion. This level corresponds to the limbic system, responsible for emotion and memory. The Perceptual-Affective level is particularly relevant in trauma treatment; affect is accessed and changed through art materials, but contained by the structure of forms and boundaries (Lusebrink & Hinz, 2016).

The Cognitive-Symbolic level emphasizes problem-solving and meaning, and corresponds to the cerebrum. Art work created on this level can be metaphoric, such as a thunderstorm representing sadness or a volcano expressing anger. Since the cerebrum is associated with higher brain functioning, this level is considered the most complex.

Teaching Students with Prior Traumatic Experiences

Trauma-informed classrooms seek to recognize, understand, and address problem behaviors within the context of the child's traumatic past. This shift allows an educator to become more sensitive to students who have experienced traumatic events, providing a backdrop to understand that problem behaviors result from past experiences rather than a fault in their character. Educators should be informed about trauma in order to provide a safe, stable, and understanding environment. By acknowledging trauma and potential triggers, as well as avoiding stigmatizing and punishing students, trauma-informed classrooms can prevent re-traumatization and promote educational well-being for these vulnerable students. Consider the following specific strategies for art education when interacting with students who have prior traumatic experiences.

Ten Teaching Tips

1 Understand your role as an art educator in order to appropriately, collaboratively, and successfully engage children with a history of trauma in the art process.

2 Remember that the art room is not an art therapy session and the role of the art teacher is to teach art.

3 Discourage students from discussing personal traumatic experiences during class.

4 Speak to the social worker, counselor, or other school professional if you have concerns about a particular student's behavior or art work.

5 Be mindful and sensitive to the nuances of the art process in order not to overstimulate or arouse traumatic memories.

6 Consider use of the ETC as a framework for artistic engagement given its relation to brain functions. Since the functioning of a traumatized child's brain is already impaired, their response to art-making may be different from their peers.

7 Provide students with a medium (verbal and/or nonverbal) to express difficult emotions. Traumatic experiences are not easy to talk about and art could provide a means by which students can express themselves. This is especially important when considering the decreased activation of the PFC and increased activity in the limbic (i.e., emotional) regions of the brain.

8 Be aware of your verbal and nonverbal communication with students. Given the literature on attentional bias towards threat and emotional stimuli, it will be helpful to approach students with a welcoming stance that invites participation.

9 Celebrate the students' art work and publically display it.

10 Make each art lesson a joyful expression and fun.

References

Belkofer, C., & Konopka, L. (2008). Conducting art therapy research using quantitative EEG measures. *Art Therapy, 25*(2), 56–63, DOI: 10.1080/07421656. 2008.10129412.

Bishop, S. J., Duncan, J., Brett, M., & Lawrence, A. D. (2004). Prefrontal cortical function and anxiety: Controlling attention to threat-related stimuli. *Nature Neuroscience, 7,* 184–188.

Blair, C., & Raver, C. C. (2015). School readiness and self-regulation: A developmental psychobiological approach. *Annual Review of Psychology, 66,* 711–731.

Briggs-Gowan, M. J., Pollak, S. D., Grasso, D., Voss, J., Mian, N. D., Zobel, E., McCarthy, K. J., Wakschlag, L. S., & Pine, D. (2015). Attention bias and anxiety in young children exposed to family violence. *The Journal of Child Psychology and Psychiatry, 11,* 1194–1201.

De Bellis, M. D., & Zisk, A. (2014). The biological effects of childhood trauma. *Child and Adolescent Psychiatric Clinics of North America, 2*, 185–222.

Dunn-Snow, P., & D'Amelio, G. (2000). How art teachers can enhance artmaking as a therapeutic experience: Art therapy and art education. *Art Education, 53*(3), 46–53.

Elbrecht, C. (2013). *Trauma and Healing at the Clay Field: A Sensorimotor Art Therapy Approach*. London: Jessica Kingsley.

Fuster, J. M. (2003). *Cortex and Mind: Unifying Cognition*. New York: Oxford University Press.

Hinz, L. (2009). *Expressive Therapies Continuum: A Framework for Using Art in Therapy*. New York: Routledge.

Kagin, S. L., & Sbrink, V. B. (1978). The expressive therapies continuum. *Art Psychotherapy, 5*(4), 171–180.

Kramer, E. (1974). *Art as Therapy with Children* (2nd edition). New York: Schocken Books.

Kramer, E. (2000). *Art as Therapy: Collected Papers*. London: Jessica Kingsley.

Lusebrink, V. (1990). *Imagery and Visual Expression in Therapy*. New York: Plenum Press.

Lusebrink, V. (2004). Art therapy and the brain: An attempt to understand the underlying processes of art expression in therapy. *Art Therapy: Journal of the American Art Therapy Association, 21*(3), 125–135.

Lusebrink, V., & Hinz, L. (2016). The expressive therapies continuum as a framework in the treatment of trauma. In King, J. (Ed.), *Art Therapy, Trauma, and Neuroscience: Theoretical and Practical Perspectives* (pp. 42–66). New York: Routledge.

Malchiodi, C. (2002). *The Soul's Palette*. Boston: Shambhala.

National Child Traumatic Stress Network (2017). Retrieved on September 5, 2017 from nctsn.org.

Romens, S. E., & Pollak, S. D. (2012). Emotion regulation predicts attention bias in maltreated children at-risk for depression. *The Journal of Child Psychology and Psychiatry, 2*, 120–127.

Saunders, B. E., & Adams, Z. W. (2014). Epidemiology of traumatic experiences in childhood. *Child and Adolescent Psychiatric Clinics in North America, 2*, 167–184.

Shackman, J. E., Shackman, A. J., & Pollak, S. D. (2007). Physical abuse amplifies attention to threat and increases anxiety in children. *Emotion, 7*, 838–852.

Shackman, J. E., Wismer Fries, A. B., & Pollak, S. D. (2008). Environmental influences on brain-behavioral development: Evidence from child abuse and neglect. In C. A. Nelson & M. Luciana (Eds.), *Handbook of Developmental Cognitive Neuroscience* (2nd edition; pp. 869–881).Cambridge, MA: The MIT Press.

Shonkoff, J. P., Garner, A. S., & Committee on Psychosocial Aspects of Child and Family Health, Committee on Early Childhood, Adoption, and Dependent Care, and Section on Developmental and Behavioral Pediatrics (2012). The lifelong effects of early childhood adversity and toxic stress. *Pediatrics, 129*, e232–e246.

Teicher, M., Samson, J. A., Anderson, C. M., & Ohashi, K. (2016). The effects of childhood maltreatment on brain structure, function, and connectivity. *Nature Neuroscience, 17*, 652–666.

Trickett, P. K., Gordis, E., Pechkins, M. K., & Susman, E. J. (2014). Stress reactivity in maltreated and comparison male and female young adolescents. *Child Maltreatment, 19,* 27–37.

Van der Kolk, B. A. (2006). Post-traumatic stress disorder and the nature of trauma. In M. Solomon & D. Siegel (Eds.), *Healing Trauma: Attachment, Mind, Body, and Brain* (pp. 168–195). New York: W. W. Norton.

Van der Kolk, B. A. (2014). *The Body Keeps the Score: Brain, Mind and Body in the Healing of Trauma.* New York: Viking Penguin.

Part II

Art Education in Practice

11 Creating a Safe and Supportive Classroom Environment

Beverley H. Johns, Donalyn Heise, and Adrienne D. Hunter

Safety is a critical prerequisite before learning can take place (Sadowski, 2016). Students are unable to focus on what is happening in the art room, or any classroom, if they do not feel safe.

A major principle in trauma-informed educational practice is the development of a safe environment because many traumatic experiences threaten a child's safety, and it is critical that we avoid re-traumatizing individuals. Children who have experienced psychological trauma must know that an expectation for all students in the school is to be safe. However, these children will need additional support, such as advanced warnings of transitions and specific changes in routine (Cavanaugh, 2016).

Schools must create environments where students feel safe asking questions and sharing their concerns. When teachers exhibit unsupportive behaviors, they cause even more stress for students. Demaria and Schonfeld (2013–2014) state, "Students won't feel safe if they believe an adult does not understand them" (p. 15). Teachers are role models and should be encouraged to share their own feelings with students when appropriate and model positive coping skills. Teachers model how to show emotions without being ashamed. Students and families look to our schools for stability and security if they have experienced trauma (Demaria & Schonfeld, 2013–2014).

Bath (2008) explains the three pillars of trauma-informed care as being safety, connections, and managing emotions. Safety is a core developmental need and safety is the first imperative in schools. Safety is multifaceted and includes consistency, reliability, predictability, availability, honesty, and transparency. Some of the challenging behaviors of the students elicit controlling and even punitive responses from the adults in their environment, and it is this phenomenon that then can create an unsafe environment for students. Positive and supportive relationships are needed to ensure safety for the students.

Children who have experienced trauma operate in survival mode as exhibited by hypervigilance and hyperarousal. They continue to look for danger, and instead of focusing on learning tasks, they are scanning the environment and are easily distracted. Nonverbal messages generated by eye contact, voice tone, and even proximity to others can be perceived by the student as danger (Fecser, 2015). Punishment-based discipline triggers flight, fight, or freeze reactions, which make matters worse (Fecser, 2015). Therefore, it is critical that the educator maintain a calm and confident demeanor and build in structure, predictability, and routine.

In one school in the State of Washington, it was reported that when a trauma-informed approach that included a positive school climate was utilized within the school, suspensions dropped from 798 to 135 and written referrals were cut in half (Stevens, 2012). When we ensure the physical and emotional safety of our students inside the school, on the bus, and on school grounds, the power of relationships is acknowledged and practiced (Walker & Cox, 2013).

When children worry that they are not safe and think the world is out to get them, they are fighting for their lives. Trauma overwhelms their capacity to cope (Wright, 2013). Any new or unexpected stimuli will send them running for cover or can result in a flashback of the trauma. Things like a loud noise, a teacher raising his or her voice, an unexpected announcement, will result in these children fearing for their safety. Unfortunately, these students who are most in need of supportive environments may be expelled from classrooms because they are too difficult and cause too much trouble (Wright, 2013). Providing concrete examples, discussing the reason for rules, repeating information, and communicating the same information in multiple ways contributes to the student feeling safe in the environment (Wright, 2013).

The two best predictors of poor post-traumatic outcomes are the absence of social/familial support and the failure of child caregivers to recognize the distress the child is facing (Marans, 2013). Teachers must be able to recognize a child's distress and provide support.

With 26% of children in the United States having witnessed or experienced a traumatic event before the age of 4 (Craig, 2016), it is critical that teachers understand that some children with early trauma experiences have a compulsive need to re-enact past traumas. The child is looking for a parental or authority figure with whom they can replay past traumatic experiences in the hope that the outcome may be different. Teachers have to be trained to recognize these behaviors as bids for re-enactment. If the teacher responds with anger or by feeling victimized by the child's behavior or rage, the child's behavior will re-escalate. Teachers must redirect children's behavior calmly and respectfully.

The following are factors that must be considered when determining how to help students. These factors include age and developmentally related considerations for children and adolescents, extent of trauma, proximity of trauma, losses, prior experiences, prior mental health symptoms, family support, and community support (Osofsky, 2005).

Indirect exposure to material that is traumatic is associated with high rates of post-traumatic stress disorder symptoms. This indirect exposure is known as vicarious trauma (Carello & Butler, 2015).

Harris and Fallot (2009) identified five principles that are critical in creating and sustaining trauma-informed settings. These principles are ensuring safety, establishing trust, maximizing choice, maximizing collaboration, and prioritizing empowerment. Carello and Butler (2015) believe that ensuring emotional and physical safety is the most fundamental because safety is a necessary precondition to an environment that is conducive to learning. Their perspective is from the college setting but can certainly be applied to elementary, middle, and high school environments. They warn that in virtually every classroom some students will be at an increased risk for re-traumatization or vicarious traumatization as a result of their history or experiences. Therefore, it is critical to preview material and eliminate content that may shock or disturb the student. Assignments should also be reviewed for their potential to disturb or trigger students. An example would be assignments that might require personal disclosure. Carello and Butler (2015) also warn that the behavior of some instructors may be activating to students. Educators should avoid coming up from behind the student. Educators should use neutral language and a strengths-based perspective. Educators must also watch closely the behavior of other students within the class. Physical features within the classroom can also be triggers for a student, such as a change in lighting or sound levels. We also recommend modeling self-care so students learn how to take care of themselves appropriately.

An art class can provide a safe and supportive environment for all students, but is especially effective for students who have suffered trauma. It can provide a safe space for both visual and verbal expressions. Students who have been exposed to trauma may not be able to process their trauma, or they may feel powerless. Providing choices in the art-making process can empower them to have a voice or to reframe a negative narrative to one that recognizes individual strengths and assets. For example, during a lesson on identity, students drew self-portraits and created a background with colors, text, symbolic objects that visually communicated something about their interests, hobbies, activities, or things they valued. This provided opportunities for students to make choices in their artistic expression. In addition, many art classes allow students to demonstrate their ability to be a responsible learner, allowing them to get up and move about the classroom to get needed supplies when necessary. This can be especially beneficial when a student feels powerless to control their immediate environment. However, it is very important to have an efficient system to keep track of all tools in the art room. Students who have experienced trauma may feel depressed. They can injure themselves or others with common tools. Counting tools before and after distribution is essential. Having visuals that quickly let the teacher see that all tools have been returned before class is dismissed can be life-saving.

Some students who have been exposed to trauma withdraw, while others act out. Therefore, it is important to avoid punitive measures without first trying to understand what is going on in a student's life. Respectful rapport and establishing a level of trust can assist in this effort. Consulting with the school counselor or school social worker can provide specific information that can guide curriculum and instruction. However, even if a student has confided in the counselor about their trauma, this does not mean they are ready to disclose anything to anyone else. Some children want to come to art, forget about their trauma for a while, and just be a kid. One elementary student who had experienced the effects of extreme poverty and homelessness said he just wanted to have fun and get away from "it" for a while. He wanted a place he could smile and not feel like "the homeless kid." Art provides an opportunity for students to reframe their narrative, casting off negative labels and replacing them with the mastery of an artist.

Another child who had an incarcerated parent experienced success in creative activity and sometimes used art as a vehicle for articulating his dreams. After a class discussion on metaphors, students were asked, "If you could be anything, what would you like to be and why?" This young man drew a leaf floating in the air and explained that he wished he were a leaf so he could float in the sky to the prison to be with his dad. This demonstrates that even young children can use metaphors to create meaning and to deal with uncomfortable situations.

Art encourages students to take risks, to explore a variety of artistic processes as they discover boundaries. Students who have experienced trauma may have trouble controlling their emotions, sometimes crying or getting upset in the middle of class for seemingly no reason. Choosing art media wisely can help students feel secure and in control of emotions. Creating lessons that include boundaries and predictable media, such as pencils, markers, and crayons, can help. Media such as these create a predictable line, and therefore can help the student consistently create. Instructing students to draw whatever they want may create a sense of confusion. Providing some parameters can help students be creative within boundaries. For instance, having students draw their ideal backyard, or their ideal bedroom, allows them to visualize their own ideal space.

Art processes can also encourage students to find boundaries, making it easier for them to then work within those boundaries. Asking students to create clay animals that are structurally sound is easier to accomplish if they first manipulate the clay to the extreme, causing it to fall apart. This enables them to know the limits the clay has before proceeding. Another example is having students paint with tempera until they weaken the paper so much that a hole is formed. Then the teacher can cheerfully congratulate them on knowing the limits of paper and water, making it easier for the students to work within that boundary in the future. Students can begin to understand that every failure can be a learning experience. It also encourages risk-taking in a safe environment without fear of ridicule.

When teaching color theory, especially to students who have experienced trauma, a fun way to explore color is to create a kaleidoscope-like spinner. Using a 9" cardboard circle disk, the student traces a variety of smaller, differently sized circles (jar lids are great for this) onto the cardboard, overlapping the circles, making the circles concentric, and at other times creating negative space by letting the edges of the circles touch each other. Next, the student is to mix colors for painting in the spaces, changing color every time the circle line changes. Having the students create names for the colors they mix is especially fun. The teacher could present nail polish colors, or paint chip colors (from the paint store), to get the ideas flowing. Finally, by placing the dried, painted cardboard disk on a flat surface, the student can spin the disk using their hand, and watch the colors whirl around. This project relieves the student of the burden of "drawing something," while allowing him or her to create an original design and paint with colors which were personally mixed and chosen. Naming the colors adds another element of creativity. Spinning the disk also reminds everyone to have fun and enjoy!

Other students may withdraw and struggle to express emotions, and therefore struggle to develop creativity. Art media and processes that encourage unscripted movement and exploration can help students find joy in that freedom. Aesthetic expression involving freely interacting with art media such as splatter painting, action painting, or finger painting can provide an element of surprise in a safe environment. Wedging clay is great for relieving anger because the student physically slams the clay to remove air bubbles. Because it provides kinesthetic repetition, clay can also be therapeutic for children who have withdrawn: It can be soothing.

Students sometimes struggle with the uncertainty in their lives and find it stressful when they cannot predict what they might experience on a day-to-day basis. Watercolor painting, while difficult to master, can be presented in a non-stressful manner. It is comprised of art media and processes that can provide an opportunity to explore and discover, as well as predict and anticipate what will happen next. Instead of teacher-directed watercolor painting lessons, such as demonstrating, telling them, and showing them exactly what happens with new techniques of watercolor painting, an art teacher can use inquiry to guide students in making predictions. This allows them the joy of seeing what happens. For example, after practicing wet on wet technique, the teacher can ask students, "What do you think would happen if you drop salt crystals on a wash of watercolor paint on wet paper?" Students can predict, experiment, then observe, and finally, students can discuss why the process makes a speckled effect. The teacher can guide them to make interdisciplinary connections to science as they discuss topics such as chemical reactions and resist. Another variation is to guide students in prediction, observation, and discovery, by dropping small amounts of alcohol on wet paper washed with color, or applying crinkled plastic wrap to wet watercolor. They can also brainstorm as a group about how these techniques can be used in various paintings to create an effect of snow, or bubbles in an underwater scene, or whatever they can imagine. Having used this process with students who have experienced trauma, we have found students who were once numb with pain come out of their shells, become active participants, and feel safe with uncertainty. A follow-up discussion with the students on these artistic processes can be beneficial and therapeutic.

Another art focus that can help students who have experienced trauma is printmaking. Printmaking requires discussion on the value of a work of art, the value and definition of an original, and reasons for creating multiple copies/prints. Dialogue about what is worth repeating and what is not can transfer to things in their lives, such as thoughts and actions that are worth repeating.

One art activity that has helped students feel more in control in their lives is altered books. Taking an old book that was destined for the trash and transforming it into a work of art can be healing. It allows students to alter the text and images, using additive and subtractive methods to create an interactive or sculptural work of art. Focusing on inquiry prompts such as, "What is something in your life you want to change, and something you want to stay the same?" can provide a starting point for students to create images and text to represent their ideas. Students are empowered to change their own narratives. While it is important not to encourage students to share their traumatic stories, they can process trauma in healthy ways by recognizing the strength they had to survive one or more challenging events.

Art education is more than making art objects. It also includes looking at art, talking about art, interpreting art, and make critical judgments. Sometimes students who have suffered psychological trauma feel that the incident was their fault. Practicing critical thought processes that have young people observe, make judgments, and defend their judgments with evidence can be beneficial. The following aesthetic art activity provides a framework for enhanced perception and developing critical thinking. In this student-centered activity, the teacher shows the class an art image and asks these three simple questions: "What is happening in this picture? What do you see that tells you that? What else do you see?" This activity requires observing, making judgments about the art, and stating criteria that justify their opinion. The third question is asking them to look even closer at the art to enhance perception. The teacher guides the dialogue, accepting all students' responses, while encouraging them to recognize the multiple perspectives that inevitably emerge. Sometimes different people can look at the same image but see different things. This may be because of the person's previous experiences or attitudes. Understanding multiple perspectives can help young people see things differently.

Self-care is especially important for students who have experienced psychological trauma. Self-care is an active choice to engage in activities that contribute to overall health and well-being. It includes physical, social, and emotional health. Learning to replace negative thoughts and actions with positive ones contributes to well-being. As evidenced above, art content and processes can help all students realize their own resources and develop resilience when facing challenges in the future. Art lessons that help them brainstorm, compile, and visually articulate their resources and sources of joy: people they can turn to, people who inspire them, places they love, things that bring joy, and things and people in the community who help in times of trauma. Knowing their resources can be essential for youth who experienced trauma in the past and may experience trauma in the future.

Many times, teachers do not immediately realize the importance of the impact of teaching, both positive and negative, on students as they struggle through difficulties. It is so crucial to be mindful of students so that the impact is positive. Sometimes a student repeats a teacher's directive, offers a constructive suggestion to another student, or even says something like, "That's OK. Miss can fix that." These are "ah-ha" moments! Teachers do make a difference. Or maybe a teacher meets a student years later who offers to exchange a big hug, saying "You meant so much to me 'back then.'" A student may not remember a teacher's name, but they never forget the impact that positive experiences made.

Ten Teaching Tips

1 Learn to recognize a child's distress so that you can provide necessary support.
2 Avoid re-traumatizing children who have experienced trauma by providing a safe and supportive classroom.
3 Remain calm when a child exhibits negative behavior and respectfully redirect them.
4 Provide supports such as repeating clearly defined instructions and verbal reminders of time remaining, to help student transition to a new task.
5 Encourage children to ask questions and share concerns.
6 Model positive coping skills.
7 Provide choices wherever possible to empower students.
8 Safely store art tools, implement and practice responsible distribution and retrieval of art tools that promote safety.
9 Choose art media wisely to help students feel secure and in control of their emotions.
10 Use art to help students visually identify their resources.

References

Bath, H. (2008). The three pillars of trauma-informed care. *Reclaiming Children and Youth, 17(3)*, 17–21.

Carello, J., & Butler, L. (2015). Practicing what we teach: Trauma-informed educational practice. *Journal of Teaching in Social Work, 35(3)*, 262–278.

Cavanaugh, B. (2016). Trauma-informed classrooms and schools. *Beyond Behavior, 25(2)*, 41–46.

Craig, S. (2016). The trauma sensitive teacher. *Educational Leadership, 74(1)*, 28–32.

Demaria, T., & Schonfeld, D. (2013–2014). Do it now: Short-term responses to traumatic events. *The Kappan, 95(4)*, 13–17.

Fecser, M. (2015). Classroom strategies for traumatized, oppositional students. *Reclaiming Children and Youth, 24(1)*, 20–24.

Harris, M., & Fallot, R. (Eds.) (2001). *Using Trauma Theory to Design Service Systems.* San Francisco, CA: Jossey-Bass.

Marans, S. (2013). Phenomena of childhood trauma and expanding approaches to early intervention. *J Appl. Psychoanal. Studies, 10(3)*, 247–266.

Osofsky, H. (2005). The essential elements in dealing with trauma in children and adolescents in the context of conflict and terrorist incident. In J. Donnelly et al. (Eds.), *Developing Strategies to Deal with Trauma in Children.* Amsterdam, Netherlands: IOS Press.

Sadowski, M. (2016). More than a safe place. *Educational Leadership, 74(1)*, 33–38.

Stevens, J. E. (2012). Lincoln High School in Walla Walla, WA, tries new approach to school discipline—suspensions drop 85%. Retrieved from http://acestoohigh. com/2012/04/23/lincoln-high-school-in-walla-walla-wa-tries-new-approach-to-school-discipline-expulsions-drop-85/.

Walkley, M., & Cox, T. (2013). Building trauma-informed schools and communities. *Children and Schools, 35(2)*, 123–126.

Wright, T. (2013). "I keep me safe." Risk and resilience in children with messy lives. *Kappan, 95(2)*, 39–43.

12 Routines, Relationships, and Reinforcement

Kari Caddell

Imagine walking into a classroom with bright florescent lights. The window shades are pulled and there is no natural light. The tables are crowded together and offer very little working space. Piles of student art work and supplies clutter nearly every counter top. There is a sense of chaos and confusion.

Now imagine walking into a classroom where the lights are dimmed, window shades are open, tables are spaced apart, and counter tops are cleared off. Student art work is displayed on top of the cabinets. Each student has a pencil box of supplies, and his or her own place to keep art work. There is a sense of clarity and order.

Most people would choose to walk into the second classroom. The sense of order that it provides does not feel overwhelming, nor is it anxiety-provoking. It is imperative that a school art space be set up in a way that not only provides structure, but encourages safety and security, both physically and emotionally. Children living in chaos and uncertainty thrive on knowing what to expect at school. They need consistent and predictable structures to feel safe. This chapter focuses on routines, relationships, and reinforcements that are essential in promoting a safe environment for all students in which to create. Presented in this chapter are representative ideal situations. When faced with a less than ideal art room, the art teacher can make adaptations and still utilize some of the recommendations in this chapter and book.

An art teacher who had to teach art in a different school every day was assigned to the gymnasium in one of the schools. She shares this story:

> First, it was required that the art teacher cover the floor with heavy tarps which then had to be removed when classes were over for the day. Second, she had to fill water buckets for the students to clean paint brushes and hands. Third, there was a large container of basketballs which, when she asked to have it removed, was told could not be done because "there was no place else to store them." As one might expect of teenage boys, they immediately grabbed the basketballs the minute they arrived in the gym and proceeded to shoot baskets. When she told her supervisor about this issue, she was told "to just write up the students." Not wishing to discipline the students for acting like teenage boys, the

art teacher came up with a solution that fostered respect, cooperation, and set up a routine. She allowed the students to shoot baskets for five minutes and then they willingly unrolled the tarps, carried buckets of water to the gym, and settled down and began the art lesson. One condition was that the students had to teach the art teacher how to shoot baskets, which they thought was hilarious.

Setting Routines

When working with a group of students, it is important to let them know that they are expected to get their supply box and their art book before sitting in their assigned seat. Each supply box contains markers, colored pencils, a pencil, eraser, pencil sharpener, and glue stick. They are numbered, and match the corresponding number on the table. The matching numbers help keep students accountable for the supplies; this way, they can let the teacher know if any supplies need to be replaced or are not working properly. Pencils may break or markers may not work, so the teacher should emphasize that it is important and kind to notify him or her in order for the next student to have working supplies. When discussing supplies with students, it is important to talk about respecting each other as well as the supplies themselves. Teachers should give them visual examples of the correct and incorrect use of supplies.

One idea is to begin the year by having each student create an art portfolio. The teacher can discuss that art portfolios are large folders used to keep their art work safe. No one is allowed to touch someone else's art work or look through the portfolio unless the student gives permission. This again helps to build trust and respect among the group, and strengthens rapport with each student. Students must feel safe at school. Establishing a safety rule in the art room can help create respect and a peaceful classroom. Having students draw what they think is safe or not safe and posting those in the room will serve as helpful reminders to everyone. Posting a statement about safety, such as "We are all safe in the art room. Our bodies, our ideas, and our art work are all safe," can also support the idea of being safe. Each group of students can create their own expectations for the group to post. This gives them more ownership and responsibility to abide by those expectations, rather than the teacher telling them.

Teachers can also start each class by working in an art book that students have created at the beginning of the year. This gives them ownership over something, and an organized place to create art. The students are given a prompt, such as "create a picture using only your favorite color," or " make a picture of your favorite kind of day," with three to four minutes to work on the image in their book. This helps transition students into the group setting before the teacher begins the day's lesson. Students are given the opportunity to share what they drew in their book, which also helps build community and group cohesion.

When working with students on an individual basis, a teacher may want to consider having a slightly different routine. Students can be asked to sit at a circle table in the room. Working at a round table provides a sense of community, and gives the teacher the opportunity to create bonds and build trust with students. Each student is also able to choose a shelf on a book shelf for storing their personal art work and supplies.

Presenting Art Materials

Basic art supplies should be presented in a way that is organized and easily accessible. It is helpful to keep art supplies orderly, and offer only the necessary supplies for each project. If the art room is chaotic and cluttered, it can be overwhelming for students who live in crisis. It is beneficial for students to have structure at school while also having some flexibility and control.

As professionals working with a wide variety of art materials, keep in mind that different media provoke different kinds of messages and responses. For example, finger paints are extremely fluid, which can be too much of a challenge for a student who is acting out. On the other hand, a depressed student might find some release using finger paints. There are a variety of factors to consider when selecting materials for projects, especially the developmental stage of most of the students. Is there a need for comfort, organization, or mastery? Do the students need to broaden their outlook or self-reflect? Can the students tolerate the challenge of a new material? Will the material be too threatening or create regression? Touch and texture are important factors to consider when selecting materials. Paper is a common material with a multitude of tactile qualities. Think of the difference between construction paper, oak tag, tissue paper, magazine, newsprint, notebook, and drawing paper. Each has a distinct touch and feel.

There are risks involved when using various art materials. Some students who worry about making mistakes are eventually able to capitalize on accidents to create something new. The concepts of decision-making and flexibility are inherent and a built-in process with many art activities.

The Learning Environment

The best way to build rapport with students is to get to know them as individuals. Learn their names and make connections with them. It could be as simple as giving them a compliment, saying "Hi" in the hallway, or asking about some of their favorite things, like sports, video games, food, or music. Talk to them about something other than school in order to strengthen the connection as a trusted adult in their lives.

It is also valuable to set up a learning environment where it is okay to make mistakes without the fear of being judged. Accept each student for who they are and make each moment count. Most students are not used to having a class or place where there is no wrong answer. Let students know that it is okay to experiment with supplies and that their curiosity and ideas are valued. Give students freedom and control over how they create each project. Of course, this does not mean giving them free reign over what they do; there still needs to be some set of guidelines or directions for each project. An example would be to give them a topic, such as creating a self-portrait, and then allow the student to choose between various materials to create it. Another example would be to give the students paper and drawing materials and ask them to make a picture of their favorite activity. In both examples, the teacher is guiding and giving directions to students while also giving them freedom and control. Allowing students of all ages and backgrounds to have control is important. Students living in uncertainty may not have much control of anything in their lives. Giving choices and letting them make decisions can be helpful as they develop and grow.

The teacher's own behavior also makes an impact on the students. Body language and nonverbal communication say a lot to a student. Teachers should use good eye contact and a calm, quiet voice. Children inherently absorb how you treat them, and may notice how you treat other students and everyone's art work. It is important to give students positive feedback on a project, and try to reach each student during a given class period. Feedback should be specific and descriptive such as, "Josh, I noticed you filled all of the space with color. I see you used your favorite color, blue, a lot." This type of feedback is much more meaningful and effective than saying "Nice job."

When looking at students' art work, try to get direct information from them about their thoughts or the meaning behind the work. Encourage students to talk about their art creations by gently asking questions. The teacher can have them write about the art work or tell about it. It is unfair to a student if you jump to conclusions about what they have created without getting their perspective. This also helps avoid misinterpretation of the art work or its meaning. It is important to listen with interest and respect their skills no matter their age, artistic level, or academic level.

In addition, establish a rule that students may not throw away their art work. If a student is frustrated or upset and throws their art in the trash, take it out of the trash before they leave the room. It is imperative to let them know that they matter as a person. Their art work is an extension of who they are. Many of these students have little self-esteem or self-worth. They often struggle in other areas of school and feel inferior. No matter how big or small, anything a teacher can do to show them and help them realize that they are important and matter in this world is worth it. This is also a good opportunity to ask a student what they would change about the art work and initiate problem-solving to alter the creation to their liking. Students are aware of whether or not others cherish their art work. Visual displays are memorable and a public way to demonstrate their achievements.

Showing appreciation to the student for positive participation, being a helper or role model, is also valuable. It offers encouragement and support with hope for success in the future. Also educators should demonstrate compassion and forgiveness to show students that each day is a new day with a new beginning and a clean slate. This sends a powerful message of working through challenges and bouncing back. When you get through tough days or situations with students, they can be grateful you did not give up on them. This is particularly true for students in crisis and with attachment difficulties.

Unexpected changes and transitions can be challenging for students in crisis. Preparing them for upcoming changes or transitions can go a long way. For example, using a chime can be helpful to signal to students that they need to pay attention or it is time to clean up. Letting students know what the next project will be or if there will be a new seating chart the following week will help ease their anxiety about the upcoming changes.

These are some questions to consider about how to create a classroom environment: Is the atmosphere warm and accepting? Does it build students' self-pride? Is there freedom of expression and creativity? Are self-confidence and self-respect nurtured? Are there opportunities for decision-making? Are students sharing successes? Are students' efforts valued? Do students feel respected? If the art educator answered yes to most of the questions, then he or she is providing wide opportunities for students to be successful and for reaching a wider array of students.

Engaging the Student through Art

Many students are willing to engage in making art. Art is a comfortable and familiar activity to so many students. Art is unique from other school subjects because, whether a student is willing to try something new or stay within their comfort zone, they are still engaged in learning. Students are more willing to take risks and try new art techniques or materials if it is connected to real life. It is also important to give students opportunities for success with "no fail" projects such as those that encourage all students to actively engage regardless of art skill and ability.

Some possible projects are:

> Students can create a CD cover about their favorite music, a comic book cover for their hero, or a box for a game. In this way, they are able to use their own life experience as the subject matter. This gives them a sense of pride and helps increase their self-esteem.

> Tissue paper collage provides mastery and competence. It is abstract and requires a student to glue vibrant torn shapes together, thus creating a visually pleasing product. This project eliminates the "I can't draw" syndrome.

> A found object collage or sculpture is a way to help students evaluate their world, to show that things that may seem useless can be rediscovered and used in a new way. This concept can be particularly helpful to students who feel abandoned or rejected by their family or society. It demonstrates that what others consider "junk" not only has value, but provides a way for creating a new identity.

Using a multisensory approach to instruction is also more likely to engage students. This includes hearing, touch, sight, and smell. The more senses you can involve when teaching art, the more students will be engaged. Some senses are naturally incorporated based on the selection of materials. For example, clay may have a distinct smell and texture. Integrating music while creating art can also be engaging and motivating. Use creativity to involve students in a wide variety of activities. Sometimes an art project lends itself to a food connection.: After making pinch-pot tea sets, students held a tea party, or after studying Chinese art, students enjoyed traditional Chinese food.

Summary

There are many factors to incorporate into the art room to help students be successful. Set clear procedures and routines for students to follow, so they know what is expected of them. Present the art materials in a way that is organized, and consider various responses that art media can provoke when selecting materials for specific projects. Making personal connections is truly an invaluable tool when working with students. Be aware of personal verbal and nonverbal communication as well. Give students the ability to have flexibility, freedom, and control within the art room to help increase their confidence and self-esteem. Doing success-oriented projects will also give students pride and encourages them to take risks. Be sure to let students tell their story through their art work without making assumptions or judgments.

Ten Teaching Tips

1　Provide a sense of order within your classroom.
2　Provide a comfortable and non-threatening environment.
3　Establish clear routines for students so they know exactly what is expected of them.
4　Avoid unexpected changes and prepare students for transition.
5　Encourage students to talk about their art work by asking gentle questions.
6　Know student interests and make connections based on that information.
7　Teach students to turn any mistakes made in an art project into something new.
8　Provide positive and descriptive feedback.
9　Encourage no-fail projects such as those that encourage all students to actively engage regardless of art skill and ability.
10　Involve as many senses as possible.

13 Integrating Art and Academics

A Collaborative Approach

Donalyn Heise, Adrienne D. Hunter, and Beverley H. Johns

I had a 16-year-old student in my alternative education art class who was a very good artist. I noticed that he did a lot of graffiti, and I was intrigued by his very ornate lettering style. I asked him if he would share his alphabet with me and he agreed. As I looked over his alphabet, I realized that a few letters were missing. I asked the young man to go over his alphabet with me, and he began to sing the alphabet song as he pointed to the letters. Much to my shock and surprise, he had learned the song incorrectly, and indeed was missing letters! I thanked him for sharing his alphabet with me, and didn't mention the missing letters. At lunch, I approached the reading teacher with the graffiti alphabet and asked if she was aware of his situation. She told me no, but that she wasn't surprised since he only read at a second-grade reading level. I checked his school records and found that he had been experiencing some degree of homelessness most of his life. He had changed schools frequently, sometimes several times a year, probably causing him to have gaps in his education. The next day, I approached the young man with a lettering book with many types of alphabets, from Old English to Greek. I asked him if he would be interested in trying out some of the other alphabets, and making me a few signs, in his spare time. He agreed, and he really seemed to enjoy drawing the letters, especially the Old English letters. Before long, other students started asking him to write their names for them, and he did, asking them to write their names down for him "for when he could get to them." He became very popular, very prolific, and very proficient. One day, I noticed a big smile on his face as he was working on his lettering. It was as if a lightbulb had gone on over his head and suddenly all the letters strung together made sense. Suddenly he could spell, and ultimately, he learned to read.

Adrienne D. Hunter

Students who have experienced psychological trauma can struggle academically and often lack a desire to learn. Some accumulate excessive absences and others lack motivation to complete assignments. Many drop out of school altogether, while others may contemplate suicide. How can teachers and school professionals increase desire for learning necessary for academic success? We know that art connects to other subjects, allows students choice in the learning process, and can help make learning relevant to students' lives.

This chapter emphasizes a collaborative approach to enhance learning for students who may have experienced violence, neglect, abuse, homelessness, and other forms of psychological trauma. We begin with research that provides a rationale for integrating art with other academic subjects, then suggest a nurturing environment for students who have experienced trauma. We provide a framework for collaboration between art teachers and teachers of other academic disciplines, and conclude with teaching tips for educators and collaborators. Throughout the chapter, we provide best practices that have been used by art teachers working with children who have experienced psychological trauma that can be incorporated into virtually any classroom setting. Many of these practices are presented as classroom vignettes, which will explain how and why these practices are successful.

Rationale for Integrating the Arts

The effects of art education on academic achievement is prominent in today's literature and presents a strong argument for integrating arts and academics. The President's Committee on the Arts and Humanities focused on data that shows the effect of arts education on academic achievement and creativity. According to the Committee: "[T]he arts is an effective way to equip students with the skills they will need to succeed in the jobs of tomorrow" (President's Committee on the Arts and Humanities, December, 2011, p. 29). It sees the arts as an effective tool in school-wide reform. Children who practiced a specific art form developed increased attention skills and improved their general intelligence (President's Committee on the Arts and Humanities, 2011). Despite the research supporting the arts, many school districts do not promote the arts.

With the emphasis in today's schools on academic standards, it is critical that art educators and general education teachers understand how they can help each other and how they should work together. Students may struggle with the math standards but be motivated to illustrate a concept with a drawing. Students may struggle with reading comprehension and may not be able to answer questions, but can produce an illustration that depicts what they have read. Arts-based instruction has been shown to increase academic engagement and reading skills (Rose & Magnotta, 2012). Understanding artistry involves cognition and contributes to the growth of mind because it requires many forms of thinking (Efland, 2002). Adrienne Hunter describes one of the first lessons she learned in her first college art history class:

> Art is a record of history! Before there was a written language, before there were books, before there were cameras or TV, before there was the Internet and social media, there was art. I remember that "ah-ha" moment as my professor, Dr. Rossi, explained how we read a work of art. I learned how the man in the portrait was dressed in a suit with frilly lace around his cuffs, so obviously he was wealthy and didn't get

his hands dirty working, there were books in the background, so he was obviously educated, and to make a long story short, this was a man who commissioned a portrait that portrayed his wealth, education, and social standing in society. It was as much of a vignette of his life, as were the early petroglyphs of the Stone Age. Many times in our classrooms, students will consciously or subconsciously share with us nonverbal vignettes of their lives by the doodles, drawings, or graffiti they add to their papers, desks, or school environment.

While art educators have had the advantage of learning art history, they also have an understanding of how art relates to the world. More importantly, they have the opportunity to guide students in meaningful learning, discovering creative connections between life and art. Art is everywhere around: from the graphics on the cereal box on a kitchen table, to clothing, cars, the color of paint on the walls of homes, to the shape of a piece of furniture, the patterns made by shadows on the ground, the texture of the bark on a tree, the movement of water as it flows around stones in a stream, and the forms of clouds in the sky. Art educators also have an understanding of the mathematics used in art—the scale of objects or the ratio of pigment to binder in paint; and the science in art—like the chemical make-up of the materials used, or the scientific process of making handmade paper. Some people create graphic outlines from which they then create written stories such as graphic novels; others create cartoons to express a humorous idea or a political comment. The youth of today have greater exposure to all forms of art through television, computers, the Internet, mass media, and digital imagery. It is important to embrace these multiple modes of visual communication to motivate and educate all students.

According to Smithrim and Upitis (2005), students involved in the arts exhibit higher academic achievement than their peers who are not involved in the arts. In schools where the arts disciplines are integrated with other subjects, students have a tendency to have an academic advantage over students in schools where this is not the case. Student involvement in the arts has a positive relationship with higher student achievement at some level (Melnick, Witmer, & Strickland, 2011).

In a study of the use of art to assess reading comprehension and critical thinking in adolescents, students in the 11th grade English class read and discussed a novel together. They were given a choice of painting, drawing, sculpture, or photography to demonstrate their understanding of the concepts in the novel. Of the 21 students in the project, 14 produced work that showed connections to things, people, and places within the realm of their experiences beyond the illustrations, and ten created work that showed metaphorical connections demonstrating a clear understanding of thematic concepts from the text (Holdren, 2012).

Many teachers of academic subjects may see "art as the icing on the cake," like the cover design for a book report. They may consider art nice, but an added extra. They may even walk past an art room and see students out of their seats, moving around, talking to each other, and think the art room is "out of control." Therefore, it is more important than ever to not only teach our students about art, but to educate colleagues and administrators about the power of art for integrated authentic learning.

Nurturing the Environment for Learning

The art room setting in general may be intimidating to those not involved in the art-making process. What many non–art teachers (and other observers) may not understand is that art teachers expect their students to be responsible learners. This means getting out of their seats without asking for permission, to get their own supplies as they need them, change their paint water, or wash their hands. Art teachers want students to be active in the learning process, learning from peers as they walk around to look at what their fellow classmates are creating, discussing their ideas with each other, relaxing and talking quietly while they are making art. This is not to say that the art room is a lawless land of chaos. There are rules and expectations; they are simply not the same as the rules found in other subject classrooms.

Sometimes fellow teachers really are not sure how or if they want to collaborate with you. When approaching reluctant teachers, it is helpful to have a dialogue to better understand their concerns, and to offer a rationale for why collaboration might be mutually beneficial for the students and for each teacher. Collaboration should encompass a shared vision, shared planning, and planned decision-making. After each participant offers insights and suggestions, the role of each participant should be articulated, as well as an estimate of the time and effort required. Participation will be discussed later in this chapter.

Inspiration for Designing Art Collaborations

How does one begin to design an integrated lesson? First, there must be an idea or a concept which will translate into an integrated lesson, whether it originates with the art teacher or an academic teacher. Sometimes ideas seem come out of the blue, and other times ideas are triggered by something encountered, whether consciously or subconsciously. For example, one art teacher revealed:

> I was at the Statue of Liberty when I came up with one of my biggest big ideas, which led to the Great American Depression project. I was on Ellis Island and they had a display where you push a button and recorded voices of actual immigrants shared their experience entering Ellis Island. I thought, "I'd love to do something like that with my students." When I returned to school, I shared my experience with the history teacher, and asked her what she was teaching this semester.

She said, "The Great American Depression." The history teacher, English teacher, and I discussed the Works Progress Administration (WPA) and the Civilian Conservation Corp (CCC). We talked about how we could incorporate the local projects of the WPA and CCC into a unit for our students. We realized that we had access to senior citizens in our neighborhood who could share their personal experiences with the students, and thus began a new journey in the art room.

(Gerber & Guay, 2014, p. 53)

This demonstrates collaboration that started with an idea and resulted in learning which was meaningful for the all students, including students who have experienced trauma. And it required no extra time from the history teacher or English teacher. The collaboration prevented learning in isolation, and linked academic subjects with art and life.

Sometimes ideas come from the students themselves. For instance, after 9/11, after creating a memorial with the Statue of Liberty, students in an Alternative Education high school art class decided they needed to add a painted mural of the New York City skyline to hang behind it.

(Gerber & Guay, 2014, p. 52)

Teachers might get ideas from brainstorming with other teachers. Inquiring about curriculum plans for the semester or year is a good place to start. By providing the vehicle to merge the subject areas, the art specialist often offers the "glue" to integrating the lesson. Events and media are also great sources of inspiration for collaborations. Just as "who, what, when, and where?" are used in writing, think of them in terms of art-making. Ideas are everywhere; all it takes is imagination!

Structuring a Collaboration for Student Participation

Once there is an idea or concept for collaboration, the next step is to structure the lesson so that the students are eager to participate. When working with students who have experienced psychological trauma, keep in mind that many of these students have a variety of reasons why they may not want to participate, and many times they will not express these reasons in a rational manner, but rather choose to act out.

One way to plan for success and factor out failure is to be mindful of some of the reasons students choose not to participate in art projects. Although it might seem like a good idea to remind art students that this is a great opportunity to use the knowledge and skills that they have learned in their other academic classes, this approach may also backfire as some art students consider art their "safe haven" where it is "OK" if they don't have strong academic skills. Conversely, not every student loves art, and many are not willing to take the risk of making art if they feel they cannot do so competently.

Another area of concern for students is the materials that they will be using. Students who are homeless, students living at or below poverty level, or students who suffer abuse will often be very careful of their clothing since they will "get in trouble if they get dirty" or know that they will not have the opportunity to launder their clothing. The teacher should wear an apron to model that everyone should wear an apron or other type of protective clothing, like an oversized shirt, and make them available for ALL of the students. (Disposable plastic aprons are an option, and aprons can be easily made from old towels.) If this is an ongoing practice in the art room, no one will think anything of it.

Teachers asking students to bring in materials to contribute to a project should be considered carefully. While you may wish to suggest that students are welcome to bring in something to contribute, it should be clearly stated at the same time that it is not necessary to bring anything because you will have a multitude of materials for everyone to use. Despite appearances, do not make assumptions about a student's ability to materially contribute to a project.

There is a level of trust that all teachers, especially art teachers and others who work with students exposed to trauma, build with their students. When something changes in the class, such as the introduction of another teacher/partner/volunteer, or even a change of location, some students may become anxious, fearful, or even resentful. This is particularly true of students who have experienced psychological trauma, so the teacher must be cognizant of this possibility and be prepared to address this *before* it occurs, by investing the students in the project prior to the beginning of the project.

One way to get students invested in the collaboration is by making the project meaningful. Making the project meaningful can be done by planning a collaboration that involves doing something they would not ordinarily get to do, a departure from the norm, and an experience they will remember years later, such as painting a mural, building a seven-foot-tall totem pole, or making a quilt that will be donated to a sick child.

Another way to motivate the students and facilitate meaningful learning is to make the project relevant to their lives in some way. By this, we do not mean personal details about their lives, but rather what music they listen to, what they read or watch on television, favorite foods, specific celebrities they admire. Occasionally a student will ask, "Why do I need to learn this? When will I ever need to know this?" Sometimes the project is related to something they are learning in another class, or maybe it is related to a current event. Whatever the impetus for the collaboration, it should be a skill and a concept that can be generalized into their daily lives. If the students are working together to make a quilt, they are learning to sew, which means they will now be able to repair their clothing. They are working together, each person doing a small part of a whole, which is teaching them to be part of a team and that they are a worthy member of the team. They are going to donate the quilt, so they are learning to volunteer and give back to the community. Above all, it should be fun and impart the joy of learning so that students will embrace education.

The project also has to be attainable. Sometimes students, especially students with limited experience with success, will want to participate but will refrain because they think they "can't do it" or "will mess it up." Sometimes students think a project is just too big or complicated to even try. By giving a clear explanation of what the project is, how it will be done, and a demonstration of how to safely use the materials, the students will know what to expect and have an idea of how to proceed. The students will appreciate knowing that the teacher will help them if they need help and will guide them as they "fix" or "solve" any problems that they may encounter. Explaining the project to students in a manner in which they believe that they can succeed will excite them to participate in the project.

An art teacher shares her experience after the September 11th attack on the World Trade Center:

> I was working with adolescents in a shelter school. As they discussed what was happening, in real time, the students couldn't understand the significance of the World Trade Center being attacked, as opposed to the Statue of Liberty, or the Washington Monument, which they more readily identified as symbols of America. In the course of the discussion, they decided to make a life-sized (student-sized) Statue of Liberty. Once they decided to build the Statue of Liberty, I explained and demonstrated how to make the form and paint it, essentially, breaking it down into steps that they could not only readily follow, but also be willing to undertake. Explaining that we would make a mummy-like body for the statue, I spoke about using a plaster-gauze material similar to a cast you would have on a broken arm. I further explained how they would all choose a job for themselves and work together. This demonstrates that providing choices when possible can empower students and increase levels of engagement.

Using the above example, this is how the lesson might be built for success. There may be students in the room who are homeless (you know that they will not want to get dirty because they do not have access to much clothing or to do laundry) or who have been abused (mentally, physically, and/or sexually and may not want to be touched by or to touch anyone). A volunteer must lie on the table, body (not head) covered with plastic and newspaper, while members of the class apply this messy wet plaster-gauze material onto that volunteer's body to make a mummy-like form. It may seem that no one would want to volunteer, but that is probably not the case. This is a position of leadership, of status, of attention, and also a job that requires absolutely no artistic ability. This student will have bragging rights for years and will live on in infamy. First, provide aprons to ALL of the students. Since the art teacher always wears an apron, this does not make

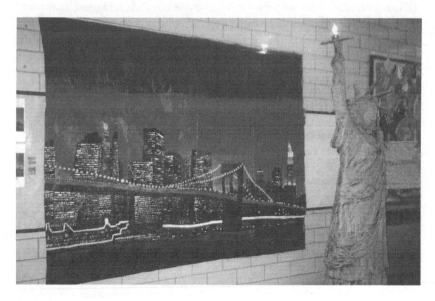

Figure 13.1 "Statue of Liberty"

anyone stand out. Then pass out plastic garbage bags and demonstrate how they can slip one on each leg, securing them with masking tape to keep shoes and pants tidy. The teacher might even make a comment about how it will help keep them from tracking plaster down the hallway when they leave the room. Next, recognizing that some students do not want to be touched or to touch others, and some will not like to get their hands wet or dirty, describe several jobs from which they can choose. One, they could help cut the plaster-gauze material strips into manageable sizes; two, they could help wet and hand the strips to others; three, who would apply the strips to the mummy; and four, since it is such a messy project, it would really help if someone would help by cleaning as everyone works. Also ask for a volunteer to help document the project, taking pictures and keeping the bulletin board in the lobby updated. This gives everyone a comfort zone from which to participate. Some of the students might even venture out of their comfort zones when they see how much fun everyone is having.

When the statue was completed, the students decided they wanted to paint a New York City skyline. The photograph they chose is not what is actually seen behind the statue, but it is what they most related to.

Art teacher Adrienne Hunter offers examples of how collaborating can be achieved in a variety of subjects:

With the Statue of Liberty project, I realized that it was an opportunity to invite the other faculty to participate or collaborate. I went to the social studies teacher, who promptly told me that he had no artistic ability at all. I told him that was not a problem, but it would be really helpful if he could cover the history of the Statue of Liberty and the events of the September 11th tragedy. "Easy, peasy," he said, "Sure, I can do that!" Next I went to the English teacher. I explained that we were building a Statue of Liberty and asked if she might be willing to work with her students on "The New Colossus" by Emma Lazarus, which is engraved on a plaque on the base of the statue. No problem I was assured. The math teacher came on board first with the Roman Numerals etched on the tablet (July IV MDCCLXXVI: July 4, 1776). We collaborated on a lesson on scale: A small photo of the New York skyline was divided into a grid; each student then enlarged a square of the grid to draw what was to become the painted mural background for the statue. She also came up with some great trivia facts about the real Statue of Liberty, like the size of the feet and who modeled for the head and face. The science teacher was ready for me. He told me that he would teach them about the patina of copper on the Statue of Liberty AND he helped the students actually wire the statue so that the torch would light up. This is a great example of challenging the definition of art, through culture and education!

It is important to keep everyone informed. Keeping everyone in the loop may help with problem-solving related to scheduling or other potential challenges. Do not forget the school support staff, such as counselors, security staff, custodians, and food service. They are an integral part of students' lives in school. With the myriad of problems these students face in life, the support staff love seeing and hearing about the positive things the students are engaged in. It would also be a good idea to give the custodians special thanks for putting up with the art room messiness.

Share your students' successes! Invite the other faculty into the art room to follow the progress. Take photographs to document student progress and post them on a bulletin board in the lobby of the school. Share information about the project and photographs of student work in school/district newsletters. (Confidentiality of using photographs of students will be discussed later in this chapter.)

Involve Community Participation: Utilize Resources

Sometimes, teachers have a tendency to just look at the space around them and forget that there is so much more out there: new materials to use, other people to work with, experiences that have not been encountered before. If the budget is limited, sometimes your community can help. Be certain to find out the district's policies pertaining to solicitations and grants; the district may already be asking the same people for a big contribution and does not want to burden the same donor with multiple requests.

Sometimes a teacher can offer students more than what he or she is able to teach by seeking volunteers and partnerships. These outside resources can provide a great way to expand school programs beyond the confines of the classroom.

An art teacher shares these examples:

> We needed a lot of newspaper for this big project, so I put the word out to the staff that I needed them to bring in their old newspapers. Boy, did I get a ton of paper!
>
> On a different project, the students were making a group quilt in the fashion of the Gees Bend's Quilters, from Gees Bend, Alabama, a small remote African American community. We decided to make the quilt using old blue jeans, just as the quilters did. The problem was, I was working with alternative education teens. Many of them were couch surfers (sleeping at a different family member's home each night), some were from group homes, and all were at or below poverty level. None had any extra clothing to donate. I sent an email out to the school staff that I needed old jeans and why. As an added aside, I mentioned that I was sure that some of them had jeans stashed away that "might fit again someday." We got a wonderful assortment of colors and sizes of jeans for our quilt. (I also silently noticed a few of those jeans went home with a couple of students.)
>
> Sometimes you have to go beyond your school for donations of materials. I have a friend who worked at the *New York Daily News*, and every year he gave me a new apron that I wore in my art rooms. It became my trademark apron. (Just a note: I was not teaching in New York.) One day I mentioned to him that I needed to make aprons for my students to help them stay clean. A few weeks later, a big box showed up from the *New York Daily News*. It was a box full of aprons for my students to wear in art class! The students loved them! We took pictures with the students clowning around and posing in their aprons, and sent the pictures with our thank you note.
>
> I have had a shoe store donate shoes for one of our projects. I have had my dentist donate false teeth samples and rat mandibles. (Rat jaws— who knew? Apparently they practiced on them in dental school.) I have had a box-making company donate cardboard. Anytime I solicit donations, I always send a thank you on school letterhead along with photos of the completed projects. Sometimes the students will write thank you notes—a great learning lesson. When I sent the thank you and pictures of the completed shoe project to the shoe store, they invited us to display the redesigned shoes in the store window. The store contacted the newspaper and we had a write-up in the news. The store owners also came to our school to meet the students and handed out T-shirts from their store. The students really felt that their art work was valued and that they, themselves, were a valued as part of the community
>
> (Gerber & Guay, 2014, p. 50)

The following vignette of an art teacher's community involvement has an important lesson to share:

> Working in an art room, roughly the size of a shoebox, I had my students hand-build clay vessels. We didn't have a kiln to fire the pieces, so I asked an art teacher in a different district to fire our projects. I learned from this teacher that our local center for the arts had an artist who would come to schools and do a Raku firing. I was able to work with this center to have the artist come to my alternative education school to set up a Raku kiln and work with the students on the process of Raku firing. A high fire kiln was set up on the school lawn and the students placed their air-dried clay pieces in the kiln. Each student had to remove his or her red-hot piece with long tongs, and proper protective gloves and aprons, and place it in a 55-gallon drum that was filled with combustible newspapers. Flames and smoke billowed, creating suspense. As the pieces cooled, they were then placed in water baths and the excitement of seeing what was created emerged.
>
> As a young teacher, this experience taught me some very important lessons. If you approach people about helping your students, you can enrich the learning experience beyond what you are able to teach them, and sometimes you can even get fees waived or reduced. I learned from this experience that some students, and especially inner city youth where fire can take out a whole city block at a time, are terrified of fire. Many of them have experienced the tragedy of fires of their own homes or those of their neighbors. Some students may have been burned, either by accident or at the hand of an abuser.

This vignette emphasizes the importance of being mindful of your students and carefully preparing them about the activity you are planning. It also reinforces the need to be sure that the outside service provider is prepared for your students.

Creating Partnerships with Outside Agencies

There are many organizations willing to work with teachers. This is especially important when working in high poverty schools, or working with students who are in non-traditional school programs that have little or no parental support, such as a PTA or PTO. Many schools lack funding for field trips and other extra activities. Outside agencies, such as art or history museums, colleges, and universities, are often willing to partner with teachers. For example, many museums have special programs to help with the price of admission and some have funds to pay for bus transportation. Many have docents and outreach programs that educators can utilize. Some art museums have internships for students that provide leadership opportunities, with students serving on museum education boards or as docents.

Some internships solicit student input when designing art packets for museum visitors. Some museums even have a lending program for their education resources. The following vignette reveals a history museum that provided valuable resources to an art class.

> I was able to borrow a taxidermy owl from the Museum of Natural History when I was doing a project on *Owl Moon* by Jane Yole. Having a real, stuffed owl gave the students an opportunity to see an owl up close and personally. They were able to see the colors and patterns of the feathers, without the owl flying away. They were able to look at the beak and talons without fear. It was a chance to really see and imagine the owl in the story before they created their project.

These types of collaborations are important because they provide meaningful connections to the community and enhance learning in the classroom. In art, part of being able to draw, paint, or sculpt something is first being able to see it to know what it looks like.

In addition to partnering with agencies in the community, local citizens can be a great resource. Educators can invite individuals in the community to collaborate and share their insights or expertise. In one urban middle school, an art teacher with no parent participation sent an email to the entire faculty, asking for volunteer grandparents to come and mentor students on a collaborative art project. She had enough volunteers for each sixth-grade student. Visual depictions of stories shared were combined to create a collaborative paper quilt, which was proudly displayed in the school. Benefits of this collaboration were intergenerational learning and ongoing meaningful relationships.

In another community collaboration, the art teacher invited individuals from the community to serve as volunteer speakers to share their experiences and insights of the decade of the 1950s. She collaborated with the science and history teachers as the students studied the context of the times, the styles, the music, and current events of this decade. Other teachers asked to be part of this project. The language arts teacher introduced literary works and had students research the fashion of the times. The music teacher focused on music trends, and the physical education teacher taught dances of that era. This unit resulted in a culminating community event that celebrated the decade, including a concert and dance. Several car collectors gave rides in their antique cars. Student visual and performing arts were prominently displayed. This collaboration appealed to a wide array of interests and ability levels, and helped provide authentic, meaningful learning that linked art to culture.

The following excerpt provides another example of a community collaboration that provided meaningful interaction between art students of an alternative high school and senior citizens:

During our Great American Depression project, my students interviewed senior citizens about their experiences during the depression. We were able to invite the senior citizens from our local senior citizen center to come and be interviewed by our alternative education students. This sharing of experiences moved beyond the art project when the students realized they shared many of the same experiences today as the senior citizens had experienced during the depression. Many of the senior citizens maintained their relationships with the students long after the art project ended. It was not unusual for them to stop by to say hello and pass the time of day (Gerber & Guay, 2014, p. 53)

Colleges and universities are another great resource for partnerships for students. They can provide mentors for K–12 students, space for showcasing student art work, and expertise in a variety of areas. Sometimes, partnering with colleges and universities can have additional benefits, such as motivating students to aspire to higher goals. For example, one community art program involved middle school children who were homeless or who had family members who were or who had been incarcerated, work creatively alongside college students. All of the students were considered "at-risk" and attended a neighborhood school where the majority did not complete high school. Art was created and displayed at the local elementary school, at the family emergency shelter, and at the university. The middle school students attended the opening reception at the university; most had never been on a campus before or had ever thought of continuing with higher education. After the collaboration, many of these students enthusiastically communicated their new desire to attend college one day.

Other partnerships to consider are businesses, local organizations, and national organizations. An example of a partnership shared by an art teacher:

In one of the shelter schools where I taught art, there was a walled in area outside of the science room that was just wasted space, filled with weeds. The science room had a door that opened out to this space. The art students designed, drew, and painted a mural on the wall of what was to become an outdoor science center. We contacted our zoo and were able to work with the aquarium staff and a zoo horticulturalist to create an outdoor science center, complete with a fish pond and landscaping appropriate for the planting zone of our area.

An Important Note about Volunteers

Be sure to follow your district's policies pertaining to volunteers. Proper background documentation is essential. Always be sure that volunteers understand the nature of the school program and describe to them the less than stellar behaviors that they may encounter from students. Volunteers must be comfortable working with ALL of the students. They must also understand and accept the school rules and work within the parameters that the teacher has set. Most schools require volunteers go through background checks. Many provide training to ensure privacy and confidentiality when working with vulnerable students.

The Importance of Being Organized When Participating in an Art Partnership

Adrienne Hunter likes to tell her student teachers, "If you don't have a plan for your students, *they* will have a plan for *you!*" While this applies to any class, it is particularly important in an art class. It is especially essential to students who have experienced psychological trauma in their lives, as they can be so accustomed to failure that they have a difficult time embracing success, sometimes even going so far as to sabotage success (Johns, 2015). These students need to be empowered and receive high rates of positive interactions. High rates of praise statements include noticing improved academic engagement and reduced behavioral difficulties (Cavanaugh, 2016).

In any partnership or collaboration, all participants should share important particulars pertinent to their contribution. Organization and assessment in an art class is essential, but the elements of organization will generally differ from other subject areas as will the specifics of assessment. Starting with the lesson plan, one might find that traditional lesson plan formats are not as helpful as they need to be. For example, the art lesson may require an extensive list of materials that will be needed; or perhaps the process requires steps that may be done out of sequence to accommodate "drying time"; factoring in adequate clean-up time is important as it means stopping the lesson earlier and perhaps needing a filler project to engage students after they have completed their clean-up responsibilities. If necessary, create a plan format that works and will be helpful for all partners to understand and implement. In art, the teacher should be observing, assessing, and guiding the students continuously throughout the class.

Unless they are making a public statement, no child comes to school wearing a T-shirt that says "I'm homeless" or "I'm being sexually abused" or "I'm experiencing some sort of psychological trauma." Even if a teacher is aware that such situations exist with his or her students, the teacher should never make this information public or call attention to it in any way directly related to the student. Structuring the art lesson should incorporate techniques that reduce the stress, fears, and concerns of the traumatized student as an integral part of the lesson.

Lesson-Planning Techniques

Building a lesson for success which factors out failure requires mindful planning. The following suggestions may be of help in planning successful art lessons for students who have experienced psychological trauma.

- Part of the lesson plan should include a task analysis. The teacher is encouraged to make a sample of the art project prior to teaching in order to analyze each step and ascertain important information that will help make the lesson more successful (Gerber & Guay, 2014).

- Ascertain every single piece of art material or equipment needed. The project cannot be successful if once started, a crucial element is found to be missing. Stopping the lesson to root around for a missing component is not only disruptive to the class, but can set everyone up for failure, including the teacher.

- Determine that this process actually works. Task analysis will bring to light any frustrating steps that could be simplified or eliminated. Not only must the process work, but also question whether this is the best way to do it. Adjusting, modifying, or even eliminating part of the process without sacrificing the integrity of the project is imperative for students who have a low thresh hold for frustration. Remember to be mindful of the students with whom you are working!

- Sequentially order each step of the process, even going so far as to make step-by-step direction charts so that students can work at their own speed, independently. Recognize that time allowances may be required for projects to "dry." Rather than having "down time" have another part of the project ready to move ahead, or if that is not possible, have an alternate project available to keep your students creating positively rather than having them creating havoc.

- Following the session, assess material needs for the next session. Did any student ask for special materials? Were all of the materials appropriate for the students doing this project? Were all of the materials appropriate for creating this project? Are there any changes; things that did not work? Are you running low on any supplies?

- Assess the progress of the lesson, adjusting the timeline for the project as necessary. The completion of an art project is not a race or competition. Is more time needed to reinforce learning? Do the students need more time to work at their own pace? Should there be more time to set up or clean up?

- Assess student behavior and general difficulties: What can be done to change, eliminate, or minimize problems? Always have a plan B, or even a plan C, in case the need arises. Sometimes it is necessary to take a time out from a project, regroup, and reconsider.

- Were there any changes in the physical layout of the classroom that would better suit this project: set up workstations, create clean-work areas, and rearrange wet-work areas? Part of the art lesson should include classroom etiquette, such as being respectful to each other, working side by side without getting in each other's way, not dripping wet paint on someone else's project, offering constructive comments to fellow classmates, and always being responsible for your own materials, including cleaning up the work area.

- Finally, how can all of the partners build the most success into this activity? This includes taking your students' suggestions into consideration. An art teacher shares her story:

> I planned a field trip for a group of students in an alternative education program. We would take a public bus to the museum. On our way back from the museum, we would stop at a fast food restaurant on the bus route. As we passed through an inner-city, low-income neighborhood, I noticed that some of the students were slumped low in their seats. As it was only around 9:00 a.m., I just assumed that they were tired. The museum trip went well, and as I shared our plans to stop for lunch on the way back to school, the students very vigorously said, "Oh, no Miss! We can't eat there! We need to go right back to school." I didn't understand until they explained that we were going through a rival gang neighborhood, and just riding on the bus was dangerous for them. We went back to the school, and I ordered pizza delivery.

Earlier in the chapter we discussed how the art room environment encourages activity that could be misconstrued as chaos. The organization and preparedness of the art teacher and partners facilitates the successful collaboration between the art specialist and all parties involved in the partnership.

Documentation, Dissemination, and Advocacy

Documenting and showcasing the success of collaborations and partnerships is an ideal way to advocate for your students. As Adrienne Hunter says, "When my students are able to shine through their art work, both my program and the whole school district shine as well" (Gerber & Guay, 2014, p. 54). However, when documenting the project, it is essential to be mindful of the privacy of the students. If a student chooses not to be photographed, be absolutely certain that the student's wishes are respected. Some students may be okay about using a photo of their art work, but not their identification. Some students may be in protective custody and their privacy must be protected at all times. Therefore, it is imperative that you get signed waivers for photography; the district should have a standard waiver form. It should be noted that having permission to use a photograph in a display is not the same as having permission to post the photograph on the Internet. It may be helpful to assign a "Photography Team" of students and staff who will:

- Take photos of the art products (without students) during various stages of progress.
- Take photos of students working on the project who have signed permission waivers.
- Include willing volunteers in the photos.
- Decide if a video of the work in progress is appropriate for the project and create one.

- Take photos of completed projects with students (with signed waivers) and photos of the finished projects without the students.
- Take photos at Opening Night/Opening Day celebrations (again, remember the importance of respecting everyone's privacy).
- Arrange a photography exhibit of the project in progress.
- Make sure each student has at least one photograph of the finished project for his or her portfolio.
- Assign a "Certificate Committee" to make certificates of appreciation for ALL participants involved in the project.
- Some students who do not want their picture taken for public use may want a photo for their own personal use.

Celebrating Student Success

At the conclusion of a project, stage a "Grand Finale" or some event to celebrate student success. Closure is an important aspect of any collaborative project. Getting to the end of the project without quitting may be a new experience for some of the more reluctant learners. Closure validates the project, and it validates the participants involved in the project. While a final critique with the students and other participants is essential, it is an assessment tool. The participants should be able to move beyond the classroom, receiving praise, expressing pride, and reminiscing about interesting parts of the experience with others (Gerber & Guay, 2014). Validation of the project can be accomplished in many ways. The following questions and suggestions might be explored:

- Is this project something that can be displayed as an exhibit?
- Do any of the works of art need to matted or framed?
- Can you hold an artists' Opening Night/Opening Day party to showcase the completed project?
- Can you invite family, other students, school personnel, partners, and community members? You might even consider inviting School Board members!
- Can light snacks and beverages be arranged?
- Can certificates of appreciation be awarded to all participants?
- Can media coverage be arranged? Some newspapers are very supportive of positive school news. Again, be mindful of participants' privacy!

A final evaluation of the collaboration/partnership as well as the actual project is essential. This should include an evaluation from the students and an evaluation from the partners/collaborators. Even if you think you are not going to ever repeat this particular project, the feedback may be invaluable for planning future projects. When designing the evaluation form, be sure to take your students into consideration, phrasing your questions so that the students can give suggestions from the "student point of view" and not just

"I liked it" or "It was OK." The evaluation for the art teacher and partners/ collaborators should be introspective and give specific information about the strengths and weaknesses of the program.

Being mindful of the students in your class who may be experiencing or have experienced psychological trauma will enhance not just your students' learning experience, but your teaching experience as well. The evaluation presents the art teacher and collaborators with the opportunity to really think through the way they spoke and worked with the students. Ways in which all were challenged to be creative and to put forth efforts to really have a positive impact on the students' desire and ability to learn are thus highlighted. Collaborating with others gives the students an important message that they are not alone, that they are an important, valuable part of a team or community, especially when the emphasis on testing students has been so strong that many teachers have had to eliminate the fun projects because of time constraints.

Ten Teaching Tips

1 Be mindful that there may be students who have experienced psychological trauma.
2 When planning a collaboration or partnership start with a BIG idea that will excite even the most reluctant learners.
3 Get students invested by making it meaningful, relevant, and attainable.
4 In planning a lesson, task analysis is key to building success and factoring out failure.
5 Get organized and stay organized.
6 Involve your school, community, and outside resources.
7 Documenting the project is advocacy for art and these students.
8 Celebrate the conclusion of the collaboration as a means of validating student success.
9 Make it fun, and reintroduce the joy of learning to all students.
10 Educate others about how your art projects are connected to academic skills.

References

Cavanaugh, B. (2016). Trauma-informed classrooms and schools. *Beyond Behavior, 25(2)*, 41–46.

Efland, A. (2002). *Art and Cognition: Integrating the Visual Arts in the Curriculum.* New York: Teachers College Press.

Gerber, B. L., & Guay, D. M. (2014). *Reaching and Teaching Students with Special Needs through Art.* Alexandria, VA: National Art Education Association.

Holdren, T. (2012). Using art to assess reading comprehension and critical thinking in adolescents. *Journal of Adolescent and Adult Literacy, 55(8)*, 692–703.

Johns, B. (2015). *15 Positive Behavior Strategies to Increase Academic Success.* Thousand Oaks, CA: Corwin.

Melnick, S., Witmer, J., & Strickland, M. (2011). Cognition and student learning through the arts. *Arts Education Policy Review, 112*, 154–162.

President's Committee on the Arts and Humanities (2011). Reinvesting in arts education. *The Education Digest, December*, 29–35.

Rose, D., & Magnotta, M. (2012). Succeeding with high-risk K–3 populations using arts-based reading instruction: A longitudinal study. *The Journal of Educational Research, 105*, 416–430.

Smithrim, K., & Upitis, R. (2005). Learning through the arts: Lessons of engagement. *Canadian Journal of Education 28(1/2)*, 109–127.

Sotiropoulou-Zormpala, M. (2012). Aesthetic teaching: Seeking a balance between teaching arts and teaching through the arts. *Arts Education Policy Review, 113*, 123–128.

14 Building Relationships through Art

Understanding the Potential of Art-Making for Students Experiencing Psychological Trauma

Lisa Kay and Susan D. Loesl

We are both art therapists/art educators who have worked in special education and regular school settings. This chapter sets out our reflections from our experiences as art teachers in creating environments in which students exposed to trauma feel safe expressing themselves. One of us has worked as an adaptive art specialist/art therapist for a large urban school district; the other as an art therapist in a special education school and a researcher in private schools within residential treatment centers serving adolescents. Collectively, we have over 60 years of experience working through art-making with students who have experienced a range of adverse childhood experiences, including psychological trauma. This chapter shares personal stories, professional experiences, successful strategies, and effective techniques for building relationships and supporting students in the art room.

A representative illustration is of a fifth-grade student who was somewhat oppositional, yet he seemed engaged while each activity was introduced. However, when the students were directed to start the designated art activity, he would pull out a piece of paper and begin drawing what he wanted rather than what the teacher had directed. The art teacher was frustrated, as it appeared this student was able to do what he wanted but everyone else had to do the presented project.

About four weeks into this behavior, the teacher felt she needed more support, so she contacted the adaptive art specialist because of her expertise in art therapy. The art teacher explained that she did not know much about the student because she had two schools with seven classes most days. Her concern was that this student might be experiencing something in his life that was manifesting in the art room. Because the adaptive art specialist was notified, she wanted to help.

This situation is not atypical. More and more students are coming to school ill prepared to deal with the realities of their own lives on top of having to learn things that may not seem important in relation to what is currently happening to them. A student may experience trauma in response to an accident, a witnessed or participated-in situation at home, a sudden loss (family member, friend, or pet), homelessness, or an illness causing an emotional weight. The student may exhibit behaviors unusual for them: verbal outbursts with little to no provocation, physically acting out by hitting a table, or limiting interactions with others when they are usually quite social. Students may feel puzzled about why people are saying they are "different," especially when they think "nothing is wrong."

Students come to school with many different challenges and may not often share the issues with others (Malchiodi, 2015). In some cases, children are in a quandary about whether to put their allegiance with their parents or their teachers. Often, they want to tell their teachers something, as a way to help their parents, but their parents tell them not to say anything. This hiding and secrecy "threat" can also be part of the trauma (Summit, 1983). How does a child deal with this conflict? Students are often given specific directions, but the resulting art may instead be spontaneous and uncensored by a student; students may not be prepared for what is created when fullfilling the assignment. Art teachers are faced with bridging what they are trying to teach their students in art class with what may spontaneously be created. Unfortunately, information related to the trauma may come out in a variety of ways, and when it is depicted in art, often the art teacher is unexpectedly the recipient. The images may show up anonymously on a teacher's desk, be left behind on a table or counter, be in a journal, or be turned in as an assignment. The spontaneous images may, and do at times, frighten and concern peers and art teachers. Art teachers do not want to overreact to images, nor do they want to miss opportunities to support troubled students. When art teachers encounter such images, it is their responsibility to determine whether the image requires further engagement or is of no concern.

Unfortunately, there is no handbook to help determine when an image is of concern. Determinations may be based on responses to the art work turned in by other students who more closely followed the directives; art experiences from communication with other art teachers regarding "unique" art images; or even just a teacher's "gut reaction" that cannot be explained. The art teacher should survey the student's past work and seek out consultation with mental health professionals, such as the school psychologist or art therapist. By collaborating with other professionals, the art teacher may learn that the student is dealing with personal challenges or that the imagery is an indication of a previously unknown challenge that the student may be facing. The art teacher is not trained as an art therapist, social worker, or counselor and should not engage in a therapeutic discussion with the student regarding the art work. It is the responsibility of the art teacher to identify resources within their school/district when concerns with students arise—before it becomes a crisis situation.

Students in crisis or exposed to trauma are not always aware that they are in crisis, as it may be *their* norm. Often, visual art is a way for the student to communicate what is inside; they may need help to make sense of what they are feeling. Often, the images can be paired with behaviors that seem incongruous to the student's previously known behaviors and may be manifested in ways that appear similar to children with specific behavioral or emotional disabilities. Students in crisis may be experiencing thoughts and feelings new to them because until this point they may have been capable of successfully handling issues in their home, school, and community environments. As a means of coping, they may draw favorite images or symbols on whatever paper is available. Chances are the student is not cognitively aware that he or she is starting to process the experience through the art. Ideally, by the student sharing the art with an adult, the student can work through this experience of the trauma.

Physical, emotional, and social reactions may also occur in tandem with art-making, so again noting changes in the student can be crucial to the student's progress. One does not have to be an art therapist to be conscious of and responsive to changes in student behaviors and to act upon the indicators with the support of school and other professionals as necessary. In situations where the student begins to spontaneously share personal information about the issue during class, a good response may be to approach the student, using proximity control, and quietly say, "Why don't we talk about this in private later?" The teacher then needs to use the "steamroller effect" and quickly move the class along so that the other children do not pick up and respond to the personal statements.

However, it may be somewhat challenging for the art teacher to find an opportunity to discuss the observations with the student, as confidentiality needs to be respected. A note to the student to stay a few minutes after class, a quick "Can you come by for a few minutes during third hour?" or "Do you have a little time to meet after school today?" may help to set a time to address the potential concerns. Not responding or waiting until something more overt occurs can be the worst thing to do. The art teacher can listen to the student and then must consider seeking out support or helping the student make an appointment with the school psychologist, school social worker, or guidance counselor, for not only the student but also for the art teacher.

Cristina was one student in crisis whose art teacher, one of the authors, other school faculty, professionals, and family members were noting behaviors of concern. Here is her story:

It was October when Cristina, age 17, transferred to the special education school. She entered the art room wearing an oversized shirt, tail out, and black leather platform shoes. She appeared depressed, discouraged, and anxious—in her words, "hopeless."

Cristina told me that she had been in and out of hospitals since the age of 13. She had spent a year in "rehab" and her "Sweet 16" in a children's psychiatric facility. Many medications were prescribed to treat numerous diagnoses: manic depression, conduct disorder, oppositional defiance, and depression. She reported having few, if any, girlfriends and said she had experienced abusive relationships with boyfriends. Cristina had been sui-cidal and self-destructive; she had difficulty trusting anyone. She said she had a Hispanic background and her family was close knit, although her parents were divorced.

Cristina loved art. She spent a lot of time in the art room as a work/study student and in a girls' art group focused on women artists. She enjoyed a variety of media and was skilled in art techniques. Cristina liked to work large; her art work was profound with bold, exquisite colors. However, she did not talk much about her work or its meaning.

Things changed when six pieces of Cristina's art work were submit-ted for the book and juried exhibition *Childhood Revealed: Art Expressing Pain, Discovery and Hope* (Koplewicz & Goodman, 1999). This project, sponsored by New York University's Child Study Center, highlighted the mental health needs of children and adolescents. Artist statements were required with each submission. For the first time, Cristina con-nected emotionally and verbally with her art work. Of 600 submissions, 100 were selected and two were Cristina's. She was ecstatic! Not only would her work be published in a book and travel in a show around the United States, she would attend the opening at the Whitney Museum in New York. This was an incredible opportunity that boosted her self-esteem, changed her outlook on life, and gave her self-confidence. This experience was a turning point.

After attending the exhibition, Cristina and the art teacher worked together weekly for six months. Inspired by an art education journal arti-cle, Cristina chose to work with plaster craft, mixed media, and a large recycled 4' x 8' canvas. Cristina had developed a trusting relationship with the teacher that allowed them to make molds of Cristina's face, neck, and arms. She also took materials home and made castings of her legs and knees. Her final assemblage was titled "The Time of My Life." As they worked together, she talked about herself; the art teacher listened and witnessed her creative process. As she attached new parts to the canvas, she shared more personal experiences.

Cristina was almost ready to graduate. She was excited to share that she had applied to art school in Chicago. She wanted be an "art therapy teacher" so she could work in art with kids who had problems, conjuring an image of her wearing an oversized paint shirt, leather platform black heels, and her ID badge reading: Miss Cristina, Art Teacher.

Cristina's story is phenomenal. She struggled with psychological and family problems. Through her art work and writing, she expressed her feel-ings, examined her life circumstances, and saw herself in a new way. More importantly, four important lessons emerged. First, building relationships takes time and so does discovering and recovering oneself. Engaging in art-making with a sensitive art therapist or art teacher can support this process. Second, labels can be deceptive. Students may have been given diagnoses that are not always accurate. Students are more than the label. Third, making art is not enough. Students need to reflect and write about their art work. Fourth, sharing with others is critical—exhibiting students' art work is essential.

Cristina's opportunity to have her work published and exhibited in a museum was remarkable. However, students can co-curate art shows for their peers, parents, school staff, and community. These exhibitions can take place in the art room, in the school, or in community venues. It is important to share the work of all students regardless of their talent and ability. Some images may be inappropriate for display due to content or school rules, so the art teacher should use discretion regarding what to display. Students may be re-traumatized by others inquiring about their art when it is displayed. However, exhibition opportunities allow others to witness students' creative efforts and understand their "pain, discovery, and hope" (Koplewicz & Goodman, 1999), which can affirm self-worth and build self-esteem.

Students experience adverse life events that may impact their ability to focus on the lessons taking place in the art classroom (Garbarino, Kostelny, & Dubrow, 1991; Steele, 2002). Often, in the art classroom, art teachers become privy to some of these concerns, either while students are just talking or when working on their art assignments. Art teachers should feel confident in their understanding of appropriate interactions with students when such concerns present themselves. The student's well-being must be considered before any intervention, even when a private discussion between the art teacher and student occurs.

It can be empowering for the student to realize other adults are aware of the circumstances, as happened in Jim's and Chad's cases.

Jim, a student in an eighth-grade art class, admitted he had heard gun shots quite a bit over the past couple of years near his home. He said that this really didn't bother him until he saw one of the "neighborhood guys" get gunned down on the sidewalk after being wrongly accused of stealing money. Jim was traumatized by this event and was unable to deal with the stress. It worked inside him in small ways; at first: he was quieter in class than normal, wanted to be alone more than usual, and finally, he seemed to fade into the woodwork of the classroom.

As time went on, Jim became vocally short-tempered when asked about his homework, snapped at other students when they got near him in the halls, and started drawing in his textbooks during class, on the bus, or at home when he took his books home. His classroom teachers noticed these images; some were doodles, some were words and images, and some were images from video games. The classroom teachers took the images to the art teacher, as they thought he might have a clue to this behavior. The art teacher had no idea that there was such a proliferation of images. No one had actually asked Jim about his images, so none of the teachers was truly aware about the specific circumstances that had led to their creation.

Jim was referred to the school psychologist, who requested that an adaptive art specialist/art therapist be a part of their meetings. At first, Jim was reluctant to discuss his art, stating that the images were "just pictures." When the school psychologist noted she was aware that he lived in a very high crime area where a number of shootings had recently occurred, he admitted that it "sorta bothered him." However, he stated later that he felt better when he was drawing and had actually drawn a picture of the shooting incident a number of times; he brought four pictures to the sessions. Over the course of about two months, Jim began to return to his previous behaviors and was able to overcome other effects of the stress caused by the event that was affecting his participation in school. Months later, he was observed often carrying a sketchbook and would occasionally stop into the school psychologist's office to show off his drawings.

Another student, Chad produced a particularly provocative piece of art work that met the requirements of the texture drawing art assignment and scored high on the assessment rubric, especially in the area of rendering. This posed a dilemma for the art teacher. From a glance, Chad's art work resembled a knight's horse covered with face armor, but closer examination revealed something quite different. This piece of art work was packed with all kinds of weapons—brass knuckles, firearms, handguns, knives, and grenades—imagery often censored in schools (Kay, 2008). In Chad's self-critique about this particular assignment, he wrote about his perceptions of violence in our culture and stated these weapons were some of the "things" that he sees in his world. This opened up a dialogue between the art teacher and Chad. While she understood his intent, they discussed the fact that his imagery was not appropriate for school and would not be displayed on the bulletin boards outside the classroom. She also contacted his mother and the principal to have a meeting about the imagery. This meeting was helpful in securing a psychological evaluation and subsequent psychiatric hospitalization for this student (Kay, 2008). Art teachers need to be aware of what is acceptable for display in the school and still be able to support a student's creative efforts. Art work like Chad's often provides evidence of more serious concerns that needed further intervention.

This chapter demonstrates the importance of an art teacher's ability to realize that images a student creates may reflect issues the student is dealing with regarding personal crisis or trauma. It also develops an awareness of potential need for support from other professionals to help the student and the art teacher. The importance of acknowledging the student's art and the art teacher's concern about the student's best interests is integral to the student's ability to use art as a means to express him or herself when in crisis. As art teachers reflect on their own teaching scenarios, ten tips are included to summarize the most important aspects of this chapter. Ideally, these tips will provide the structure for art teachers to create safe environments for their challenging students to be creative.

Ten Teaching Tips

1 Build relationships with students that nurture creativity and self-expression: artistically, nonverbally, and verbally. It takes time and so does discovering oneself through art.
2 Understand that students may have been given diagnoses that are not always accurate. Students are more than the label or diagnosis.
3 Provide an environment in which students feel that they can be creative without fear of being interrogated about their art as they work.
4 Provide opportunities for students to reflect on and write about their art work.
5 Realize that art-making provides opportunities for students to express themselves in nonverbal ways that may be hard for them to understand.
6 Trust intuition or "gut reaction" when an image appears too different from previous art teacher experiences.
7 Feel confident in the understanding of appropriate art teacher interactions with students when concerns over images present themselves.
8 Collaborate with other school and mental health professionals to increase understanding and support the student in crisis.
9 Know what is acceptable to display in the school but still be able to support student creativity.
10 Encourage art-making outside of class by providing sketchbooks and a variety of art materials to take home.

References

Garbarino J., Kostelny, K., & Dubrow, N. (1991). *No Place To Be a Child: Growing Up in a War Zone*. New York: Lexington.

Kay, L. (2008). Art education pedagogy and practice with adolescent students at-risk in alternative high schools (unpublished doctoral dissertation). Northern Illinois University, DeKalb, IL.

Koplewicz, H., & Goodman, R. (1999). *Childhood Revealed: Art Expressing Pain, Discovery and Hope*. New York: Harry N. Abrams.

Malchiodi, C. (2008, 2015). *Creative Interventions with Traumatized Children* (1st and 2nd editions). New York: Guilford Press.

Steele, W. (2002). Trauma's impact on learning and behavior: A case for intervention in schools. *Trauma and Loss Journal, 2(2)*, 1–16. Retrieved April 1, 2006, from http://tlcinstitute.org/impactarticle.html.

Summit, R. C. (1983). The child abuse accommodation syndrome. *Child Abuse and Neglect*, 7, 177–193.

15 Yellow Bricks

An Approach to Art Teaching

Lisa Kay

In this chapter, transformational art pedagogy, an approach to art teaching with students who have experienced psychological trauma, is defined and described (Kay, 2008). The use of a quintessential story, *The Wonderful Wizard of Oz*, as a framework for teaching reflection and art-making with students who have experienced trauma is introduced. Questions are posed for the art teacher to consider along with Oz lessons, which can be discerned from teaching stories. *Yellow Bricks: An Oz Art Program* (Kay, 2004) for children and adolescents is outlined through a series of art-making directives that are drawn from the powerful metaphors in Baum's beloved fairy tale. This transformational approach to art pedagogy can assist students to metaphorically find "home" through an educational practice that offers students a sense of identity, a sense of place, and a sense of hope (Giroux, 1992).

Transformational Art Pedagogy

Transformational art pedagogy is an approach that can be used by art educators because it combines art, education, and therapeutic elements. It can be defined as an approach to teaching art that addresses issues related to students' identity and personal beliefs, sense of place, feelings of empowerment, and personal growth through art-making, the creative process, reflection, and dialogue. It is a way of teaching art that incorporates feminist principles (Collin & Sandell, 1996; Garber, 1992; Kay, 2008; Kay & Arnold, 2013). This approach to teaching art offers a fluid, flexible, personalized, student-centered art-making curriculum focused on self-expression and self-identity. Art educators can adopt this transformational approach to art teaching that addresses social and emotional aspects of learning like feeling–identification, identity exploration, and personal concerns. Through practicing transformational art pedagogy, teaching about making and learning about art can occur while dealing with complex social, emotional, personal, and cultural issues.

The Oz Story

The Oz story and the metaphor of the "yellow brick road" are powerful when considering ways to think about working in the art classroom with students who have been traumatized. As art educators, we can metaphorically walk with our students—just as Dorothy did with her companions—to face challenges, recognize the students' strengths, and achieve artistic, academic, and social success. Creativity is at the core of art-making; creativity involves courage and taking risks (Bayles & Orland, 2001; May, 1994). Art education can facilitate creative growth in much the same ways that Dorothy and her companions developed courage, kindness, and wisdom as they journeyed through Oz.

Questions and Lessons for Consideration

The following six questions are important for art educators to consider and guide their work with students who have been exposed to trauma.

First, how has each of us has been personally affected by trauma? We have all had traumatic experiences and stressful times in our lives. We have experienced adversities, dealt with loss, and coped with illness, which are all human experiences. By creating art work and reflecting about experiences, art teachers can gain empathy and understanding for their students who are experiencing difficulties in their lives. The Oz lesson is that by making our own art work and reflecting about personal encounters and feelings about crisis, illness, and trauma, we can gain awareness and understanding of our own experiences and discover that we are not really that different from others.

Second, how can we be fully present to our students who are impacted by these traumatic experiences? Dante's story below is one example.

> Dante was homeless. Peers called him "worthless" because he did not have a place to live. "Living on the streets ain't safe," they told him. When the art teacher asked why he took construction paper from the art room without permission, he answered, "'Cause I don't have that stuff to make stuff." [Knowing he was homeless, perhaps the art teacher should not have expected students to furnish materials from home.] Once his art project was finished, Dante was asked to take his art with him. He remarked to his art teacher, "Forget it. I ain't got no place to put it. Keep it yourself," which she did. [Again, the teacher might have asked whether he wanted to take it with him or leave it in the art room.] In response to another student asking why he was just sitting and not working on his art project, he said, "I don't like making art. What good is it anyway? Ain't got nowhere to put it." The art teacher contacted the classroom teacher to offer support for Dante. His teacher explained that the student had reported he had not seen his mom in a few days, that she could be at the hospital because she gets paranoid. As he had said, "She ain't right when she ain't on her meds."

The Oz lesson is that students have many traumatizing life circumstances over which they may not have control. These situations dominate their reality, influence their self-image, and their ability to function in school. We cannot always change the situation but we can be present, listen, and provide emotional support.

Third, how can we make meaningful connections with our students? Where are those points of connection? Here is Mike's story.

> Mike enters the art room and sits down quietly. He appears discouraged and withdrawn. He puts his head down on the table. He doesn't say hello. He answers questions with monotone, one-syllable words "yes" and "no." I sit beside him and draw his portrait. After finishing it, I hand it to him and he accepts my gift drawing. He silently leaves the art room. During our next class time Mike is more animated and responsive.

The Oz lesson shows that art teachers must give students the time and space that they need to engage with others—listen visually and reflect on what can be seen in a drawing. By doing this simple gesture, the art teacher can communicate that he or she accepts the students just as they are. It is crucial for art teachers to be authentic and sensitive to a student's needs and where they are at the moment.

Fourth, how can art teachers better understand their students' energy levels, behavioral cues, and respect students' personal space? The following two students' stories offer important insights.

> Jake, an energetic nine-year-old African-American boy came in the art room. He was very stimulated by what he saw and wanted to do everything. We walked around the room together; initially I paced my movements with his. Then I slowed down my pace and he began to slow his pace. I invited him to sit down with me. He looked around the room and remained unfocused. I gave Jake a multicolored chunk of crayon and a piece of paper. I asked him to scribble on the paper as hard as he could. He complied. Jake thought that the scribbling was "silly and fun" and said his scribble was a "wild man" just like he was. After scribbling, he was now more relaxed and calm and able to focus on his art assignment.
>
> Jazmin is a 15-year-old Latino female who was guarded, yet very social. She came into the art room. I walked behind her table, reached from behind her and put materials on the table. She jumped and said, "Don't do that—it makes me nervous." I apologized for invading her personal space and moved around to the front of the table. Jazmin selected her art materials and began to draw.

The Oz lessons here demonstrate that students will usually calm down and be ready to listen and focus on tasks when the art teacher models a slower, more relaxed pace and breathing pattern. Some students may require more personal space, especially students who have been abused. Standing or sitting by a student's side when talking or giving art materials is preferable to standing over them or reaching from behind and over them.

Fifth, how can art teachers use what they know about developmental stages in child art to understand and support their students? Noting significant changes can be useful clues to share with parents and counselors. Jennifer's story is an example.

> Jennifer had been a talkative, friendly, and precocious eight-year-old little girl. She loved making art and talked a lot about becoming a big sister while in the art room. Her art work appeared to be what you would expect for her age, and she could focus when presented with highly structured assignments and guidance to stay on task. During parent–teacher conference, she was proud to show her parents her work and the art room.
>
> Jennifer's art work started to change, and she was more aggressive with people and the way that she used art materials. This prompted a discussion with the school social worker and her parents. Her parents expressed concerns about Jennifer's learning and behavior issues. They were noticing changes, especially after the birth of her brother. She was having greater difficulty processing language, concentrating, and paying attention. Her parents were encouraged to have Jennifer evaluated.

The Oz lesson is that even though art teachers are not art therapists or mental health professionals, they have access to important information about their students. Understanding the stages of visual artistic development helps teachers know what to expect, where to begin planning and adapting lessons, and developing teaching strategies. It also provides helpful evidence that can be used to get support services for students who need it.

Sixth, how can we make art a normalizing experience? Why is this important?

Christopher's story is a poignant example.

> Christopher was a curious, inquisitive, creative, bright, and outgoing 11-year-old boy who I met while directing a pediatric play therapy program. He was admitted to the hospital because he complained of headaches. After coming in as a day patient for an MRI, it was confirmed that Christopher had a malignant brain tumor. Over the next 11 months, we worked together in art every time he came in and out of the hospital. During this time, he missed a lot of school. As the tumor grew, Chris lost the ability to do many things; his vision became impaired, and the right side of his body became paralyzed. However, a constant in our experiences together was his desire to continue to create art, despite his limited skills and weakened abilities. Chris wanted to do things like his peers were doing at school. Making art

(paintings, drawings, tissue-paper collages, constructing kaleidoscopes, and other special objects) provided Christopher with a sense of normality despite the fact he was dying.

The Oz lesson here is that students who have experienced psychological trauma (accidents, illness, loss, poverty, homelessness, or abuse) are coping with serious life and death issues. They want to be like everyone else; they want to be normal and to be seen as normal as possible. Art-making can have a normalizing effect, like it did for Christopher, even in the most abnormal circumstances.

Yellow Bricks: An Oz Art Program

Classic literature and folktales can be instructive and have therapeutic value when paired with art-making. Such teaching stories provide rich images and themes that can be structured to an art-making process for a lesson plan or an entire curriculum. The resulting art work can mirror a student's current experience, progress, and/or mastery over personal loss, crisis, and trauma in creative and imaginative ways. Many stories can be used this way: *The Wonderful Wizard of Oz, Alice in Wonderland,* and/or *Harry Potter and the Sorcerer's Stone,* to name a few. What follows is a series of art directives that are drawn from the powerful metaphors in Baum's fairy tale. Like Dorothy in the story, these art-making activities present a step toward "home"—a place where students of all ages, with a range of issues, concerns, and needs—can find the "brains, heart, and courage," just like the Scarecrow, Tin Man, and the Lion.

While this program was initially designed for and implemented with students in a K–12 special education school, it can be easily applied to any other art room, or after-school or summer program. For example, this particular program was adapted as an after-school community art program in rural libraries over the course of one year in celebration of the 100th anniversary of L. Frank Baum's *The Wonderful Wizard of Oz* (1900). Art directives, activities, and materials were adapted depending on the ages and developmental levels of the students or participants in the class or group. To set the stage, each session began with a reading from the story or a clip from the movie. Next, an art directive or lesson with art materials was introduced to guide the art-making process. Using this format, the art teacher can motivate students to create individual and collaborative art work that has the potential to engage students indirectly with the healing or transformational lessons in the classic story.

"Yellow Bricks" was a therapeutic art curriculum originally designed for students in a therapeutic day school identified with social and emotional disturbances, who had experienced adverse childhood experiences including multiple traumas. However, this story and sequential "artivities" offer a strong metaphoric strategy that can be used with all students.

Yellow Brick 1: Building and Constructing Home[1]

What does home look and feel like? What does your fantasy home or the home of the future look like? Home is both a literal and metaphorical place and space within the self. The inside/outside of the house can correlate with actual perceptions of how children perceive inside and outside of homes, and imagine what they would like "home" to be. This can also represent inner and outer perceptions of the "self."

Materials: 12 × 18 white paper/cardboard, mixed media, found objects, adhesives

Directions: Fold paper to create a free-standing 3D house; collage or embellish with mixed media/found objects to create outside/inside of house.

Yellow Brick 2: Tornados/Rainbows

This is a metaphorical exploration of representation of conflict/chaos and positive calm after the storm.

Materials: Black paper and multicolored chunks of crayons, magazine images, mural paper, glue, pastels.

Directions: a. For young children: Create tornado drawings, cut in a spiral, and move like a tornado.

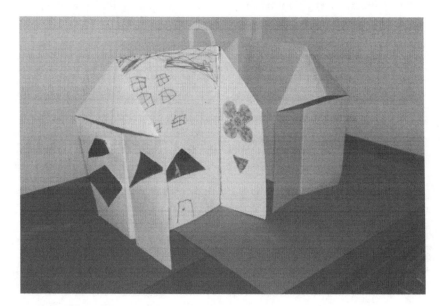

Figure 15.1 "Views of a House"

b. For adolescents: Create an "Over and Under the Rainbow Mural." Draw a large rainbow on paper. Attach black and white images from magazines to represent conflicts/chaos under the rainbow. Add colored images to represent solutions to problems, hopes, and discoveries over the rainbow.

Yellow Brick 3: Shoes

Shoes have many purposes. Our shoes offer support and ground us to the earth beneath us. They carry us throughout our daily travels and take us many places.

Materials: Shoes, found objects, mixed media, hot glue gun and glue sticks, paint, glitter. (Consider asking local shoe stores to donate shoes, as used shoes may be unsanitary.)

Directions: Paint, decorate, and/or embellish shoes.

Yellow Brick 4: Bricks/Brick Road

Bricks are the metaphoric building blocks to help us create and follow our life path by teaching how to set goals and create a path step by step.

Materials: Clay, clay tools, rolling pins, stamps, objects and fabric to press into clay.

Directions: Roll out clay to create slabs. Cut into 4" × 8" bricks. Make a "goal brick" of something the student wants to accomplish. Carve and engrave words or details. Glaze or paint with acrylic paint after they are fired. When students are all finished, construct a collaborative brick road with finished clay pieces.

Yellow Brick 5: Glasses

Help students, by peering through "lenses," to see themselves in creative ways, from different perspectives, vantage points, and points of view.

Materials: colored and manila folders, colored cellophane, scissors, mixed media, glue, stickers, and confetti

Directions: Construct your own set of glasses. Trace a template or draw a design for a pair of glasses. Add colored lenses. Decorate with mixed media and found objects.

Yellow Brick 6: Hearts' Desire, True Colors, and Passions

Materials: Pre-cut cardboard hearts or heart boxes, scissors, mixed media, glue, found objects, yarn, hot glue gun and glue sticks, paint, glitter, magazine images

Directions: Each student decorates his or her heart with their choice of collage materials, considering the color of their hearts, thinking about their hearts' desires or needs. What is inside and outside their hearts?

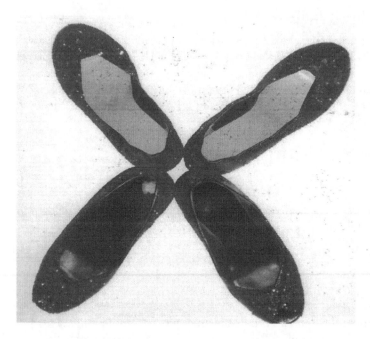

Figure 15.2 "Ruby Slippers"

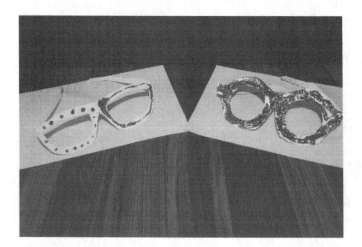

Figure 15.3 "Emerald City Glasses"

Yellow Brick 7: Award Ribbons

Ask each student to think of something that they do best? Materials are provided for students to make awards or ribbons for something they do well. This capitalizes on their strengths and reinforces their positive abilities. At the conclusion of the program, the focus is on strengths and accomplishments. As in the Oz story, a certificate of completion is awarded at the end of the semester or the culmination of the program.

Materials: Colored ribbon, scissors, paper, glue, paint, glitter

Directions: Each student will create an award for him or herself to recognize something they do well. "Give yourself an award."

The activities included in the "Yellow Bricks: An Oz Art Program" are well within the boundaries of any art educator's practice. These activities have therapeutic potential for students; however, they are not art therapy. They do provide students opportunities to create meaningful art work that connects to their lives in non-direct ways. The program offers art teachers a structure for lessons based on a classic story that helps students who have experienced trauma or may face challenges by recognizing their strengths, helping them to grow creatively, and achieving artistic, academic, and social success.

Concurrently, art educators can adopt a pedagogical approach that is between traditional art education and art therapy, which incorporates feminist principles and a transformational approach to art teaching (Collin & Sandell, 1996; Garber, 1992; Kay, 2008; Kay & Arnold, 2013). Transformational art pedagogy addresses social and emotional aspects of learning like feeling-identification, identity exploration, and personal issues. This approach to teaching art offers a fluid, flexible, personalized, student-centered art-making curriculum focused on self-expression and self-identity. Transformational art pedagogy deals with issues related to students' identity/beliefs, sense of place, and feelings of agency through the creative process, reflection and dialogue. By incorporating transformational art pedagogy, teaching about, making, and learning about art can occur while dealing with complex social, emotional, personal, and cultural issues.

This approach to art education is effective because it can be viewed as a transformation of education. In the book *Border Crossings: Cultural Workers and the Politics of Education*, Giroux envisions pedagogy as "a configuration of textual, verbal, and visual practices that seek to engage the processes through which people understand themselves and the ways in which they engage with others and their environments" (1992, p. 3). Giroux argues, "educators need to approach learning not merely as the acquisition of knowledge but as the production of cultural practices that offer students a sense of identity, place, and hope" (p. 146). Art educators who employ transformational art pedagogy can provide such a configuration of educational practice that offers their students a sense of identity, a sense of place, and a sense of hope.

Ten Teaching Tips

1 Adopt a transformational approach to art education.
2 Employ the metaphors and stories from classic literature, like *The Wonderful Wizard of Oz*, to build curriculum.
3 Be willing to be a companion on the "yellow brick road" with students.
4 Make your own art work about personal encounters/feelings about crisis, illness, and trauma, and reflect about those experiences in written form.
5 Listen, observe, and be fully present to students.
6 Make meaningful, authentic connections with students.
7 Understand students' energy levels and behavioral cues.
8 Respect each student's personal space.
9 Know about developmental stages in child art.
10 Make art a normalizing experience.

Note

1 This art activity may be difficult for some students who are experiencing trauma, in foster care, or who have lost their home for whatever reason. It is important to be sensitive to the needs of these students and to craft the introduction carefully.

References

Baum, L. F. (1900). *The Wonderful Wizard of Oz*. Chicago, IL: George M. Hill.

Bayles, D., & Orland, T. (2001). *Art and Fear: Observations on the Perils (and Rewards) of Artmaking*. Eugene, OR: Image Continuum Press.

Collins, G., & Sandell, R. (1996) *Gender Issues in Art Education: Content, Contexts, and Strategies*. Reston, VA: National Art Education Association.

Garber, E. (1992). Feminism, aesthetics, and art education. *Studies in Art Education, 33(4)*, 210–225.

Giroux, H. (1992). *Border Crossings: Cultural Workers and the Politics of Education*. New York: Routledge.

Kay, L. (2008). Art education pedagogy and practice with adolescent students at-risk in alternative high schools (unpublished doctoral dissertation). Northern Illinois University, DeKalb, IL.

Kay, L., & Arnold, A. (2014). Order out of chaos: An arts-based approach to counteract violence. *Art Education, 67(3)*, 31–36.

May, R. (1994). *The Courage to Create*. New York: W. W. Norton & Company.

16 Non-Traditional Educational Settings, Center Schools, and Students with Behavioral Disorders[1]

Joseph A. Parsons, Adrienne D. Hunter, and Donalyn Heise

The Nature of Emotional Disabilities and What It Means for an Art Teacher

Emotional disturbance designations are wide and encompass diverse differences that make teaching a challenge. The federal government's definition of an emotional disturbance is a condition exhibiting one or more of the following characteristics over a long period of time and to a marked degree that adversely affects the child's educational performance:

1 An inability to learn that cannot be explained by intellect, memory, or health factors;
2 An inability to build or maintain satisfactory interpersonal relationships with peers or teachers;
3 Inappropriate types of behavior or feelings under normal circumstances;
4 A generally pervasive mood of unhappiness or depression; and/or
5 A tendency to develop physical symptoms or fears associated with personal or school problems.

The term "emotional disturbance" includes schizophrenia; however, the term does not apply to children who are socially maladjusted unless it is also determined that they have an emotional disturbance as listed above (Kupper, 2014).

Students with emotional disabilities come under two categories: Psychiatric disorders and behavioral disorders. Psychiatric disorders require treatment, including medications (Education Corner, 2016). Recent estimates from the National Center for Health report 7.5% of U.S. children between the ages of 6 and 17 were taking medications for emotional or behavioral difficulties (Insel, 2014). Medication usage by students with behavioral disorders in a self-contained school was 38.2%, and 16.8% were on more than one medication (Mattison, Rivera, & Michel, 2014). Our experiences in Center Schools reveal more than double these statistics. Medications may have profound effects on students' cognitive and functioning abilities. Students with behavioral disorders who have learning and/or language disabilities may be further compromised by side effects (Mattison, Rundberg-Rivera, & Michel, 2014).

Children with behavioral disorders may have been the victims of abuse and neglect, meaning abuse in the forms of emotional abuse, physical abuse, sexual abuse, and child neglect. Child abuse is a common problem worldwide. It has been linked to changes in victims' mental and behavioral development throughout their lives, putting them at risk of engaging in potentially dangerous behavior in the future (Odhayain, Watson, & Watson, 2013). Research in childhood abuse is extremely difficult for a multitude of reasons. It should be noted, however, that the factors that identify behavioral disabilities are highly correlated to those behaviors that are manifested by children who are identified as abused.

In compliance with Free Appropriate Public Education for Students with Disabilities (2010), a student must undergo an assessment to determine if the child has a disability (U.S. Department of Education, Individuals with Disabilities Education Act, IDEA, 2004). This evaluation may include aptitude and achievement tests, teacher recommendations, medical history, discovery of social and cultural background, and descriptions of a child's adaptive behaviors. It can also include a psychiatrist who will enter a diagnosis. Using the DSM-5 identification in the form of a specific number (i.e., 309.24, Adjustment Disorder with Anxiety; 296.89, Bipolar II Disorder; 293.83, Depressive Disorder NOS; or 293.81, Psychotic Disorder Due To . . .), a diagnosis is assigned to the student (Hsiung, 2015). There are many DSM-5 numbers, and some students have a number of labels. Many schools refer to these children as students with behavioral disorders.

An art class of students with behavioral disorders will typically have students with different diagnoses and will require different approaches to successfully reach and teach each one. This leads to the development of a student's Individualized Educational Program (IEP). The IEP ensures that a student receives the appropriate and least restrictive educational program through the public school system. An IEP identifies the student's needs, how the needs will be met, and drives the student's educational and behavioral goals. This process of assessment, identification, consultation with parents and educators, and ongoing evaluation guides decisions on the best educational setting for each student. Some students with behavioral disorders are educated in programs housed within a public school. Some refer to these programs as a "school within a school." Other non-traditional approaches, such as a Center School described below, provide targeted support for students with disorders so severe that success in a regular school setting is unlikely.

The Center School Advantage

A Center School is a self-contained facility, designed for a specific educational disability and provides multiple services. Different states may use different names for this type of school.

Behavior management is the critical issue for students with behavioral disorders. It is their behavior that has been recognized, documented, and evaluated and has determined that they do not behave in a normal and acceptable manner and need assistance. In a regular school setting, it is up to the individual special education teacher or the student's IEP team to develop and implement a plan for assisting the student to achieve an acceptable level of behavior. The Center School provides a significant advantage with relation to serving these students' unique needs through school-wide collaboration. Center Schools generally incorporate a Behavior Management System with these components: Rules and Expectations, Record Maintenance System, Point System, Token Economy System, Reward System, and Time Out/Seclusion.

Joseph A. Parsons, an art teacher with over 39 years of experience working with students with behavioral disorders, shares his personal perspectives on teaching art in a Center School:

> I believe a Center School is the best place to work as an art teacher of students with behavioral disabilities for a number of reasons. First, a good Center School is staffed to meet the needs of these specific students. The administration is experienced in working with the population of students you will be teaching and will most likely provide you with more support than in a regular school. Second, as an art teacher you will be working with colleagues who are trained and experienced in the education of the emotionally disabled. These veteran teachers will often provide you with a wealth of tested methods and considerations to meet the needs of these students. Third, Center Schools routinely have a wealth of auxiliary staff like psychiatrists, therapists, social workers, behavior specialists, Exceptional Students Education (ESE) specialists, speech therapists, safety/security personnel, classroom aides, and other educational professionals who can provide you with support and assistance that you would not have direct access to in a regular school setting. Fourth, class sizes in a Center School are significantly smaller than in a regular school. Public Law 94–142, IDEA, and subsequent reauthorizations of the law have specific provisions concerning class sizes. Individual states create their own class size requirements and no two states have exactly the same specifications (Jackson, 2003). Most classes in Center Schools will also have a teacher aide. In the three states I have worked in and several others I have visited, Center Schools' class size varies somewhere between five and 15 students.
>
> In summation, I feel a Center School is the best place to work and meet the unique needs of behaviorally disabled students due to the additional support, lower class sizes, and colleague understanding and collaboration.

Art Students in a Center School

A number of elements influence teaching art in a Center or other non-traditional school setting. Typically, students with behavioral disorders are expected to meet normal educational standards and graduate with a standard high school diploma. However, because of students' behavioral disabilities, like obsessive-compulsive disorder, manic-depressive disorder, paranoia, schizophrenia, or attention deficit/hyperactivity disorder, as well as fragmented exposure to art, and/or use of medication, their capability to function at the same rate of production as in a regular art class is often difficult and unreasonable. The art teacher should create a balance between covering the curriculum and meeting students' needs.

It is the students' behaviors and diagnoses that have placed them in the Center School or non-traditional educational setting. These behaviors are so severe that these students could not successfully exist in a regular school setting. Because of these student characteristics, the connection between the teacher and the student is paramount. When a teacher knows each student, their thought processes, perspectives, and reactions to their environment, the teacher will be able to recognize when negative behaviors are festering and can be proactive and thwart their manifestations before the student loses control. He or she can make appropriate choices and be able to direct the student effectively. Sometimes, students in non-traditional educational settings are very transient, and there is no opportunity to get to know students prior to class. An alternative education art teacher shares some of her expertise:

> When working with new students, it is essential for the teacher to immediately establish a rapport. This is easier said than done. Be quietly welcoming: Smile and say hello to your student, introducing yourself, addressing your student by name. Ask the student if he or she likes art, and if they are good at art. Respond positively by saying something like: "Great! I'm happy to have you in my class!" or "Then this is your lucky day! I happen to be really good at teaching art!" Recognize that your new student may not be too happy to be in your school: Don't call attention to them, do respect their privacy, and don't take their issues personally.
>
> If a student comes into your classroom angry, it is a sure bet that the anger has nothing to do with you. Instead of making it your problem, try reaching out to the student, asking how you can help make his or her day better. It is a good idea to have some alternate projects to ask this student to do while de-escalating. Such projects might be special jobs to help, like sorting papers, hanging papers on the bulletin board, or looking for pictures in magazines. This approach should help a student feel calmer, "needed," and "valued," and will avoid having an angry student destroy a project on which he or she has previously been happily working.
>
> (Gerber & Guay, 2014, p. 58)

To connect with the students with behavioral disorders, trust must also be established (Mathis, 2013). Trust is earned through a teacher's continuous demonstration of caring and a non-aggressive approach to correction and instruction. Saying, "Try it this way," is better than "You did this wrong." Asking the student questions such as "What do you think about trying this?" can also empower them as they make artistic choices in a nurturing environment. As the student learns that the teacher is there to assist and improve, not judge and condemn, their motivation to seek out assistance increases. The teacher is invited to help/educate because the student feels safe and accepts the guidance.

A uniqueness of art is that there are numbers of ways to achieve the "correct answer" to a problem. This is sometimes very confusing for students who are looking for the one and only answer. Art teachers have observed students rework and rework a painting because they think the color is not perfect or discard paper after paper because the drawing is not right. This is the perfect opportunity for an art teacher to provide guided practice. If the student is having difficulty drawing, perhaps the teacher might use the eraser on the pencil to "sketch" the problem area. This provides the student with a chance to see how the teacher would draw it, without the teacher actually drawing it. The student may then use the erasure crumbs as "guidelines," or brush them away and start drawing with a new perspective. Some students just need a departure point—they don't know where to start! If a student is having trouble painting within the lines, and this will often make them very unhappy, it might be a good time for the teacher to show the student how he or she paints on a scratch paper. For example: "Let's start by picking out the right size brush for the paint job." "Let's wash this brush to make sure it's clean and then use the paper towel to shape it into a nice point." "Painting is sort of like playing basketball—it's a wrist action—watch my hand as it moves." "If you only have a small space to paint, you don't want to press hard on the paint brush. You want to press lightly and let the paint flow gently. If you do have a big space, then you will want to put more pressure on the brush and let the brush do the work for you." And finally and importantly, "If your hand is shaky, it's OK to use your other hand to brace it and hold it steady. See, like this . . . ."

The Classroom Environment Should Also Be One of Consistency and Predictability

Consistency means fairness and equitable treatment. Arguments and disrespect have no place in a consistent classroom. Consistency in the emotional demeanor of the teacher affects the way the student responds. If the teacher gets drawn into an argument with a student, his or her voice and blood pressure can rise and credibility as a professional will be all but lost. As Dr. Phil would say, "And how is that working for you?" It is important to critically reflect on your practice to see if what you are modeling gets positive results from your students. "Setting an example is not the main means of influencing others; it is the only means" (Albert Einstein). Some children who have experienced trauma struggle with feelings of insecurity, not knowing what to expect from adults or peers. Family life may be unpredictable, making it difficult for students to anticipate what will happen next. Therefore, it is important to be consistent and develop a safe place for students to learn.

Along with consistency is predictability. Being predictable provides the trust and comfort level a student with behavioral disorders needs to appropriately participate in the classroom. If the student knows what to expect, they do not have to act out to see what will happen.

> Knowing students' special needs is absolutely paramount in a teacher's ability to connect, educate, remediate, and develop students. All these must happen to be successful in guiding their individual success.
>
> (Kupper, 2014)

> Teaching children with emotional and behavioral disorders can be extremely challenging. Remember: fostering and rewarding positive behavior has proven to be vastly more effective than attempting to eliminate negative behavior. Punishment and negative consequences tend to lead to power struggles, which only make the problem behaviors worse. It is not easy to remain positive in the face of such emotionally trying behaviors, but don't give up. Your influence could mean a world of difference to these students who are struggling with an incredibly difficult condition.
>
> (Education Corner, 2016)

Working with students who have experienced psychological trauma is not for the faint of heart. In explaining her alternative education classroom setting, Adrienne D. Hunter has said:

> Imagine the student with the worst behavior that you have ever had in your classroom. Then imagine 15 of those same students in one class. Then imagine your most difficult student, and imagine him or her being my best student. Most days, it's like walking on eggshells. You are just waiting to put out the next "behavioral fire." There is never a dull moment. It challenges me to be creative in working with my students and, ultimately, it is so very rewarding when I hear a student say, "No Miss! I can't leave now, I have to finish this!" I know that I am making a difference in their lives, even if only during my class.

The ability to survive teacher "burn-out" (Rosales, 2011) in this truly high-pressured, highly stressful teaching field is not easy. The average "special" teacher "burn-out" rate is 50% in the first five years, and of those who remain, another 50% quit between six to ten years (Ferry, 2012).

All three of the art teachers contributing to this chapter each have more than 35 years' experience teaching students who have experienced psychological trauma.

Teaching Art through Projects

Working with students with behavioral disorders requires teaching appropriate behaviors before or alongside teaching art. If not, inappropriate student behavior will continue to disrupt the teaching environment. Art projects allow for teaching behavior and curriculum simultaneously. As the art teacher in Center School settings, Joseph A. Parsons observed and taught students who had a diverse range of art skills and abilities. Over the years, he has found that the more successful art projects for most of his students are three-dimensional works. There seems to be a level of safety and capability that allows these students to pursue these projects more readily and more proficiently.

He incorporated ideas from many sources and adapted them into art projects for his students. Frequenting many art shows, Parsons looked at what the current or new trends were and designed projects accordingly. He found free materials from wherever he could, and fortunately had colleagues who found resources, materials, and ideas for him as well.

Intentionally allowing for artistic freedom with his art projects permitted each student to be involved by choosing their subject matter within the confines of the assignment. This promoted student "buy in" and lead to project success. He therefore works *with* the students' choices, since student resistance is like pushing a rope.

Art Projects

In this following section, Parsons shares some of his most successful art projects and his perspectives on how and why the students and the projects were successful. Although these projects were designed for students with behavioral disabilities, these art projects could be implemented in any inclusive art program.

Component Constructs

Using craft sticks and a hot glue gun the student constructs 30 triangles or 30 squares and then builds/creates their sculpture with these component constructs.

Crazy Birds

Crazy Birds evolved from an artist whose bird bodies were made from 60-watt light bulbs. Since light bulbs were not a reasonable option, I decided to use plastic bottles instead. I collected Gatorade, coffee creamer bottles, and similar sized plastic bottles for the bird bodies. Wood dowel rods and the other features were made from bits of wood (factory wood remnants that can be purchased for craft projects).

Students each chose a bottle shape for their bird body. Then we had a discussion of what makes a bird unique—that is wings, beak, tail, legs, and feet. The students were told to fabricate their bird parts from the given wood shapes. Wood was glued on to the bird body with a hot glue gun.

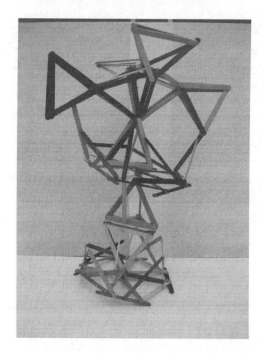

Figure 16.1 "Component Construction"

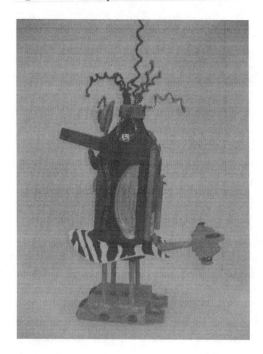

Figure 16.2 "Crazy Bird"

Completed "raw birds" were Gesso-primed and then painted with acrylics. The Crazy Bird could also be decorated using feathers, beads, and fabric. The students' Crazy Birds grew in popularity and public awareness. Student-made Crazy Birds were commissioned for two annual district P3 science award events. Being asked to produce their art work for an organization developed a true feeling of pride, worth, and success within each student, since they were recognized by others for their art work.

Coconut Fish

Coconut Fish bodies are made from the outer, intact husks of coconuts. The "fish" is then spray or hand painted with vibrant fish-like colors. The fins are usually made from trimmed palm fronds, but can be made from other materials. I found that corrugated cardboard worked for the fins and could be shaped and cut easily.

The project begins with a display of several 3D examples, as well as pictures from the Internet of Coconut Fish. The various fish structures and the types of fish fins are discussed. The student begins to formulate and draw out their ideas. Each student chooses their coconut, traces its shape and designs their fish and fins. I use a powered rotary hand tool to cut grooves into the coconut husk to attach the fins. Hot glue is applied to the fins and they are pressed into the husk. The Coconut Fish is Gesso-primed and then painted with acrylic paint. Some students choose to decorate their fish with sequins, beads, pipe cleaners, and whatever they find interesting. An eye screw is attached on the top of the Coconut Fish to hang and move freely. I have had students who were commissioned by adults to create Coconut Fish for them. These "fish" are highly personalized by the student and may convey a special theme or character. The student gains a significant level of accomplishment and realizes that art can be made from anything.

Snyder Tubes

George Snyder is an artist who has developed a unique painting style on canvas to create sculptures. To produce his sculptures, he paints a flat canvas, wraps and adheres the canvas to PVC tubes, and then assembles the tubes to create his sculptures.

I use free, 18" to 36" cardboard tubes from professional printing shops. These tubes have an 11" circumference and have removable plastic ends. The student chooses from three to five tubes of assorted lengths. Students then sketch out the desired positions of their tubes for the sculpture they will build. Each student then selects paper from a standard 36" wide paper roll and cuts 12" wide strips. This allows for a 1" overlap on the tube. The 36" × 12" paper is cut to cover each tube the student selected, and the student then colors the paper as desired using markers, paint, or colored pencils. The paper is glued around the tube. The tubes are assembled with

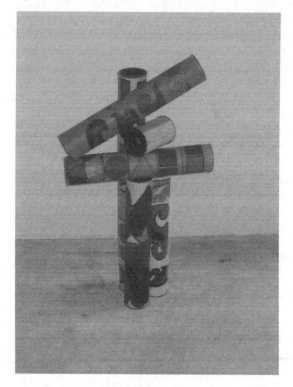

Figure 16.3 "Snyder Tubes"

¼" wood dowel rods, cut 7" long. The dowel rods are hot glued in holes drilled into the tubes at critical attachment points. Each student takes pride in his or her creation as a sculpture imitating Mr. Snyder's style. They also see that they can be successful in creating art at their own artistic level using simple and free materials.

Canvas Painting

I have students make their own stretched canvases from scratch because it improves the quality and teaches them how professionals make their own in custom sizes. I have the student use 1" × 2" pinewood at 8" lengths. The student learns how to measure and cut two 45-degree ends with one cut to save time and wood. The student also learns how to measure and cut canvas and the art of stretching canvas on a frame without wrinkles. They also use saws, miter boxes, sanders, scissors, and staple guns. Canvas sizes vary, with an 18" × 24" canvas as the standard. I have each student use Gesso as the primer and acrylics as the paint of choice. Each student takes great pride in their canvas construction and is eager to draw and paint. This is one of the most requested art projects I have used. There is something inherently motivating about a canvas painting that makes it a highly personalized project. The subject matter is up to the student. The student becomes invested in the project since it is "theirs." Their internal pride is heightened as they share their visual creation, since a painting is made to be hung and viewed by others. Many of my students' paintings have been sold outside of school.

Totem Poles

My respect for Native Americans inspired me to share their history and culture through this art project. From the Internet, I discovered that each figure carved on a totem pole has a significant meaning. The websites identified animals with the characteristics the Native Americans assigned to them. Using that guideline, I have each student design their Personal Totem Pole. I have the student list ten personal characteristics. The student then chooses their top six characteristics and matches these to the animals that Native Americans assigned with the same traits. With a little creativity, the student has the six animals that tell their personal story. The student designs their "character" animals using a variety of materials. The images are glued to a 36" printer's tube in rank order from top to bottom. One tube end is

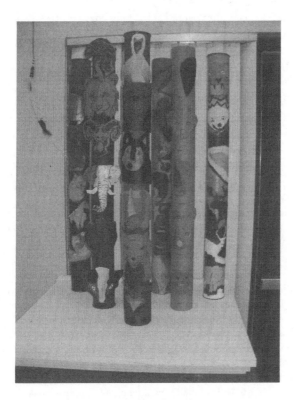

Figure 16.4 "Personal Totem Poles"

sealed and gravel added to weight the tube for vertical stability. Then the other tube end is sealed. The student learns about another culture by making a visually personal self-representation. It is rewarding when you watch a student explain their Personal Totem Pole to another person.

Ten Teaching Tips

1 Know the students—their disabilitie(s), medication(s), artistic abilities, mannerisms, behavioral triggers, likes, and dislikes.
2 Network with your peers to gain ideas about successful teaching strategies.
3 Understand behavioral motivations for misbehavior and the appropriate responses to the misbehavior.
4 Develop and implement behavioral rules and expectations for the classroom.
5 Practice consistency in your behavior which establishes predictability for students.
6 Model and practice positive and appropriate social behaviors.
7 Establish trust and respect for others.
8 Expect and plan for the unexpected. Have alternative plans B, C, and D for artistic projects and student participation.
9 Tomorrow is another day—move from the negative to the positive.
10 Have a life outside of your classroom. You will need the personal escape from the inherent pressure of your job: LAUGH LOUD AND OFTEN.

Note

1 While this chapter focuses on non-traditional settings and Chapter 8 discusses alternative education programs, both present art education practices that can and should be generalized to traditional inclusive schools. Integrating art with academics and problem-solving should be an important part of all school curriculums. See Chapter 13, Integrating Art and Academics: A Collaborative Approach.

Recommended Resources

Corey, G. (2005). *Theory and Practice of Counseling and Psychotherapy* (7th edition). Location: Thomason Brooks/Cole.

DeBruyn, R. L., & Larson, J. L. (2009). *You Can Handle Them All: A Discipline Model for Handling 124 Student Behaviors at School and Home* (2nd edition). Location: The Master Teacher "Develop. Support. Honor."

Dreikuers, R., Grunwald, B. B., & Pepper, F. C. (1998). *Maintaining Sanity in the Classroom: Classroom Management Techniques* (2nd edition). Location: Taylor & Francis.

Gerber, B. L., & Guay, D. M. (Eds.) (2006). *Reaching and Teaching Students with Special Needs through Art.* Reston, VA: National Art Education Association.

References

Education Corner (2016). Emotional and behavioral disorders in the classroom. Retrieved October 12, 2016, from http://www.educationcorner.com/behavioral-disorders-in-the-classroom.html.

Einstein, Albert. Retrieved on October, 2016 from http://quotations.about.com/cs/inspirationquotes/a/Teacher35.htm

Ferry, M. (February 1, 2012). The top 10 challenges of special education teachers. Retrieved October 3, 2016, from http://www.friendshipcircle.org/blog/2012/02/01/the-top-10-challenges-of-special-education-teachers/

Gerber, B. L., & Guay, D. M. (Eds.) (2014). *Reaching and Teaching Students with Special Needs through Art*. Alexandria, VA: National Art Education Association.

Hsiung, B. (November 30, 2015). DSM-5 diagnoses and ICD-9-CM and ICD-10-CM code, Alphabetical Listing. Retrieved October 9, 2016, from http://www.dr-bob.org/tips/dsm5a.html.

Individuals with Disabilities Education Act (1990). Pub.L. 101–476, amended (2004), Pub.L. No. 108–446 (2004), 20 USC sec. 1400 et seq.

Insel, T. (June 6, 2014). Are children overmedicated? Retrieved September 9, 2016, from https://www.nimh.nih.gov/about/director/2014/are-children-overmedicated.shtml.

Jackson, T. L. (September, 2003). Caseload/class size in special education. Retrieved September 9, 2016, from http://nasdse.org/DesktopModules/DNNspot-Store/ProductFiles/10_d2fad293-9994-4b81-b27b-a67b78a10104.pdf

Kramer, M. (2009). The top 10 challenges of special education teachers. Friendshipcircle.org/blog/.

Kupper, L. (2014). Teaching students with emotional disturbances: 8 tips for teachers. National Dissemination Center for Children with Disabilities. nichcy.org.

Mathis, M. (2013). When students need emotional support: Dos and don'ts. *K-12 Teacher Alliance*. Retrieved from www.TeachHUB.com.

Mattison, R. E., Rundberg-Rivera, V., & Michel, C. (August 1, 2014). Psychotropic medication characteristics for special education students with emotional and/or behavioral disorders. *Journal of Child and Adolescent Psychopharmacology, 24(6)*, 347–353. Retrieved August 30, 2016, from https://www.ncbi.nlm.nih.gov/pmc/articles/PMC4137357/#.

National Dissemination Center for Children with Disabilities (2010). Emotional disturbance, disability fact sheet #5. Retrieved from nichcy.org.

Odhayani, A. A., Watson, W. J., & Watson, L. (August, 2013). Behavioral consequences of child abuse. *Canadian Family Physician, 59(8)*, 831–836.

Rosales, J. (2011). Surviving teacher burnout. *NEA Today, Today's News from the National Education Association*. Retrieved from neatoday.org.

U.S. Department of Education, Office of Special Education Programs, Individuals with Disabilities Education Act (2004). Building the legacy: IDEA 2004. Retrieved from www.idea.ed.gov.

U.S. Department of Education (2010). Free Appropriate Public Education for students with disabilities: Requirements under section 504 of The Rehabilitation Act of 1973. Retrieved from http://edpubs.gov.

17 Art and Youth Who Are Incarcerated

Adrienne D. Hunter, Beverley H. Johns, and Donalyn Heise

The year was 1974. It was my first day teaching in a juvenile detention center. In filed my class of adolescent boys, and WOOOSH! slammed the door, and CLICK! went the lock! Suddenly I realized that I was locked in my classroom with no key to get out! How, in all of the interviewing and hiring process, did no one think it was necessary to explain this part of my work environment to me? I was 24 years old, too naive to be afraid, and too idealistic to do anything but get busy teaching art! And teach art I did. But sometimes I wondered, if there ever was a fire, would anyone run up three flights of steps and have the key to let us out?

Adrienne D. Hunter

Incarceration

In 2010, there were over 70,000 juveniles either committed, detained, or in a diversion program, with more than 68% of them placed in a facility because of a court-ordered disposition (Murphy, Beaty, & Minnick, 2013). In 2013, approximately 2.3 million youth under the age of 18 were arrested, with 130,000 placed in either detention or juvenile correction (Underwood, Phillips, von Dresner, & Knight, 2006). Adolescents in these situations are often frowned upon by society. One of the common denominators for these individuals is low self-esteem. As a result, art has been found to be an effective medium in meeting their needs (Murphy, Beaty, & Minnick, 2013).

Meeting the needs of incarcerated juveniles is even more complex, because beginning in the 1990s, there has been an increase in the number of juvenile offenders with mental illnesses, and this increase continues today. Juveniles with mental health issues are overrepresented in the juvenile justice system (Underwood, Phillips, von Dresner, & Knight, 2006). The mental health needs of youth in the juvenile justice system are at least twice as high as in the general population of youth (Cocozza & Skowyra, 2000), while the needs of females in the system have been overlooked or minimized; they have higher rates of mood disorders, sexual abuse, and physical abuse (Underwood, Phillips, von Dresner, & Knight, 2006).

Over the last 60 years, the understanding of the relationship between delinquency and trauma has evolved: It is now known that exposure to acute and chronic danger shapes a child's personality structure, behavior, and beliefs. Most offenders have been exposed to trauma and that trauma exposure is linked to criminal behavior. Many juvenile offenders have been exposed to numerous traumatic events, leading to the development of post-traumatic stress disorder (PTSD). Hypervigilance and arousal may lead to aggressive patterns. Protective factors that assist against the development of PTSD are a well-developed sense of self and family and community support (McMackin, Leisen, Sattler, Krinsley, & Riggs, 2002).

Strength-based approaches have been longstanding in the juvenile justice system, dating back to the late 1800s. However, they have not been practiced consistently (Oesterreich & Flores, 2009). There are not many art programs for incarcerated juveniles, but those that do exist indicate decreased recidivism and reduced behavior problems as well as an increase in positive social and personal identifiers (Miner-Romanoff, 2016).

Trauma treatment groups with incarcerated juvenile offenders conducted by McMackin and colleagues focused on the use of cognitive-behavioral and expressive arts techniques. When group participants were able to share their trauma experiences, both directly and symbolically, they came to recognize the relationships between their trauma and their criminal acting out (McMackin et al., 2002). Visual arts was seen in this study as a strength-based practice that allowed young men who were incarcerated to be engaged in connection, community, contribution, concentration, and completion.

A qualitative case study known as "The Artist Inside Program" was conducted over two years in a juvenile correctional facility. The arts projects were not viewed as one ending and another beginning but rather an opportunity to build upon those that had gone before. The program recognized that everyone has artistic abilities that can lead to imagination, visualization, and creation. The youth were exposed to a variety of art media and techniques. Each class was designed around a particular medium (Oesterreich & Flores, 2009).

Another project is known as "The Emanuel Project." The project was named after Emanuel Martinez, who as a youth drew with matchsticks in his cell during his incarceration for over a year. Martinez now goes into facilities and paints "murals of hope" with juveniles who are incarcerated. The juveniles paint 80% of the mural on their own, and teachers are also provided training. Some students are given art supplies to use in their classrooms to complement their academic curriculum. The project increases students' self-esteem. As of 2013, 25 murals of hope have been painted in eight states. It was found that there was an increase in student self-esteem as measured by before and after surveys (Murphy, Beaty, & Minnick, 2013).

"Voices from Inside" was a partnership between Franklin University and the Ohio Department of Youth Services that sponsored three exhibits. The resulting research and interviews that accompanied this project showed support for art classes for incarcerated youth and the public display of their art. The art from the exhibits was donated to a charity, chosen by the youth, that enhances social bonds and provides the community with a means to develop new knowledge and more positive attitudes about youth who are incarcerated (Miller-Romanoff, 2016).

Personal reports from teachers who work in prisons convey their optimism about the potential for changing their students; this differs from the perceptions of many members of the public who support policies that focus on punishing rather than rehabilitating those who have committed crimes. The teachers see their students not as criminals but as students and focus on educating them and improving the quality of their lives (Michals & Kessler, 2015).

Teaching Art to Students Who Are Incarcerated

In many ways, teaching art to students who are incarcerated is different from teaching art in public education. For safety reasons, the art teacher must be aware of potential danger to the student, other students, and staff. Social, emotional, and behavioral issues should be considered in designing and implementing appropriate and meaningful curricula. This section provides educators with information on types of detention and programs for youth in the juvenile incarceration system, which we have gleaned from years of teaching, followed by sample instructional ideas and teaching tips.

All youth are entitled under federal law to a Free and Appropriate Public Education (FAPE), with some form of education, either classes or tutoring. The 2004 federal Individuals with Disabilities Education Act (IDEA), requires that juveniles in correctional facilities receive special education.

Juvenile law is different from adult law; that distinction is made known here, not to discuss the law, but to create an awareness of the fact. Juveniles are determined to be "delinquent" rather than found guilty and do not serve a "term" but are re-evaluated every six months, with the age of 18 as the final end of incarceration. These six-month reviews are usually held via video conferencing: A youth may come to art class extremely angry because he or she wanted to talk to the hearing officer in person, not on a TV, and was not allowed to say all that he or she wanted; the youth may think their lawyer does not know what was important, is lazy, and does not care; or perhaps an over-due review has not yet been scheduled.

There are various forms of juvenile incarceration. In the pre-adjudication process, the youth might be detained in a juvenile detention center, but depending on the alleged offenses, is more likely to be released into society with or without a tracking device. This means that teachers in public schools may have a youth, with or without a tracking device, in the class and not be aware of this student's legal issues. If the juvenile is retained in a detention center, it should be noted that a juvenile detention center is just that—a place to detain or hold youth until adjudicated, that is, a court has determined their delinquency.

If a youth has been adjudicated and found delinquent, then again, depending on the charges, they will most likely be put on probation; however, those with more serious situations are placed in a correctional program such as an alternative education program, a court-mandated after-school program, a minimum-security program, or a maximum-security program. It is not uncommon for a youth to wait for an opening in a placement, during which time he or she will usually remain in the detention center and continue to attend school there. These court-mandated programs are known by a variety of names such as youth development programs, youth training centers, and juvenile correction facilities.

Sometimes a youthful offender will be charged as an adult, in which case, he or she will be placed in a juvenile section of an adult jail, if there is one, or remain in the detention center until the court hearing. Again, all youth in this situation are still entitled under FAPE to some form of education, either classes or tutoring. These adolescents have not yet been convicted of a crime; however, if they are found guilty, they will be sent to an adult prison. While an adult prisoner is entitled to an education until the age of 18, this is usually part of a General Education Degree (GED) program, which may or may not offer art classes as part of the school program.

Detention Centers

While these facilities may not provide a behaviour-management program *per se*, they do have strict rules and regulations, which in turn provide a degree of behavior management. Students are given credit both for the work completed and the days in class toward their attendance requirements in their home schools.

A detention center education is a very transient and disrupted learning environment. New students come in every day and leave every day. Additionally, students may be called out of class to speak with their advocates, lawyers, caseworkers, or probation officers. This transiency and class interruption can cause challenges for the art teacher. A teacher will not have the continuity of the same group of students in class each time, so teaching styles should accommodate the lack of continuity. Individualized lesson plans work well in this environment. They allow the students to work at their own pace. Another advantage of the individualized lesson plan is that the students cannot compare their progress with that of other students. An example of the importance of this strategy might be a lesson for a 16-year-old student reading on a third-grade level because he or she has educational gaps due to traumatic events, such as homelessness, moving from school to school, and chronic truancy.

Because of the transient nature of the attendance, there will be a higher number of projects that will never be completed. This equates to a large hit in a supply budget; therefore, careful planning of materials needed for projects and a recycling plan are important. Every institution has its own rules regarding school policies and materials. A teacher must be aware of these rules. It challenges the art teacher's creativity to find materials to substitute for forbidden art materials. Adaptations and modifications can be made without sacrificing expectations for student achievement.

Most students absolutely do NOT like to finish other students' art work. Some teachers have found that if they ask a student how long they think they will be in the detention center (students almost always know the exact date of their court hearing), they can offer the student a project choice that will be more attainable and budget-friendly.

When a student is pulled from class for a meeting with a probation officer, case-manager, advocate, or lawyer, they are often returned back to class. Be prepared for a change in temperament and behavior, especially if the meeting upsets or angers them. Provide the student with a safe area in which to de-escalate, rather than insist that they "get back to work." Sometimes giving the student paper and a pencil and suggesting that they write a letter to their judge (or parents, best friend, whomever) helps them sort out their feelings.

Never ask the student questions about his or her case. Adrienne Hunter shares this experience and then explains what to do instead:

> I was working with a juvenile offender who was pre-adjudicated for a murder charge. The student came into the room very angry, and I asked him what was wrong. He then proceeded to tell me specifics about the murder, how he planned it, and how he wasn't happy with the outcome because, although "the guy died," he didn't feel that the "guy suffered enough." He ended his story by telling me that next time, he would do it differently. While I finally calmed the student down, and got him engaged in making art, I was very disturbed by the conversation. When I later reported the conversation to the school counselor, I was told not to repeat the story, as I could be accused of leading the student to make a confession without his lawyer or parents present, and that could change the outcome of his trial. The counselor also said that there was a possibility this may even have been a manipulation attempt by the student to affect his case. The counselor assured me that the court-appointed psychiatrist would gain this insight from his sessions with the student.
>
> This is not what to do. If a student who is incarcerated begins to offer information about their case, the teacher should immediately insist on a change of topic. This is important, as the student is confessing and the teacher CAN be called to testify against them. A teacher does not have a confidentiality privilege as does a lawyer.

Safety should be the number one priority. The teacher must be constantly mindful of what is going on in the classroom and strive to create a safe haven for all students, as discussed in the following section.

Youth Development Centers (YDC), Youth Training Schools (YTS), and Maximum-Security Facilities

YDC and YTS programs may be minimum-security, which allows some degree of freedom for the students, or maximum-security, which are very structured and very controlled locked facilities. All of these types of programs begin with an in-take process which usually includes a series of assessments of the juvenile. Generally, there are comprehensive screenings including medical, psychological, and educational testing. The goals of these programs are rehabilitation and restitution rather than punishment. Depending on various factors, the commitment is of an indeterminate length, from as little as three months to retention until one's 18th birthday. As with the other types of programs mentioned earlier in this chapter, the students are entitled to a FAPE, and IDEA applies to any student with special needs.

The longer stay of students in a YDC or YTS eliminates some of the art room difficulties discussed in the above detention center section. Working with longer-term students gives the art teacher an opportunity to get to know the students and offer them projects that can be developed into more serious works of art.

There are many similarities in teaching art to students who are incarcerated and students who are in alternative education programs. The first of which is that upon entering the program, the students do not want to be there and do not want to do anything constructive. This brings up two important issues: Safety and motivation. No matter whom you are teaching, safety should always be your most important concern. The importance of safety will be stressed repeatedly throughout this chapter because of the serious implications for teaching art in a maximum-security facility. Students who are facing long sentences for very serious offenses may not feel that they have anything to lose by getting into further trouble. Many students who belong to gangs may feel that they need to exact revenge on other students of a different gang. Some students with psychological problems may not be getting or taking their medications; some students are just plain angry and are determined to act out as extremely as they can.

As an art teacher in a YDC, YTS, or maximum-security setting, you will be addressing safety from many directions, including classroom management, behavior management, the materials you are permitted to use in the classroom, the non-toxic ratings of the materials you order for your classroom, the lessons you develop for your students, the way you present your lessons, and the constant awareness of your surroundings.[1] There will be occasions when dangerous situations may arise from routine classroom activities. One art teacher in a detention setting was asked to remove the student-made masks that were hung on the classroom walls because they could be used as a weapon. The electric pencil sharpener had to be kept in a locked drawer because students sharpened the ends of paintbrushes in the pencil sharpener, and the paintbrushes became weapons. Other art supplies that might ordinarily have been left out for class use had to be scrutinized to determine if they should be limited in use and accountability (such as counting total number in use and being aware of these items at all times) or even not used with certain students.

An art room should be a neutral zone, a safe haven, a place where inmates can just be art students. Sometimes students do not want to think about or deal with their infractions or their legal issues, and do not want to feel the stigma associated with negative labels such as "delinquent" and "criminal." They just want to paint or enjoy the feeling of clay in their hands. They want to learn about artists and envision themselves as capable, creative individuals who are able to master art techniques. Other times, students seem to want to talk about their conflicts. Curriculum starters can help develop positive identity formation without discussing their crimes or trauma. For example, an art teacher had students reflect on one thing they had done that made them proud. "What about you makes you a person admired by someone who is at least five years younger?" she asked. "What do you admire about them? What about them makes you feel worthwhile? What do you think makes them proud?"

Adrienne D. Hunter shares this story:

I was teaching art in a juvenile program in the county jail. Most of my students were involved in gang activities and the art room became a battleground. I had to find a way for these students to work together and re-establish peace in the art room. I began by planning projects that eliminated color, such as using clay, because different gangs have different colors. I appealed to their need to "leave their mark" by then having them work on a mural using colors their gangs would never use. I chose Ancient Egypt as the theme, because I felt that these students had unresolved issues about death and dying and that they could relate to the culture of Ancient Egypt. They had to use the colors that were used by the Ancient Egyptians.

I motivated the students to participate in the mural project, which we named "Road Map for the Spirits," by allowing the students to paint the names of their deceased loved ones in the border of the mural. The catch here is that I only allowed them to write these names using Egyptian hieroglyphics. This eliminated the gang graffiti. Of course, I had to monitor the "names" for curse words and threats. Working together was very difficult at first. The students had difficulty working side by side, banging elbows, reaching across each other, sharing materials. They also had to agree upon the images that they would draw on the mural. Some of the more talented students didn't want the less skilled students to "mess up their work." Soon the more talented students, who now held a level of respect from all because of their "mean art skills" became the "art directors," drawing areas for others to paint or "fixing" up areas that were "butt ugly."

It was like a miracle: for the duration of class, these warring factions of students were able to not only co-exist, but actually enjoy themselves. One student remarked to me that he "couldn't believe he was having so much fun in the art class." He said, "I never could have been friends with these kids before."

Unfortunately when they left my class their real world returned, but at least the art room had become "neutral turf" and a safe haven to enjoy being creative.

(Gerber & Guay, 2014)

This vignette shows how a teacher can change the climate of a classroom by planning art projects that help to establish common ground between warring factions of students. In dealing with unresolved issues of death and dying, but not engaging in counseling these students, Ancient Egypt presented the perfect culture to study. This culture placed great emphasis on death and dying, indeed planning burial sites almost from birth. Ancient Egypt, with its pyramids, sarcophagi, and wall paintings, told the life story of the deceased. Using the colors of Ancient Egypt became not a battle over colors but a tribute to the dead. By substituting an appropriate alphabet for a street alphabet, graffiti was eliminated, an ongoing battle, which also brought the students together in using entirely different symbols. By allowing the students to make this mural as a memorial to their loved ones, the mural became sacred to the students. More than a strong motivation not just to participate, it was an incentive to invest in doing the project beautifully. In the process of creating this masterpiece, the students became more interested in the project than in who was working next to them. The students forgot themselves while they were engaged in painting or drawing, and became engaged in conversations about the work and then about other topics in general. Art brought the students together using artistic expression and creation.

Recognize anger and fear; many students act out their fear through anger. Fear turned into anger was one aspect of the gang members' behavior at the beginning of the Ancient Egypt project. Students must be in a learning mode to learn. If a student is angry and acting out, he or she is not in a learning mode. The teacher must find a way to de-escalate the student's anger and reduce his or her stress before the student can be engaged in an art project. Otherwise, the teacher will be adding to the student's stress and the lesson will be unproductive. It is not uncommon for an upset student, who has worked hard on a project, to sit down to work on that project and "ruin it," whether intentionally or subconsciously.

Providing positive motivation for a student who is uncertain about his future will require a degree of trust. Trust starts with respect, and respect is a two-way street. If you want your students to show you respect, then you must be prepared to model that respect for them. For example, if a student is using bad language, instead of making a big deal out of it, you might calmly and quietly say something like, "I don't talk like that to you, I would appreciate it if you wouldn't talk like that to (or around) me." Sometimes the student will even apologize and admit that they didn't even realize they were cursing. Cursing has become such an integral part of youthful expression that many students aren't even aware of the words they are using.

Never lose sight of the fact that, as art teachers, we are there to teach art, not to be therapists and not to pass judgment.

Motivation can be achieved by finding common ground with students. Think about the students' interests, their needs, their abilities. In choosing projects for your curriculum, think about the best way to get students interested in your objective. Think about how to achieve the chosen goal and have everyone enjoy doing it. The objective is clear to the teacher, but what will make the project achievable, desirable, relevant, successful, and fun.

Just because the available materials are limited does not mean that creativity is restricted. Scott Renk, an art teacher at an alternative education high school in a southeastern state, shares how he created meaningful art instruction with limited supplies:

> The school counselor approached me about providing art coursework for a student who was incarcerated in a maximum-security facility and who would be missing at least a semester of school. The counselor was trying to help the student earn the credits he needed to graduate.
>
> Providing the course work was more difficult than I first perceived as there were restrictions on the materials that could be used, as well as restrictions about computer and Internet usage. Further, the lack of personal interaction, the use of teaching, voice, and physical guidance, had to be reduced to step-by-step written directions that had to be clear, concise, and yet motivate the student to complete the work.
>
> Focusing on the elements and principles of art and design, the lessons as designed would take two to three weeks at a time to complete and require only five pages of paper and a pencil. Such a lesson included a drawing by me illustrating the lesson, written information about the key concepts of the lesson, and boxes in which the student would draw, demonstrating his mastery of the key concepts. One such lesson on "shapes" involved the design of a robot along with a story about what the robot could do in terms of the design of the robot that the student drew. Another lesson taught the formula for drawing a human face: the spatial placement of facial features both male and female. The student then was to draw a male face, a female face, and a zombie face. The lessons also introduced the concept of abstract art. I demonstrated the concept of abstraction with thumbnail sketches of organic compositions versus geometric compositions. The student then demonstrated his mastery of the concept by drawing an organic composition.

Renk's vignette demonstrates a true commitment to doing anything a teacher can to get these students to graduate and learn art, even with extreme barriers placed on them. While designing and implementing these lessons takes extra effort on the part of the teacher, the payoff of having the student earn credits while being incarcerated was invaluable.

Many art teachers find that once their students have accepted and settled into their placement, they will often be a very willing and cooperative population to teach. Some students will eagerly await art class days and will even come to art class with new ideas for projects that they wish to pursue independently. Perhaps it will be gifts that they would like to make, or something they would like to learn, or something they would like to share with the art teacher. Having long-term students, particularly students who will be incarcerated for a number of years, provides the art teacher with an opportunity to really get to know the students and to help them develop their arts skills and art appreciation. Some art teachers believe that this eagerness relieves the students of tedium and boredom of being incarcerated.[2]

As a final reminder, be sure to follow the dictates of the facility. Ignorance is not an excuse, it can be life-threatening. Being incarcerated, your students will have plenty of time to think of ways to get into trouble, and they will think of things that would never come to your mind in a million years. An example of this would be taking a ball bearing out of a file cabinet, fitting it into the hole at the end of a toothbrush, and gently tapping the ball bearing against a safety glass window until the windowpane disintegrates.

As Adrienne Hunter has often said, "When you are working with incarcerated students, you have a captive audience. Take advantage of this! You can become the highlight of their week!"

Ten Teaching Tips

1 Put SAFETY FIRST always! Be constantly aware and mindful of your students and your surroundings.
2 Remember that you are there to teach art, not to be a therapist and not to pass judgment.
3 Never allow your students to discuss their legal cases in class. Change the subject.
4 Be aware of and adhere to the rules of your institution, including school policies and materials allowed in classrooms.
5 Create and cultivate an atmosphere that is a neutral zone, a safe haven, a place where your students can just be art students.
6 Consider creating individualized lesson plans because they work well for students in this environment.
7 If a student is angry, provide them with a safe area in which to de-escalate, rather than to insist that they "get back to work."
8 Motivation is achieved by finding common ground with your students. You know your objective, but what will make the project achievable, desirable, relevant, successful, and fun?
9 Trust starts with respect, and respect is a two-way street. If you want your students to show you respect, then you must be prepared to model that respect for them.
10 Strive to have your art class become the highlight of your students' week.

Notes

1 Chapter 11, Creating a Safe and Supportive Classroom Environment, of this book provides many classroom management suggestions that can be adapted to this classroom environment.
2 For a model art program for youth in a training school, please see Chapter 18, *Where have we come from? Who are we? Where are we going?* A Ceramic Mural for and by Students of the Rhode Island Training School.

References

Cocozza, J., & Skowyra, K. (2000). Youth with mental health disorders in the juvenile justice system: Trends, issues and emerging responses. *Juvenile Justice, 7(1)*, 3–13.

Free and Appropriate Public Education, 34 CFR sec. 300.101 et seq.

Gerber, B. L., & Guay, D. M. (2014). *Reaching and Teaching Students with Special Needs through Art.* Alexandria, VA: National Art Education Association.

Individuals with Disabilities Education Act (1990). Pub.L. 101–476, amended (2004), Pub.L. No. 108–446 (2004), 20 USC sec. 1400 et seq.

McMackin, R., Leisen, M., Sattler, L., Krinsley, K., & Riggs, D. (2002). Preliminary development of trauma-focused treatment groups for incarcerated juvenile offenders. *Journal of Aggression, Maltreatment and Trauma, 6(1)*, 175–199.

Michals, I., & Kessler, S. (2015). Prison teachers and their students: A circle of satisfaction and gain. *The Journal of Correctional Education, 66(3)*, September, 2015, 47–62.

Minor-Romanoff, K. (2016). Voices from inside: The power of art to transform and restore. *The Journal of Correctional Education 67(1)*, 58–74.

Murphy, A., Beaty, J., & Minnick, J. (2013). Improving self-esteem through art for incarcerated youths. *Corrections Today, July/August 2013*, 44–48.

Oesterreich, H., & Flores, S. (2009). Learning to C: Visual arts education as strengths based practice in juvenile correctional facilities. *The Journal of Correctional Education, 60(2)*, 146–162.

Renk, S. (2017). Discussion with Adrienne D. Hunter.

Shippen, M., Houchins, D., Crites, S., Derzis, N., & Patterson, D. (2010). An examination of the basic reading skills of incarcerated males. *Adult Learning, 21(3–4)*, 4–12.

Underwood, L., Phillips, A., von Dresner, K., & Knight, P. (2006). Critical factors in mental health programming for juveniles in corrections facilities. *International Journal of Behavioral and Consultation Therapy, 2(1)*, 108–141.

18 *Where have we come from? Who are we? Where are we going?*

A Ceramic Mural for and by Students of the Rhode Island Training School

Peter J. Geisser

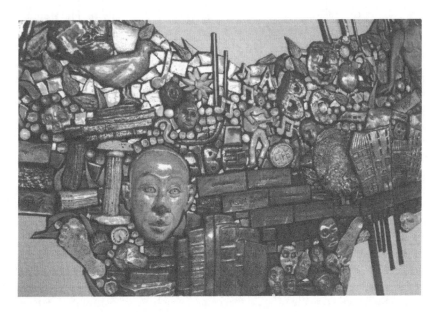

Figure 18.1 "Harry"

"Where have we come from? Who are we? Where are we going?" is the title of Paul Gauguin's masterpiece in the Museum of Fine Arts, Boston. These seemed like the perfect questions to ask the student–inmates at the Rhode Island Training School (RITS). My colleague Mika Seeger and I were asked to create a work of art there, under the 1% for Art Program of the Rhode Island State Council on the Arts (RISCA).

Societies' perceptions of young people, adjudicated and incarcerated, were revealed in the process of developing the commission for this new training school. Some people felt that because this new state facility was a "prison for youth," that it did not qualify for the 1% for Art Program that other state facilities benefited from. Rhode Island, like many states, has a "public policy that a portion of each capital construction appropriation be allocated for the acquisition of works of art to be placed in public places constructed" (Rhode Island P.L. 42-75.2-2). The director of RISCA advocated for the project and for the students in the facility, challenging that it was a school and one whose unique mission made it even more in need of art than other facilities. A compromise awarded one-half of the money required for the planned 80-foot mural.

For two years, Mika and I went into the students' regular art classes with their art teacher, Jim, and worked with clay. Each week, we would pose one of Gauguin's questions: *"Where have we come from? Who are we? Where are we going?"* Mika, a master ceramicist, and I, who had worked with students with special needs for over 30 years, were artists in residence. Neither of us had any fear of these students; we were told later that this was one of the factors that allowed us to work so successfully with them. The population was about 100 students at any given time, and they met in groups no larger than ten at one time. The students were in the Training School for some infraction of the law. These infractions could have varied from stealing to homicide, often involving some kind of violence. While all of these students were agents in crime, many were also victims of crime and physical and/or psychological abuse. Ages varied from 10 to 18, and although those in this facility were all male, we also worked with classes of young women in an adjacent facility.

The very first day we were in the art room, my cell phone went off. I answered and it was my friend Mike, a lawyer. "Yes, I can't talk right now. I'm in jail!" I said with a note of humor. One of the kids said: "You told that guy you was in jail. You are in jail," he affirmed. This student then went on to tell me how they sometimes had visitors who come to do things with them. "One time we had these ladies come in and they wanted to know what we did when we went home on weekends. 'Ha,' I said: 'Lady we are in jail so there aren't no weekends out!'" The many stories of our time with the students were amazing. Often young people who are at-risk, and who have had really tough experiences, will have deep thoughts in their art work, and are extraordinary in their visual storytelling. Although we were not trying to delve into the personal tragedies of our students, stories inevitably emerged in the clay that really answered Gauguin's questions.

"Who are you?" provoked self-portraits, but it also got students talking. Topics emerged as we created a studio atmosphere where such conversations became the background for the sculptural creations that were being made. On a technical note, we were working in stoneware that would be wood-fired along with porcelain background tiles. A unifying feature was hundreds of porcelain "finger prints" which were glazed in turquoise with a small piece of broken car glass placed in each print. The resulting tiles were a bright contrast to the earth-colored glazes of the sculptural pieces that the students made.

One day a young man, Harry, came in with a "don't-bother-me" attitude. I asked Mika if she would make a portrait of Harry. Being a model was not something that he had ever experienced. Mika worked on a life-sized relief for a couple of weeks and the finished product was an amazing likeness of Harry; I will return to Harry later in this chapter.

"Where have we come from?" brought out images of tenements, private homes in suburbia, and prison cell doors. One restriction was that there could be no gang signs. A level of trust was established, as was my expectation that they would not waste their time on gang signs was met. The staff examined all of our creations and eliminated anything that was not appropriate. After two years of workshops, we had only about 12 pieces that had to be eliminated.

One of the questions that people always ask is, "How do you manage a group of students who are incarcerated?" There is no one answer to this given all of the variables of not only students but also environments. The situation we worked in put us into an art program with an experienced teacher who remained in the room with each class. As the visiting artists, we were at once a curiosity and a challenge to the students. Outside the classroom was a security person who could be in the room in a moment if needed. All of this "teacher power," while giving a sense of security, also created a tension of "who's the boss." This is especially true since these students were in the constant presence of, and many times in conflict with, authority.

Authority is one of the pressing features in a juvenile facility, but in reality it is a major factor in working with any group of young people. Art is at the heart of "authority" in that it is about authorship, ownership, and power. One way to "control" a group of students who have trust issues is to give them trust and give them the authority that art-making can have. Rather than being an authoritarian, the artist/teacher can use their art skills to first "wow" the students. Essentially, we are talking about the old skill of redirecting students into a positive direction rather than going down the negative paths that are so often where these young people travel.

Rules? Absolutely, but use rules that make sense. You can't throw clay on the floor, not because it will somehow destroy the floor, but because we can't afford more clay. Sharp tools? Yes these are needed to work fine details in the clay or to cut the clay from a block, but because we are here in this facility we have to count the tools both at the beginning and end of a session. Materials and tools that are somewhat of a challenge to behavior can also be small paths to establishing student–teacher relationships. Here is an opportunity to build trust by asking students to assist with covering the work with plastic or other basic responsibilities. How do you trust someone who you cannot be sure you can trust? Take the chance, and if it does not work on a given day, move on and try another day. Guaranteed, things will go wrong, but that does not mean that you have failed. I have found that when there is a student who is having a "melt-down," being defiant, or just not responding to what is happening, this is not the time to panic or get hyper. Students will follow your lead and, as you focus on the person with the conflict or problem of the day, the other students in the room are taking notes on how you behave. This is again a question of trust; that you are giving your attention to one person, because that person needs the attention. "When I am done with 'Charlie,' I can work with you," can be voiced or even said with your behavior. You are showing that you are there to serve, and at this point "Charlie" is the one in need of the attention. This method assumes a level of trust that the other students are being respected, but respect has to be seen and spoken to the one who needs it most at a given time. Sometimes the group dynamics may require that you ask the larger group to "hang-in-there" while a crisis is resolved. People will ask how you can take that chance, but I believe there is no other choice but to take such a chance and give the students the expectation of respect.

At the beginning of the studio time, limit the amount of time that you spend explaining the lesson. Your students will be eager to begin and if you take too long to get them started, they will not only lose interest, but may take the opportunity to misbehave. The quality of your voice will also be very important to gaining respect. When you are not pleased with something that is happening, rather than raising your voice, as is the normal human response, lower your voice. Speaking softly can force people to listen more closely and will also turn down the volume of the students. Many of the students will have learning problems, and to speak slowly and thoughtfully is essential. It is far better to demonstrate, than to keep talking about how to do a procedure. Many years ago, I had a class of deaf students who were watching a presentation of a visiting artist. After five minutes of a very dull explanation, I asked the artist to go right to the demonstration and show the students what they were to do. One of the students said: "Why didn't you just say that?" Art is a way to "say" things, and we often undervalue that visual power we have.

There was a young man who made the most amazing dragon of clay, and then a couple of weeks later, the same guy came in with a foul attitude. One of the security people gave us a look that we'd do well to ignore him. When everyone else had begun working, I threw a canvas on the floor and started throwing clay on it, right near where this young guy was standing. He looked at me like I had three heads! When I had maybe a four square foot area covered with clay, I stood up and stomped on the clay with one foot. He laughed at me. I laughed back. "What are you doing man?" "I'm being mad." I then asked if he'd like to stomp on the clay too. Without a word, he jumped on it, pounded it with his feet, and then stood back and laughed. Mika came over and we both started marveling at the great foot textures he had made. "Yeah, that's state-issued sneaker prints," he said. Everyone laughed. Then Mika took a tool and cut the area into interlocking shapes so we could fit it into the kiln. Each week, we brought any finished clay work to Mika's studio on the other side of the state where it would be dried, bisque-fired, glazed, and then wood-fired to cone 10, 2300°F. About a month later, we brought this piece of textured clay back to the Training School with a beautiful, high-fire glaze. The students in the class were wowed by what they saw. "That's beautiful." "But it's only his angry feet." "How did you make it so shiny?" "That was ugly before and now it is really nice." The things that are to be learned with a little patience!

Portraits and masks, religious symbols, and hot autos were only a few of the directions the work took. The idea was to create a multi-layered work that you would never get bored looking at. The old folk song, "One man's hands can't tear a building down" gave birth to hundreds of "bricks" which were made in various sizes. The larger bricks had Gauguin's questions written on them, three questions in 28 different voices! In the lobby, prison bars changed from cold vertical lines to become a musical staff with birds as the musical notes.

Not every day we worked with the students was a good day, although most days we left the school inspired. A young man, who had spent weeks making a city of the future, shocked security members and his teachers with the beauty of his relief sculpture. Perhaps the biggest revelation to the staff and faculty was the quality of work that he produced. It is my strong belief that if you give young people a monumental forum, they will respond by making monumental art. One aspect of the transformative aspect of the project was a mural that had been done years before in paint in the school's former building. Because the colors in the mural were now deemed to be gang colors, this strong image that illustrated "Success" had been removed from the old school and was to be trashed. Mika and I traced and recreated the large figures in the painted mural, then turned these figures into sculptural relief. A young family, a basketball player, a soldier, and a rock singer were symbols of success on a wall in the old building, and now these same images became a focal point in the new mural in the new building. By paying homage to the art work that was part of the heritage of the Training School, we paid homage to students of years past. A small clay image of a chapel which had been the center of the facility when it was built in the early twentieth century, and other things that came from the history of the school, communicated to the students that we gave respect to the people who came before us, and that respect was given to these students as they made their mark on this wall.

As mentioned earlier, the funding for the project was half of what was needed to adequately cover the 80-foot hallway and the adjacent lobby area. To complete the project, we made an appeal to the community and were able to raise the other half of the money needed to fund the second part of the mural. VSA of RI, a Rhodes Island organization on arts and disabilities, and several businesses, as well as many faculty and staff of the Training School, contributed financial support.

We were able to add the dramatic conclusion to the mural: "Where are we going?" The spiral that brought the design to completion had the ambiguity of a beginning and an end. There was a countdown on the hallway part of the mural. It began with 24 (as in hours) and moved up the ramp in eight sections, each contributing to the countdown. The last of the numbers became part of a daily calendar "TODAY IS." There is always difficulty in using a stereotype. Things that are said well are often quoted to the point of being meaningless. On the other hand, things become stereotypes because they do articulate a message. It was interesting to hear people comment on the calendar of the mural. Faculty and staff were as fascinated with the emerging images as the students were. This common object of art created a conversation. "Today," many older people would look at this tile and comment, "The first day of the rest of my life!" Curious looks by students would begin conversations on what that phrase and the image could mean.

The installation took place in the summer of 2007. A young colleague, Dan Ryan, helped me install the mural. Our tools had to be carefully guarded, counted, and removed at the end of the work day. An hour to set up and an hour to clean up each day made it wise to work 12-hour days to get the most out of our time. We would begin work at seven in the morning as the students all walked by us on their way to breakfast, then again at lunch, and by dinner we would still be there. "Why you work so much mister?" "They must pay you a lot of money." "This is our stuff and you're making it look good."

There were sections of the mural which became memorials before they were even installed. The reality of our young artists was that some left the facility and went to college, some to work, and some to violence and violent ends. Staff and faculty were astounded at the fact that this work was made by their students. This was a part of the students that they had never seen. The students were also amazed that their work looked so good. Indeed, if there was one goal of the project that was fulfilled, it was the aim of aspiration. When students were creating their answers to Gauguin's questions, they made their very best work. Now that these small testimonials were shining out of the 24- to 30-hour wood-firings, they were brought to a level of fine art. The interplay and juxtaposition of all elements and ideas created a mysterious narrative with visual tension and response on the walls of the Training School.[1]

Perhaps the most profound moment in the art-making process came as I was cleaning our tools at the end of a long day. The door at the end of the hallway opened and all of the students came walking up the ramp past the mural. When they got to the top of the hallway, the security staff member who was leading the line had everyone stop. "Harry!" he said in a loud voice that halted all motion. Pointing to the face on the wall, he asked Harry, who was fourth person in line, "Who is that?" "That is me man!" said Harry. The security member continued, "I know, and everyone here that sees that knows that that is you." Harry stood beaming, as he understood that this image gave him a level of immortality. "Harry, tell me something," asked the staff member. "In ten years, what are people going to say about that face on the wall?" Harry looked perplexed, as the line of young men who had each created pieces of this masterwork were silent and listening. "In ten years, are people going to look at that and say 'Oh, yeah, that's Harry and he

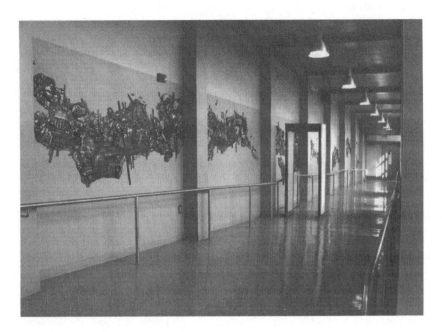

Figure 18.2 "The Hallway"

got out of here and screwed up again and now he's across the street in the big prison.' Or are they going to look at your head and say 'That's Harry. He got his sh#t together and is doing really good now'?"

"Where are we going?" is of course the hardest question of all.

Ten Teaching Tips

1   Listen and learn from the student. Young people who act out are usually doing this for a reason and the teacher should not be the reason. Patience and respect are good attitudes for the teacher to have, especially in the face of a defiant student. The normal response is to respond to negative behavior in a negative way, but if you see such behavior as the result of something in the student's past, then your understanding will hold your own anger in check.

2   Active listening may be used to engage an angry student. Making "angry footprints," as described above, was a good method to engage a student without being judgmental.

(continued)

(continued)

3   When a student is engaged in a work, the best support is to ask about their work. Supportive assistance sometimes means to ask if you can be of help. If the student responds to your request, then provide it, but if the student is content with what he or she is doing, let it be. **Showing such respect will give the student the courage to ask for help when needed.** The final product of art isn't the art object, but the path to it.

4   Walking from student to student in a studio setting and engaging in dialogue about what is happening in each person's work will give each person the authorship that art-making can provide. Remember the word "authority" comes from the word "author," so being an author can also give authority to the maker.

5   Do not teach, but rather set up situations where the student can discover. Discovery is how we all learn best, so consider that you are not a teacher, but one who sets up the students to learn.

6   Power and independence are essential to identity, but in art the real power is in authorship. Steer away from confrontations and be respectful of the student's power to create. The best way to avoid power struggles with a student is to redefine power as respect. He or she who has the most respect has the most power. By modeling humility, the student is more likely to see the power of respect.

7   Too often our lessons are restrictive. Open-ended lessons are lessons that give each student the freedom to be different. This translates into developing unique solutions in assignments that are not right or wrong but are based on the work and choices of the artist making the art.

8   Students with personal needs of food, hygiene, safety, and clothing are not in need of intervention as much as they are in need of a safe homelike environment where they can be comfortable enough to ask a trusted teacher, often the art teacher, for help. Create that environment.

9   Assess the student's needs before intervening. The old joke of the scout who walked the old lady across the street, only to find that she didn't want to go across the street, is a good lesson for teachers and of our need to be of help. If you have created that safe environment, the intervention will become a request for help.

10 Be sure that students know what is expected when they enter the art room. A young elementary teacher I observed ended each lesson by talking about what would happen the next time the class met. When the students entered the room a week later, she began with "What are we doing today?" This simple routine gave a structure that had students thinking about their art class and built an expectation because it allowed the students to think about and be better prepared for the short time they would be in the art room.

Note

1 See other images at: http://www.petergeisser.net/community_projects?lightbox=
image1mf1.

References

Geisser, P. (2007). Documentation of the mural can be retrieved from http://www.
petergeisser.net/community_projects?lightbox=image1mf1.

National Assembly of State Arts Agencies (2017). Retrieved from htttp//www.
nasaa-arts.org.

Rhode Island Public Art. Retrieved from www.arts.ri.gov/public.

Rhode Island Public Art Legislation. P.L. 42–75.2-2.

19 Prison Art

A Recreational Model

*AnneMarie Swanlek, Beverley H. Johns,
and Adrienne D. Hunter*

"On any given day in the United States, approximately 92,000 school age youth are imprisoned" (Young, Phillips, & Nasir, 2010, p. 203). As was discussed in Chapter 17, Art and Youth Who Are Incarcerated, both the Free and Appropriate Public Education and Individuals with Disabilities Education Act (IDEA, 2004) apply to all students who are in correctional facilities, including prisons. This education is generally in the form of General Education Development, General Education Diploma (GED), or Commonwealth Secondary Diploma (CSD). Art is not a required course for these programs and is not even necessarily offered.

Some correctional institutions do offer college courses through partnerships with higher education institutions. "Good Time," a reduction of one's sentence, is sometimes offered to inmates who attend post-secondary classes. For example, inmates who attend classes in the Boston University Prison Education Program can receive two and a half days of sentence reduction for every month they attend 80% of the classes held. Good Time is only applicable to those inmates not serving a mandatory sentence. College courses are paid for by the inmates, with varying prices. According to the program's website: "Rigorous study gives prisoners the intellectual leverage they need to revise their view of themselves and leave prison better equipped to contribute positively to their families and communities" (Boston University, 2017). This website offers supportive information for those interested in post-secondary prison education, faculty, students, and researchers.[1]

The Harvard University Law School's Charles Hamilton Houston Institute for Race and Justice launched the Prison Studies Project (PSP) in 2008. In addition to raising public awareness and generating discussion on justice policy alternatives, PSP offers college courses inside prisons. It is currently compiling the first nationwide directory of higher education programs in prisons in the United States. The National Directory of Prison Education Programs is online, state by state, and continually updated.[2]

Recreational art programs are often offered to inmates, financed either through the prison budget or by grants from outside partnerships.

Arts in Corrections (2017) is a partnership between the California Department of Corrections and Rehabilitation (CDCR) and the California

Arts Council. Programming is provided by professional artists who are all trained to work in correctional settings, and includes disciplines such as writing, poetry, painting, drawing, and sculpture. The program was launched in 2014 and has since reached more than 2,000 inmates at 20 CDCR institutions and is currently offered in all 34 CDCR adult institutions.

The Prison Arts Coalition defines prison arts programming as "art-based workshops, projects, and courses offered in prison. Possible art forms include creative writing, poetry, visual arts, dance, drama, and music. Yoga, meditation, and horticulture may also be considered prison art programs" (2017, p. 1). Their website has identified 48 states with prison programs listed by region and state.[3]

Located in Florida, ArtSpring, Arts for Healing and Social Change has received national recognition for longest ongoing arts-in-corrections programming. It began by teaching arts to incarcerated women. It provides arts-based educational workshops to over 600 inmates and juveniles each year. According to their website, they "maintain a faculty of artists, teaching a variety of disciplines including dance, theatre, music, visual arts, poetry and creative writing, utilizing collaborative expressive arts process based in community arts" (ArtSpring, 2017, p. 2). Their current and past programs include "Inside Out—Expressive Arts Workshops for Incarcerated Women," and "ArtSpring Visual Arts"—weekly programs taught in prisons including 2D and 3D media; contemporary art history; play to encourage reflection; and visual self-expression such as drawings, paintings, murals, thread art, and soap sculptures (ArtSpring, 2017).

Art in Pennsylvania State Correctional Institutions

AnneMarie Swalek: "Time is all inmates have when they are incarcerated."

This section provides insight into the importance of art as learned in a correctional facility but applicable to all art teachers as they work to incorporate the advantages of art in working with individuals who have suffered psychological trauma. As a teacher, a school principal, and currently the Education Administration Manager for the Department of Corrections, I have been witness to the many talented inmate artists who have turned to art as a means to deal with their incarceration.

For many of the youthful offenders, their path had been one routed straight for failure and a life in prison. Once incarcerated, they turn to other means to occupy their life once filled by the culture of gangs, drug and alcohol abuse, or abusive home environments.

Some of the activities inmates are given opportunities to do to fill their time while incarcerated include: work inside the prison, attend academic or vocational classes, participate in mandatory or voluntary groups, attend religious services, go to medical appointments, spend time in recreational activities, and go to meals. Then there is the rest of the day or night . . . and art is one of the avenues that some young inmates turn to when filling time.

Art Does Not Discriminate

One place most people never expect to find beautiful works of art is in a state correctional institution. Some people would like to believe that youth in our country do not commit terrible crimes and are not sentenced as adults. The reality is that youthful offenders do commit these crimes and are sentenced as adults. But as strange a pairing as it may seem, art sometimes becomes the outlet for them to deal with the stress of their incarceration or the crime that they have committed.

I am always amazed when students tell me they never read books, took school seriously, or had any interest in art other than tattoos and graffiti. Now they find themselves reading books and going to school to get their GED or CSD. Even more amazing is how many of them have been able to self-teach or learn from adult inmates how to paint, sculpt, thread, and draw. In the education library, there are many books available to borrow on famous artists, how-to art books, or art magazines. Art and books can serve as tools to keep their minds off the correctional environment they are now sentenced to live in.

Art Promotes Imagination

Since most artists in prison have limited access to art supplies, an inmate must make the best out of their "art tools," such as the ball point pen and generic colored pencils. But prisoners somehow find other creative ways to make drawings and paintings that mesmerize art lovers and people all around the world. Artistic inmates adopt the culture of prison life and select art as a way of expressing their anguish and loneliness.

When I started as a new teacher at a state prison that was originally designed to house youth 21 years and younger, I was first introduced to "panos" art. The word panos (Spanish for cloth or handkerchief) has come to mean the art form itself, a ballpoint pen or colored pencil drawing on a handkerchief. It customarily takes a prisoner weeks to complete one. Just imagine using a ballpoint pen to carefully shade a cloth handkerchief with the delicate stroke of a pen. My students would show me colorful handkerchiefs with Disney characters, flowers, hearts, religious symbols, or a drawing of the person to whom they were sending it. They would show me the picture of their mother and the resemblance they drew on the handkerchief was amazing. They would then mail them out to their family or a girlfriend. This was especially popular around Christmas and Valentine's and Mother's Day. Scholars have yet to determine the origin of panos art, but some believe that it emerged in the 1940s among Chicano prisoners in the southwestern United States who drew on their handkerchiefs or torn bed sheets.

When I became the principal at another state prison, the teachers had a holiday door decorating contest every December. My door was bare, so one student gave me a panos to hang, with a jolly Santa Claus holding a bag overflowing with gifts, while a little girl was leaning over and kissing him

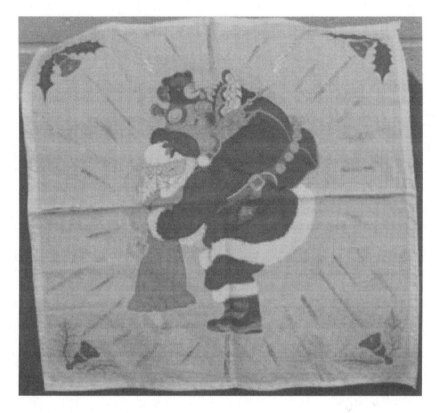

Figure 19.1 "Santa Claus *Panos*"

on the cheek. It was done in colored pencil, and I asked the student how he was able to get such vivid colors. He told me about a technique he had learned in prison to get maximum color out of the colored pencils sold in the prison commissary. He had learned to add just a dab of baby oil or petroleum jelly, allowing the pigment to attach to any surface as easily as any quality colored pencil. I still have that handkerchief and hang it on my office door every December.

Art Can Unify

At one prison where I worked as a school principal, there were both youthful and adult inmates. The Program Service Building where the education area is located is near the center of the prison. It also holds the chapel, library, barber shop, and gym. The only things on the walls were signs and posters for rules and policy procedures, mission statements, and schedules. The Activities Department asked if anyone was interested in having murals painted on the walls. I immediately emailed back, yes, for the barber shop, the hallways by the library, and an academic/vocational classroom.

Inmates are given the opportunity to work for a small wage so they can pay for commissary supplies, medical appointments, photo-copying, postage, and toiletry items. One of the more popular areas to work is in the Activities Department. There they can assist with indoor and outside recreational activities. They also assist with photographing, videotaping of inmate activities, or painting murals. The inmates or staff can suggest ideas for the type of art work or designs or words for the murals, but the administrative staff has the final say in what is permitted.

The barber shop was first. Along the walls is now a timeline of the history of barbering. It starts with a drawing of barbering services being performed on Egyptian nobility with crude instruments. Barber-surgeons of the Middle Ages are depicted not only shaving, cutting hair, and hair-dressing; they also are shown dressing wounds and performing surgical operations. Next is a scene showing how the barber pole evolved from the practice of blood-letting. Clippers, lathers, barber chairs, barber smocks are all part of the mural which wraps around the room.

I came to work one day to see a busy hub of activity across from the library where the walls were being washed and painted white. A few days later, there was a group of inmates with an overhead projector, a sketchbook of drawings, and a box of pencils, paints, and brushes. They were busy sketching or tracing large letters on the wall, which was about 30 feet long and 9 feet tall. Each day brought the art work and designs to life. I would stop to admire the work in progress, ask a question or two, and then move on to my office.

The inmates painted and drew for about three weeks, young and old, from different cultures, races, and neighborhoods . . . united together as artists in which they designed selected areas of interest that impacted their lives in the prison environment.

Let me describe the finished project. There are three large books titled "Parenting from the Inside Out," "The Wizard of Oz," and "Black's Law

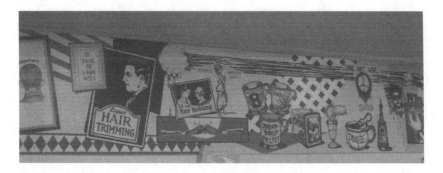

Figure 19.2 "Barber Shop Mural"

Dictionary." Then there is an open book with a large black and red dragon starting to fly out of it. After the dragon is a black hand holding up a magnifying glass toward more open books with beautiful art work. Depicted are: Botanical Science with flowers and birds as an illustration; Paleontology with various dinosaurs; The Arts with Pablo Picasso's *Weeping Woman* (1937); followed by Music, Kurt Cobain. This is followed by a large world globe and two more open books: Ancient History with a painting of the "Library at Alexandria," and a book on African History. Next is the rendition of the Blind Lady Justice complete with scales and a sword.

This is followed by the United States Constitution with the following rights noted (a little ironic inmate humor): #1 Freedom of Religion, Press, and Expression, #4 Search and Seizure, #5 Trial and Punishment, #8 Cruel and Unusual Punishment, and #14 Citizen Rights. Then red ink lines and scribbles lead to a white hand holding an ink pen, followed by a drawing of "The Thinker," a close likeness to the original sculpture by Auguste Rodin.

On the bottom of the wall is a James Allen quote running the entire length of the wall, in block letters, weaving through the mural: "Mind is the Master Power that molds and makes, and Man is Mind, and ever more he takes the Tool of Thought, and shaping what he wills, brings forth a thousand joys, a thousand ills—He thinks in secret and it comes to pass; Environment is but his looking-glass" (James Allen, 1902, p. 1).

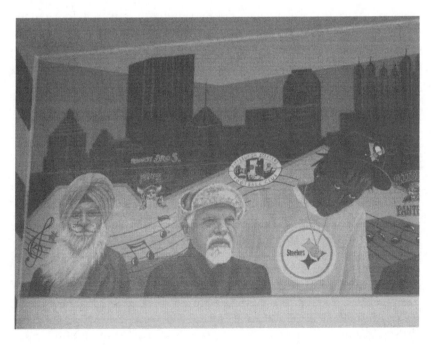

Figure 19.3 "Pittsburgh Proud"

Inmates and staff all can enjoy the colorful, realist renditions of the art work they had selected, the books that inspired them, the tools they needed to defend their rights, and just the enjoyment of art.

In the education hallway, powerful educational words are painted: "Knowledge," "Never Quit," and "Think." Black and white silhouettes of students in graduation caps and gowns, a young man leaning against a stack of books taking a nap, the light bulb going off when an older man grasps a complicated math concept are also painted on this wall. Then there is my personal favorite, which they surprised me with: the word "Principal" (which is often spelled Principle when students send me requests slips) was painted outside of my office with a yellow background in a black frame . . . they knew that I am an avid Pittsburgh Steeler fan.

Art Can Reform

A Therapeutic Community (TC) is an intensive treatment modality, self-contained and semi-autonomous, with shared responsibilities by staff and inmates. This program was developed to treat inmates who meet the diagnostic criteria for dependency on alcohol and other drugs. TC participation provides an opportunity to focus on learning and behavior changes on a 24-hour-a-day basis. In a TC, cognitive behavioral therapy (CBT) concepts are not just taught in group sessions, but are carried through in individual counseling sessions, in regular conversational contacts, in other group activities, in homework assignments, and in learning experiences. Inmates are expected to demonstrate, in all daily activities, what they are learning in the program through observable attitude and behavior changes. There are three phases to the TC. Therapy groups are to run on the CBT 30/30/30 model of providing 30 minutes of homework/journal review followed by 30 minutes of new topic presentation. The remaining 30 minutes is to be used for in-class assignments, role playing, and process sessions. A TC is comparable to inpatient treatment in the community. The standard duration of a general population TC is six months (Pennsylvania Department of Corrections, Standardized Programming).

Why do I mention the TC in an art chapter? Amazingly, therapeutic art is encouraged as part of this community, to deal with issues such as the inmates' alcohol and drug abuse history that may have led them to a path of crime.

Before me I have five handmade invitations to attend a TC graduation ceremony. Each invitation is unique, hand drawn art in colored pencil. I always thought it was a shame to throw them away after the graduation, so I have placed them in the subsections of my window in the hallway. There, anyone walking in the hallway can see the art work of those invitations.

The first invitation I receive is titled "The Recovery Games" and has three parachutes with a small box tethered below; inside each of the parachutes is a drawing showing what the box is carrying—various TC Tools. Then the invitation itself has bright yellow clouds on the inside.

The second invitation is titled "Living Clean . . . The Journey Continues." This handmade card has a road that divides into two paths, with a sign in the split of the road. One side says "Relapse" the other says "Recovery."

The next one I receive has a black tire with a spinning green rim. Inside some abstract shading highlights the names of those who are graduating.

Then there is the Sargent's Stripe with a fancy scroll wrapped around the top and bottom of the arrow, spelling out Therapeutic Community, with a pair of military dog tags on the bottom. On the corner is Victorian-style edging that continues on the inside.

The last and most recent invitation is a tombstone next to a sign on two boards attached to wooden posts. The names of this graduation class and the dates they attended are placed inside this rustic frame. A star, a cloud, and a grassy hill complete the image, with multi-colored shading announcing the details of the graduation.

These young and older inmates who were unwilling to seek help are now, through their incarceration, getting the help they need to deal with their drug and alcohol issues. The goal is to have them return to their communities and families with the tools needed to not relapse into substance abuse. To me, the art drawn on their invitations displays their internal reflections that helped them address the reasons they turned to alcohol and drugs and then to recovery. Current members and former graduates of the TC are happy to know that I have kept their invitations. Or, as one inmate told me, "Someone here cares that we are trying to heal."

Art Teaches Responsibility

The Activities Department at one prison where I worked offers a planned schedule of recreational and therapeutic activities, including art classes, to the inmates. The program serves artists of all media and skill levels. If an inmate is involved with something positive, their mind is positively occupied. A mind that is not positively occupied may lead to issues and destructive behavior. The following is what is sent to interested inmates who wish to participate in an art program or class.

Inmate Orientation for Art Classes.
State Correctional Institution (SCI) Somerset offers three structured art classes. These classes are designed for the beginner, intermediate and advanced artists. All the classes are led by inmate mentors and supervised by Activities Staff. Please watch for announcements for upcoming classes. Note: Inmate artists that wish to practice artistry in their cell must obtain an art permit to do so. Also, it is required that you have an art permit to purchase art supplies from an outside vendor. You are required to have an art permit to possess or to purchase art supplies. The permit must be renewed yearly and it is your responsibility to request a renewal. Art permits are free and may be obtained by submitting a request to the Activities Department.

Guidelines for any Art Contest Entry Presentation: The privilege of participating in an art contest includes acting responsibly in the presentation of that art. Responsible presentation takes into account the diverse make up of inmates and staff. Art presentation should also reflect consistency with the treatment goals and objectives found in SCI Somerset's treatment programming. In order to insure the presentation of art work is in good taste, not unnecessarily offensive, and consistent with treatment programming offered by the DOC; the following guidelines are established for art work being presented publicly in contests.

1   Art work depicting violence and/or bloodshed is prohibited.
2   Art work glorifying or encouraging violent acts or the results of violent acts (i.e. cut throats or body parts, dismemberment of body parts, etc.), whether towards males or females, is prohibited.
3   Art work consisting of the erotic display of male or female personal parts or the implied impression of those parts is prohibited.
4   Art work depicting sexual exploitation or violence is prohibited.
5   Art work depicting a sexual act is prohibited.
6   Art work promoting or encouraging racial, religious, or other forms of discrimination is prohibited.

These standards are designed for art contests and are not intended to replace other DOC policies regarding the use and possession of pornography or publications. All art work will be reviewed by members of the Activities Department and other staff as needed prior to submission to any contest.

Example of an announcement for an art contest:

In observance of National Hispanic Month, the 3rd quarter art contest is themed "Energizing our Nation's Diversity." There is a limit of two pieces of art work per inmate. Entries must be submitted by Friday, October 9th, 2015. Art work must be in good taste and abide by the contest rules (airing on channel 11). Art work entries will be voted on by Department of Corrections (DOC) staff and chapel volunteers in the Officer Dining Hall.

Example of an announcement of an art class:

2014 Watercolor Paint/Watercolor Pencil Class. Anyone wishing to enroll in this art class should submit an inmate request to the Activities Department. This class is committed to watercolor paint and watercolor pencil medium only. Classes will be held Tuesday through Friday from 0900-1045. The deadline for submission is Monday, June 30, 2014.

Art Helps as Psychological Escape, but Not Actual Escape

I have worked at a state prison with many terminally ill inmates where one of the education classrooms was used to hold the art classes. More and more prisons are creating time for artistic expression to help prisoners deal with their individual situations. The funding and grants that once permitted talented artists from the community or colleges to teach actual classes are often no longer available, so activities departments attempt to fill the gap by holding art classes and contests to allow inmates an avenue from which to benefit. It should not be surprising that prisoners are interested in art. Many great artists have spent time in prison.

> "We artists are indestructible; even in a prison, or in a concentration camp, I would be almighty in my own world of art, even if I had to paint my pictures with my wet tongue on the dusty floor of my cell"— Pablo Picasso.
>
> (Frank, 2014, p. 1).

Prison violence is universal; despite the most stringent measures, weapons are still found, often in the most unlikely places, and made from even more non-weapon-type materials. This includes art materials such as colored pencils, paint brushes, and pens. So while corrections facilities want to encourage art as a therapeutic means of escape, they also need to be careful that the artists' tools are not used as a means of actual escape or weaponry.

While encouraging the development of a creative arts program, correctional facilities also must ensure the security of art supplies so they are not used as weapons that could harm staff or other inmates. All art supplies and materials have to be inventoried so that inmates can work on their art work in their cells.

While we need to be careful that inmates do not use art tools as a method of creating any type of security risk, most inmates use art work to escape the long hours of time served. As noted earlier, I was surprised by how much attention to detail was present in many of the works of the prisoners serving time and doing time. There is a tremendous talent hidden behind prison bars and while, for some, their time is wasted or made worse as they learn more criminal ways, there are many who use the time to learn and grow.

An activities department had an art contest and displayed the art on a digital picture frame in the Officer Dining Hall. Staff were given the opportunity to vote on their favorite picture. It was hard to pick just one picture, as one image flowed to the next picture. A dog hunting a pheasant, a castle in medieval times, an elderly black couple sitting on a park bench . . . then the one I finally selected as my favorite was a watercolor of a small child playing marbles in the dirt.

Art Lets Us Develop Hidden Talents

"The deputy for centralized services wants you to stop by her office this afternoon," the school principal told me. I was a new teacher at State Correctional Institution Pine Grove, teaching incarcerated juveniles adjudicated to an adult prison due to the serious nature of the crimes they had committed. Other than the deputy occasionally walking around the housing unit where my classroom was located, we had minimal contact. I taught my class that afternoon, called her secretary to set up a meeting, and then proceeded down the walk outside to the deputy's office.

"I hear you like to plant flowers," she told me. This began the decision and then the vision she had to make the prison just a bit more colorful. She said, "I'm starting a beautification project; we're going to plant flowers and I want you to be on the committee." I wracked my brains to determine who told her that I liked to plant flowers, and then recalled a lunchroom conversation in the dining hall in which I told the activities manager that I had planted 200 flower bulbs around the fence of my house. As the saying goes at work, "There are no secrets in jail."

Before the beautification project committee could meet, I knew I had to get inmates involved in helping to design flower plots around the housing units, planting the flowers, and taking care of them. The first thing I did was post a flyer on the inmates' TV channel, asking for anyone interested in being on a beautification project to send me an inmate request. I didn't get a big response, and as one of my students told me, "No grown man wants to be on something that has the word beautification in it." So I started recruiting from my students and tutors, I stopped and talked to the inmates on the lawn/ground crews, and soon had enough names to hold my first orientation. We discussed what the deputy wanted to have done and soon the excitement spread. I started to get both young and older inmates requesting to be on the beautification project.

We had numerous meetings over the winter, and we received permission to take the 15 inmates who continued to be willing participants on a walk around the housing units. Two inmates drew up designs of the plots and where we needed to clear ground to plant flowers. Then at our next committee meeting, I showed the staff the designs, what we anticipated the cost to be, and requested that the institution's maintenance department clear some of the ground. Rules were determined, such as no shrubs or trees where there would be wood that could be made into a weapon.

So the work began, with each housing unit allotted a small diamond plot at the entrance near the walkway inside. In the larger area between the buildings was a larger circle plot. Then I had a wonderful time purchasing flowers at a local store, making sure to get a lot of perennials that would come up every year and some of the more colorful annuals. We made arrangements with security for when we would bring the flowers in, and which dates we would plant them. Maintenance staff assisted by lending me some hand shovels, which we had to account for and return each day. The inmates were placed on the "beautification call-out" that gave them permission to be released from their cells under my supervision, and away we went.

They took such pride in laying out the flowers in patterns as I explained the difference between annuals and perennials. I taught them which flowers needed a lot of sun and which ones needed more shade. In total, we planted six flower plots, with all the designing and planting being done by the inmates on what we called the "Flower Committee" per their request. Then they were assigned who was responsible for watering the plants and who was to be weeding. They would get a large 30-gallon garbage can, fill it with water in the housing unit, then use small plastic watering cans each unit was given. They coordinated with the officers on the housing unit at what times they would be permitted to water and when they could weed. The inmate enthusiasm and dedication to the project has served as its roots.

This mixed group of inmates had many talents to offer. One used to help his father with a landscaping business. Another used to help his mother plant and take care of the flowers in her garden. Some of the inmates were originally from an inner city where plants were never any part of their lives, but they made up for that by their willingness to learn. Others had an artistic eye for color and design. So we had tulips, iris, ornamental grasses, daylilies, marigolds, mums, pansies, and Shasta daisies.

The inmates came and went. "I'm getting paroled next week; can you find someone else to water the plants on B-Unit." Next, "The officers wouldn't let me off the unit to water the plants last night." What was most rewarding was, as one inmate left the committee, there was always someone willing to take his place, and we all looked forward to the next time we needed to plant and add or divide the flowers.

The beautification project, or flower project (as the inmates liked to call it), was a chance for some of these inmates to provide a little beauty and life during their incarceration for all to enjoy. It was designed and maintained by a dedicated group of inmates from behind security fences. These inmates were able to see the physical results of their hard work. They had a vested interest in those flowers, and it provided them with another artistic avenue to develop their hidden talents.

Art Can Speak Many Languages

As noted earlier, institutions are very multi-cultural and have many unique programs to help inmates be successful upon release. So I have always decorated my offices to reflect my love of art and to also acknowledge their diversity, struggles, and what they miss about "home." I am resourceful, too, as we are limited as to what we can bring inside our places of work. One of my offices was in a prison which had an arts and craft shop, so I was able to find wood picture frames made by inmates in a storage closet. I asked the maintenance department to hang them on my walls; we are not permitted any glass, so they were just open frames on cement walls. A student walking down the hall could see the five most recent TC invitations in the subpanels of my window. Then in one frame I rotated old calendar pictures (the most recent being a cat coming out of a pumpkin among fall leaves).

A Native American dream-catcher was hanging from a ceiling corner. A larger frame had my young grandson's watercolor of a tree which he drew at art camp. A small seashell sat on my computer modem alongside a small ceramic owl (an animal figurine that you used to get for free when you purchased a box of tea bags). A small American flag was on my bulletin board behind my desk (they were given out after the tragic 9/11 incidents). And there were two art pieces hanging in my office that seemed to startle students, or have them puzzled: my pair of African tribal masks.

I had inherited a large cushy maroon-colored chair with brass buttons on the arms and a large backrest, plus a typical blue cloth-covered office chair. A small round table was there between the chairs. My pencil/pen holder sat on my desk, with the pen wrapped in white thread with "Ms. Flick is the best teacher" in red thread. The students would sit in the maroon chair, and that surprised them as it is very comfortable, then when they looked up behind my desk they saw the two authentic African tribal masks hanging on the wall. I worked at State Correctional Institution Cresson which closed in 2012. After helping to empty the education building, sending books and other items to other institutions, I found the masks sitting on a library shelf. The chapel director told me that they used to hang on the library walls. He had made a pilgrimage to Africa, purchased them there, and donated them to the library. Since no one else had taken them, I brought them both with me to the prison I was transferring to. The students asked in wonder or disbelief, "What are those? Are those African masks?"

According to the National Museum of Ghana, "In most traditional African cultures, the person who wears a ritual mask conceptually loses his or her human identity and turns into the spirit represented by the mask itself" (National Museum of Ghana, 2017, p. 1). I took them with me as I appreciated the art work and the details carved into them. The other art work in my office got its fair share of attention, and even staff had commented about some of the art work I display. So why did I make sure to have a variety of art work in my school principal office? I like to reference a saying by Joseph Addison, one of my favorite quotes: "What sculpture is to a block of marble, education is to a human soul" (1711).

Art Helps Heal

At State Correctional Institution Pine Grove, the inmates approached me to see if I could get permission to start an inmate newsletter. We got through all the red tape and finally received permission to publish. There were articles that they felt would help make a difference in their lives. "Staff that Makes a Difference" was one article in which they would select and interview a staff member. "Educational Merits" would note those who had received a Commonwealth Diploma or passed their GED test. Original articles were written about personal experiences, relating inspiring stories on how to get out and stay out of prison, and providing tips about how to deal with the stress of incarceration. Original poetry and art work were always popular. There were a lot of black-and-white drawings of animals, loved ones, or funny cartoons.

My first job as a school principal was at State Correctional Institution Cresson. As I was making the transition from teacher to principal that first year, I was introduced and asked/told to continue the annual December holiday program. My education staff told me it had started as an in-house education program, for which each class did a skit, sang a song, or provided some kind of entertainment. It quickly grew to be very popular, was moved to the chapel, and opened up to the inmates and staff to attend the program. It evolved into a short holiday play, choral songs, and band selections. When there was grant money, the Activities Department was able to hire musical artists to teach inmates how to sing or play instruments. Then the grant money was eliminated, but the deputy wanted to continue the annual tradition. Saying that it was such a special event, unique to the institution, and that she had never seen anything like it in her career, she and the Activities Department continued to make it happen. So with some big shoes to fill and with no prior experience, I appreciated it when the education staff came to the rescue. One of the teachers who sang professionally in a community chorus agreed to lead the choral group. Another teacher volunteered to find a skit that would be appropriate for the holiday program. Others volunteered to help make theater props that would pass security guidelines, and of course the inmates themselves were eager to sign up and be part of the program. So I would sit in my office or walk around during rehearsals, listening to the singing and acting.

Now my biggest contributions were to organize the big rehearsal in the chapel, get permission to sign out the drums, speakers, keyboards, and other music instruments, and arrange for refreshments (cookies and punch) for afterwards. I coordinated with security to have extra officer coverage for the actual program, got an open all-call for the inmates housed there, meaning anyone could attend, and made sure that the theater props would be approved by security. But as with any theatrical production there were also a number of mishaps: A frantic call from one teacher that security had an issue with inmates using the wrapped fake presents, and another call that the kitchen was not sure that they could have the cookies and punch delivered prior to 1:00 pm. The worst crisis was that one inmate, who was a lead vocal and the only one who could play the keyboard for the songs, violated policy and was sent to the Restricted Housing Unit (RHU).

The singer/keyboard player was able to be released from the RHU days before the program. The cookies would be delivered during the event and set up. The fake presents were approved. The inmates set up the chapel for the skit and choral concert, including all the background props.

One of life's greatest gifts is the fact that life is difficult. The chapel quickly filled up with staff and inmates . . . then the magic began. It really was magic! For that brief hour, you forgot you were inside a prison, that the actors and choral participants were wearing brown uniforms with large white DOC letters on the back, and that the artistic props were very basic due to security restraints.

Those inmates, young and old, from inner city and rural communities, mentally ill and recovering addicts, swayed to the lively Hispanic choir's rendition of "Feliz Navidad"; the staff tapped their feet; and at the end everyone joined in and sang "Jingle Bell Rock." We all forgot where we were: It was joyful, funny, out of tune at times, lively music, and it was that special time of year when there is forgiveness and healing.

In dealing with life's difficulties, we build strength. This strength enables us to be successful, fulfilling our deepest, most meaningful purposes. For the inmates housed there, we were able to truly matter. This was a special magic, unique to that institution that I have never seen at any other prison where I have worked.

Art for Inner Peace

In most prisons, there is a special group of juvenile and adult inmates sentenced to life. When you are sentenced to life in prison, it is easy to give up hope.[4] Part of their search for inner peace can be found through art and being part of the Activities Department mural art crew. While I was a principal, we had an educational audit. When the superintendent of the prison came to my office for the exit interview, he told the auditor the story of the inmates on the mural art crew asking if they could do something for the community. After contacting various civil groups, he was told by the Somerset County Humane Society that they could use something for their walls as they were just bare painted cement.

The inmates were excited, but then came the bad news; due to the budget the institution would not be able to fund this through the Activities Department. The mural art crew later went to the superintendent and said they would like to use their own money to purchase the art supplies needed for the project. At the end of the audit meeting, we stopped by the superintendent's office to see two of the four mural panels they were painting which would be hung in the Humane Society.

I have to be honest here, it is easy to become cynical working in a prison. But when I took the auditor to view these panels . . . well, they were so beautiful . . . I thought of how they used their own money to purchase the art supplies and tears came to my eyes. One was a painting of a chalk board with pictures of drawings on white paper taped to the chalk board. You had to touch it to realize it was not a real chalk board, that it was not real masking tape holding those pictures of animals to the board. The other was more whimsical using the Johnny Depp movie *Alice through the Looking Glass* (2016) as their theme, with all sorts of deserted animals frolicking in the garden, happy to have a home.

As artists, how do we inspire our children and youth to take up the practice of peace? If nothing else, we must remember that art is derived from the freeing up of all boundaries combined with the ability to imagine something new, and the ability to recognize the humanity of others. Who else, therefore, is better suited than the artist to inspire alternatives and alternative ways of thinking?

(Golden, 2013, quoting Children's Peace Theatre)

This passage sums up art in a correctional setting: handkerchiefs, thread-wrapped pen, murals on the walls, African tribal masks, plays, doodling, soap carving, music, landscape gardens, newsletters, paintings, and drawings. Art is a way to deal with time and express oneself in prison; art-making is a natural human impulse and everybody has the potential. So during incarceration, art can become a means to survive, hope, and dream.

Ten Teaching Tips

1 Be aware of and follow all institution regulations regarding teaching art in their facility: FOLLOW ALL INSTITUTIONAL RULES AT ALL TIMES.
2 Remember your role as art teacher. Maintain confidentiality and don't pass judgment.
3 Make your classroom environment a peaceful and SAFE haven for your artist inmates.
4 Seek opportunities to have the inmates work together as a group to foster a sense of community.
5 Introduce art appreciation through multicultural projects.
6 Showcase the inmates' art work to foster success, pride, and personal accomplishment.
7 Encourage your students to participate in art shows, challenges, and/or competitions.
8 Research grant opportunities, in conjunction with your facility, to raise funds for projects not covered by the budget.
9 Research partnerships in conjunction with the facility.
10 Help the students embrace the joy of creating art by being enthusiastic about teaching them art.

Notes

1 Retrieved from: sites.bu.edu/pep/.
2 Retrieved from: www.prisonstudiesproject.org
3 Retrieved from: http://theprisonartscoalition.com/programs/.

4 The United States Supreme Court in *Montgomery v. Louisiana*, 577 U.S. _____ (2016) struck down mandatory life sentences without parole for crimes committed while a juvenile, granting either parole or resentencing hearings. During a hearing, an inmate's characteristics can be considered in order to issue a fair and individualized sentence. While awaiting these hearings, the inmate remains in prison and even after a hearing the juvenile or former juvenile may be resentenced to life in prison. In Pennsylvania, of the 517 juvenile lifers, thus far 70 men and women have been returned to their communities (Melamed, 2017, p. 1).

References

Addison, Joseph (1711). BrainyQuote.*com*. Retrieved July 3, 2017, from https://www.brainyquotes/quotes/quotes/josephaddi121289.html.

Allen, James (1902). *As a Man Thinketh*. The James Allen Free Library. www.james-allen.in1woord.nl, p. 1.

Arts in Corrections. Informational flyer. Retrieved July 4, 2017, from arts.ca.gov.

ArtSpring. Retrieved July 3, 2017, from artspring.org

Boston University Prison Education Program (2017). Retrieved July 4, 2017 from sites.bu.edu/pep/.

Frank, Priscilla (2014). Inspiring HOPE art challenge turns former current and former inmates into artists. Updated October 1, 2014. Retrieved from m.huffingtonpost.com/us/entry5900456.

Free and Appropriate Public Education, 34 CFR sec. 300.101 et seq.

Golden, B. (October 15, 2013), quoting Children's Peace Theatre. Finding inner peace through art. Retrieved from https://www.beverleygolden.com/finding-inner-peace-through-art.

Harvard Law School, Charles Hamilton Houston Institute for Race and Justice (2008). Prisons Studies Project. Retrieved from www.prisonstudiesproject.org

Individuals with Disabilities Education Act (1990). Pub.L. 101–476, amended (2004), Pub.L. No. 108–446 (2004).

Melamed, S. (September 7, 2017). *Pittsburgh Post-Gazette*. Pittsburgh, PA.

National Museum of Ghana (2017). Traditional African masks: Ritual and social meanings, para. 1. Retrieved from http://nationalmuseum.ghana-net.com/traditional-african-masks.

Pennsylvania Department of Corrections. Standardized Programing. Retrieved from http://www.cor.pa.gov/Inmates/Pages/Treatment-Programs.aspx.

Prison Arts Coalition (2017). Retrieved July 4, 2017 from http://theprisonartscoalition.com/programs/.

Prison Studies Program (2017). Retrieved July 4, 2017, from www.prisonstudiesprogram.org.

Young, M., Phillips, R., & Nasir, N. (2010). Schooling in a youth prison. *The Journal of Correctional Education, 61(3)*, 203–222.

Part III

Identifying Future Directions

20 Pre-Service Art Teacher Preparation and Professional Development

Juliann B. Dorff, Lisa Kay, Lynne J. Horoschak, and Donalyn Heise

Meeting the needs of students who have experienced psychological trauma can be challenging for experienced teachers and mental health professionals, and particularly difficult for those in the process of becoming art teachers. This chapter presents four models of pre-service education that can prepare pre-service art teachers for teaching children who have been exposed to trauma.

Model 1: Juliann B. Dorff

> Teaching this week, I found that these students value when they are trusted, for most of the time their actions have been seen as wrong. I found the good in all of my students this week and I could tell they felt good in return.
>
> (Sedar, 2012)

Model 1 of this chapter will review the experience of pre-service educators who teach at area detention centers as part of their field experience class. It will cover their preparation, personal reflections, and curriculum development strategies. In order to meet the needs of children who have experienced trauma, it is important that art teachers are acutely aware of student needs and take the time to consider all possibilities.

Experience is very important. A large Midwestern public university requires a six-week field experience teaching in area juvenile detention centers as part of its art education undergraduate program. Not only does this provide these pre-service educators with the opportunity to practice teaching high school students, it also breaks down their preconceived concepts about youth in the juvenile detention system. The experience has four distinct features: Personal Investigation of the Pre-Service Educator's Personal Teaching Philosophy, Understanding the Needs of the Students, Creation of Appropriate Curriculum, and Teaching and Reflection.

Field Experience at Juvenile Detention Centers

Investigation of the Pre-Service Educator's Personal Teaching Philosophy

> You have to make a commitment based on faith that all human beings have capacities and abilities that are not always visible. Your most fundamental job as a teacher is to find the unlimited potential that you assume every child has. You assume it: They don't have to show it to you.
>
> (Ayers, *How Can a Teacher Help Students Find Their Best Selves*, para. 2, 1998)

On the first day of class, pre-service educators are naturally wary about the teaching experience before them. They are divided into teams of two: In the classroom, they will take turns, with one as the lead teacher while the partner observes. Each team will teach incarcerated youth at an area juvenile detention center.

The process begins with a written exercise that asks the pre-service educators to reflect on a personal experience with a teacher. They are asked to finish the sentence, "I remember my teacher . . . ." This prompt, based on the book of the same name by David Schribman (2001), encourages the pre-service educators to review their educational experiences. They complete the sentence by recalling the first teacher from their K–12 education who comes to mind. The pre-service educators are encouraged to write freely and openly about their memories. Although they are not required to share their responses, those who are willing are asked to share. As the class members read their comments, it becomes clear how powerful one teacher can be in our lives—both positively and negatively. The exercise is a reminder of the power teachers possess.

The pre-service educators need to be acutely aware of the impact they will have on their students and of the impact these past instructors have had on them. Aware that all teachers often fall back to the practices they experienced and "teach the way they were taught," this exercise highlights how each choice the pre-service educators make will be remembered by their students. What memories, positive and/or negative will the pre-service educators' students have if asked to answer this prompt? This is an essential sentiment when approaching teaching practice, as it requires critical examination of each choice made.

After this self-examination, the pre-service educators will investigate the works of several authors/educators, both generally and regarding at-risk youth specifically, to guide their understanding of and approaches to teaching. The educator and activist William Ayers (1998) encourages the pre-service educator to consider each child as a unique and special entity. He reminds them that it is not the student's responsibility to reveal their unlimited potential; rather, it is the educator's job to uncover it.

This daunting task requires instructors to study students and uncover the keys to tapping into this potential.

To help reveal a child's potential future, Akins in her work *Simply Sacred* (2000) addresses the need to continuously respect ourselves, our surroundings, and others in all we do inside and outside of the classroom. This respect fosters a spirit of care. Pre-service educators need to consider how they can prepare themselves for their teaching. What care do they need to take to be the best for their students? A good night's rest? Healthy food? Time to center oneself before the teaching experience? If they are willing to take the time to care for themselves, they can also consider how to care for others.

Respecting one's surroundings is also part of one's attitude toward teaching. Instructors should create an open and inviting room to engage students in learning. The pre-service educators teach in classrooms at the juvenile detention centers. These rooms are designed for typical academic instruction. The pre-service educators are "guests" in these rooms and must be mindful of the needs of the teachers who use these rooms daily. With the space and tables provided, the pre-service educators make choices regarding the room layout, traffic patterns, and available teaching materials, including white boards, projectors, lights, and sinks. They may make changes to facilitate art instruction but must return the room to its original configuration when the lesson is completed.

Akins also encourages a respect for the art-making materials. Showing care for the materials and tools used in the creative process reinforces an attitude of respect. The pre-service educators organize materials so they are safely accessible for students, teach students the proper use and care of materials, and require all students to participate in the clean-up of materials and the classroom. In order to have an attitude of respect and care for their students, the pre-service educators need to recognize that "all [people] constantly change, grow and adjust" (Akins, 2000, p. 101), and they must be ready to listen and watch for the signals of these changes. Akins also believes that students are teachers as well. This concept of shared control for teaching and learning in the classroom runs contrary to some of the negative stories told during the exercise, "I remember my teacher . . . ." but often rings very true in the positive stories. This shared classroom experience can lead to an atmosphere of experimentation and wonder.

Understanding the Needs of the Students

To examine the needs of students the pre-service educators review research on learned helplessness.

An examination of Eric Jensen's (1998) work regarding the brain and learning provides exposure to the concept of learned helplessness. Jensen discusses this concept in detail in his text *Learning with the Brain in Mind*, and gives a reason for the response from a student of "I'm stupid" or "I can't do it." Although this response occurs in a typical classroom, it is very common in a room of incarcerated youth, and becomes a major block to learning. It surfaces when a student has sustained an event where he or she had no control over what was occurring. Severe trauma from physical, verbal, or psychological abuse can cause this reaction in children. An abusive teacher who calls a student out in front of classmates, a bully in the hallway, or a parent or other authority figure who consistently tells a child he or she is unworthy and incapable of success, can all result in a student who appears to lack motivation or "isn't trying hard enough." A student with learned helplessness has literally had their brain rewired to accept failure. These students take the attitude of "Why try? I will fail anyway." They are more apt to suffer from anxiety, depression, and anger. One pre-service educator's experience was captured in her teaching reflection:

> One student had done an incredibly elaborate drawing on his idea generator sheet. He told me this was the best drawing he had ever done, and he absolutely insisted that he needed to keep it for himself. Only a couple minutes into the studio portion, this student was pulled out of the class to talk to someone. He came back in about 20 minutes later with a very defeated attitude. I could not help but feel awful that whatever the interaction he just had, had made such a complete difference in his attitude and inspiration.
>
> When I went over to speak with the student individually, desperately hoping he would at least try to do something, he threw out a countless number of negative statements like, "I cannot do this." "This is stupid." "There is no way this is going to look good." It was certainly disheartening to see this happen after he had been so in love with and proud of his drawing earlier. This also proved to me that even though his conversation likely had absolutely nothing to do with art class, it still made a tremendous impact on his ability to function in class and to use his creativity.
>
> (Romanic, 2013)

To address the issue of learned helplessness, teachers must use the variables they can control. Outside the classroom, instructors have little control over what may occur. As with all good teaching, the pre-service educators are encouraged to stand in the doorway of the classroom at the change of classes, which provides a good view of the hallway. In this posture, they are able to see what is happening outside their door. This vantage point provides the pre-service educator with the opportunity to determine the "temperature" of her or his class and also provides another set of eyes that could prevent an incident from occurring. Additionally, the pre-service educator is able to welcome each student into the classroom and make eye contact with everyone. Preparation that makes the art room a welcoming and interesting environment, and a well-planned opening activity, provide a transition for students, and prompt them to leave what may have occurred outside the classroom and begin fresh with this art lesson.

The pre-service educator must continue to work to minimize or reduce threats for all students inside the classroom. Clear expectations regarding behavior, and the consistent enforcement of expectations, ensure that students know what will and will not be tolerated. The pre-service educators must establish that their art room is a safe place where all ideas are valued. Jensen (1998) also recommends reducing threats by examining unrealistic deadlines. By providing a fresh piece of sketch paper or a few more minutes to finish a project, an instructor can help a student realize they can be successful. So often, teachers are eager to move on, convinced these are "delaying tactics" designed to "get out of work." Approaching these events with care rather than criticism can have meaningful results.

Armed with this introductory information and following a site visit, the pre-service educators are ready to prepare an art curriculum that will tap into the interests of their students.

Observational Visit and Orientation

To prepare for the teaching experience, and to begin to break down misconceptions and alleviate fears, the pre-service educators visit the juvenile detention facilities for orientation. The visit begins with the security procedures. Purses, keys, and coats are left in lockers, and each guest entering the facility walks through a metal detector. The group of pre-service educators is greeted by the coordinating teacher who will escort them to one of the four classrooms used for daily instruction. The orientation covers the facility's general rules and regulations, and provides detailed information regarding the classroom materials, dress, classroom management, and routines.

The pre-service educators are:

- welcomed and thanked for their willingness to share their love of art with this very special group of students. This will be the students' only opportunity for art instruction and they look forward to this break in their tightly structured education schedule.
- not left alone in the classrooms. The daily classroom teacher or a detention officer is present at all times.
- encouraged to enforce the established classroom expectations and add their own based on the needs of an art classroom. They are encouraged to not overwhelm the students with a lot of additional "rules and regulations." The pre-service educators create minimal but key expectations of their own, often focusing on the attainable and measurable expectation of "follow directions."
- responsible for providing an inventory of supplies brought into the center including the number of each item (pencils, erasers, brushes) and must be certain to count and leave with the same number.
- not to use contraband materials in art-making, such as art knives, permanent markers with alcohol, non-rounded scissors, paper clips, staples.[1]

- not to discuss the reasons for a student's incarceration. The pre-service educators are often curious about why their students are in the detention facility. This information is protected and must remain private for the protection of the students. This guideline is also for the protection of the pre-service educator, as any information disclosed to them by a student could require that they testify during that student's court proceedings.
- to dress professionally at all times, including no low-cut tops or midriffs showing for women, no low-riding trousers on men, no more than three piercings per ear, and no other visible piercings or tattoos.
- reminded of the mobility of their students. Each team of pre-service educators is assigned to a classroom. Although this classroom remains the same, their student population will vary greatly from week to week. The population in the classes is very transient. Students will leave the facility (released to go back home or be transferred to another, more permanent facility) and new students will enter the system. Students also may be called out of class for meetings with supervisors, attorneys, or medical personnel. The pre-service educators must be prepared to "go with the flow," adjusting by welcoming newcomers and bringing them along with a lesson that may already have started, and working to not allow these comings and goings to disrupt the lesson's rhythm.[2]
- given a complete tour of the facility. The tour is often the most profound and powerful experience of the orientation day. Locked doors separate all sections of the facility. All areas are constantly under surveillance. Each pre-service educator stands in a cell (unoccupied) becoming acutely aware of their students' experiences. The tour is an essential component to aid the pre-service educators in developing a compassionate understanding of the students they will be teaching.

After the orientation, the experience is discussed in the on-campus class. The pre-service educators examine what met their expectations and what was different. Generally, the pre-service educators expect the security measures, locked doors, and cinder block walls, but do not expect bright and open classrooms, supportive, optimistic faculty and staff, and the stark simplicity of the cells. The overarching concept that emerges from orientation regards the humanity of all students. Whether wearing the latest fashion at an area high school or a jumpsuit in a detention center, these children possess the same desire for acceptance and hopes for the future. As stated by D. Humphrey,

> I was extremely nervous going into my first day of teaching at the detention center. It is only natural. What I soon found out was that my students were not "bad kids," but rather kids that made bad decisions. They were still kids—still students—and they needed a strong teacher.
>
> (2013)

These children are no less deserving of quality art instruction than any others.

Creation of Appropriate Curriculum

To create appropriate and relatable art curriculum based on issues of emerging relevance to the students, the pre-service educators must develop an understanding of their students and their culture, identify issues of student interest, research relevant artists/artifacts addressing the issue selected, and design the art lesson from introduction to art-making.

Although the majority of the pre-service educators are traditional college students and only a few years removed from their own high school experiences, these college students are light years removed from students in middle and high school today. To prepare for their teaching experience, the pre-service educators delve into contemporary youth culture with an assignment that requires they research the issues adolescents are faced with and interested in.

A web idea generator encourages the pre-service educators to identify issues of possible interest in today's youth culture, and to dig deeply into issues and concerns. For example, a web that begins with the generalized issue of "relationships" breaks down into more specific issues of peer pressure, cliques, bullying, and stereotypes. Selecting one of these issues, the pre-service educators then research their issue in a variety of ways. They review professional articles written on the issue, talk with and/or survey teens they know, and examine visual culture (ads, movies, music videos) representations of the issue.

Research is also conducted on a contemporary artist (works created in the past ten years) aligned with the pre-service educators' chosen issue. The contemporary work provides an entry point into the issue with images that are directly identifiable and connected to the students' experiences. The pre-service educators often struggle with the selection of contemporary art works. Their studies have included a series of art history courses covering art from the dawn of man through the late modern period. They are encouraged to investigate contemporary art journals, and website sources, such as *Art in America, Artnow,* and *Art:21,* as well as museums of contemporary art. They are also encouraged to select artists who are as different from them as possible. This opens the door for artists with varied backgrounds, cultures, sexual orientations, and ages. Hopefully, this fills in gaps often missing from art education, moving beyond traditional race/ethnicity identifiers. The result is an approach connecting everyday experience, social critique, and creative expression for contemporary relevance with the students. Addressing issues and ideas that students truly care about and that are relevant in a larger life-world context, art becomes a vital means of reflecting on the nature of society and social existence (Cahan & Kocur, 2011). The use of diverse artists helps to illuminate different perspectives of an issue for students. In turn, this encourages the students to value and speak from their own perspectives and then examine critically these perspectives in light of the social issue.

The resulting research paper reveals not only the artist's methodology in creating a work, but also the artist's intent. Yet, it is essential that the pre-service educator goes beyond this and uncovers other meanings and messages presented in the work. "What personal connections does the educator have with the piece? What drew the educator to stop and look deeper into it? What imagery is present that will connect with the students the educator will be teaching?" The pre-service educator must then investigate other artists, both historical and contemporary, who have worked with the same issue(s). Focus is placed on uncovering connections with other artists based on the idea(s) of the work not the processes, style, or medium used. The result is a gallery of works (at least three) by different artists who have approached the same issue and created distinct, successful solutions.

Armed with this background research, the pre-service educator is ready to construct her or his lesson. Best practices to lesson development are used that are appropriate for the creation of quality art instruction to any population. During each step of the lesson's creation, the pre-service educator must keep their learners in mind, reflecting on the relevance of each activity, strategy, idea, image, and process to be used by her or his students. Based on research into their students' ages and stages of development, what expectations are reasonable for the population they will be teaching? This is presented in the form of a script, written as though the teaching story is unfolding. The pre-service educators are required to be playful and to present the information to their students in engaging and interesting ways. They are also encouraged to utilize a constructivist approach, remembering they are guides and co-learners in this exploration (Brooks & Brooks, 1993), and must focus on the "sacred-ness" of their students (Akins, 2001). By scripting the lesson, the pre-service educators can see the language they are planning to use and identify problem areas before they teach. Lengthy sections of scripting can be evaluated through the lens of shared learning. Lecture moments are highlighted and can be reworked. Demonstrations can be made interactive to allow for student input.

Teaching and Reflecting

After each teaching experience, the pre-service educators are required to write a paper based on their experience. This takes the form of a reflection from the lead teacher and an observation by her or his partner. Pre-service educators must complete them within 48 hours of their experience to ensure that the essential details of the teaching day are not lost. They are encouraged to focus on one or two events that occurred and expand on them. Here is an example of one pre-service educator's reflection. She had been teaching a group of incarcerated young women and one of her students had chosen not to participate. The pre-service educator had been told not to expect much from this student by the classroom teacher and support staff. She writes:

Although this was the only incident that really stuck out, and other teachers may just dismiss it with "her loss if she chooses not to participate," it left a bad taste in my mouth. I wanted her to enjoy this. I keep wondering if she was just in a bad mood, or if it was because I failed to provide enough genuine encouragement. I can't help but feel responsible, whether or not I should. It was obvious she didn't want to even try.

She seemed to be under the impression that if you are not good at drawing realistically, you should not be drawing. However, this may have had nothing to do with her skill level. Her art was about missing out on her little brother's life. She was one of the only girls that was not talking about her life before her arrest, and instead focusing on what she could not have while she was detained. Maybe she was angry because she was thinking about that. If that were the case, how was I supposed to handle it? Or, if she was simply frustrated about her art, there should have been a better way to deal with it. I wanted to motivate her.

Was I too pushy or insensitive? Or, did I not give her enough attention? Maybe she felt like I did not care. There is a line you must walk between over-pushing a student and not giving them enough attention, and that line gets incredibly thinner if they are in a bad mood. My instinct tells me she needed more attention, but in a different form. I should have been more convincing when she expressed disgust in her art abilities. I do not know what I could have said, but it felt like something more reassuring would have been helpful. She deserved to be satisfied with herself and able to take the opportunity to create.

(Ostrowski, 2012)

This reflection reveals how this writing exercise provides the opportunity for the pre-service educator to examine the teaching experience in detail. At the time of teaching, emotions and adrenaline are in full gear and often cloud the educator's ideas about the teaching day. Delving deeply into one or two scenarios encourages the educator to work through inconsistencies, rethink approaches, and troubleshoot solutions. In addition, it establishes and reinforces the practice of reflective teaching.

Reading the observations of their teaching partner also provides needed feedback for the lead teacher. While the pre-service educator will receive a written observation by the instructor and/or teaching assistant, this peer feedback is particularly helpful. Peers provide a singular voice and perspective. The peer is present for every minute of the lesson while the faculty observers may come in and out. Little details of the teaching; the inflection of the pre-service educator's voice, a facial expression, repetitive phrases, a caring and supportive comment are often picked up by the peer and sharing these with the pre-service educator not only helps to improve her or his teaching practice, but points out the many successes of the teaching day. In addition, the observer is able to dissect the teaching day and use this information once they are the lead instructor.

A sample of a portion of an observation follows:

> I feel one of the most successful teaching events occurred as a result of the various activities my partner had planned for the class. She created an introductory activity that allowed the students to get out of their seats and move throughout the room to different locations. Also, she had a worksheet activity and brainstorming activity to help generate student ideas. The videos that my partner showed the class were very relevant to the student population. They recognized the videos and were amused by them. These events were successful because they helped get the students interested in the topic for the day and held their attention.
>
> (Sloan, 2012)

In addition to covering the positive events, the partner also includes areas the pre-service educator could consider for improvement. This balanced feedback from a peer is very helpful for both pre-service educators (lead instructor and observer) to improve their teaching practice.

Conclusion

The growth experienced by our pre-service educators through their first-hand teaching opportunities with diverse populations cannot be understated. Teaching is a practiced skill. If this teaching practice does not include all children, the pre-service educator is truly not prepared to teach in our diverse and gloriously inclusive world. This practice provides pre-service educators with an enthusiasm and confidence that can only be achieved by trying, occasionally failing, learning from failures, and having success. The following is an excerpt from a student's field experience reflections addressing this notion of practice:

> When I left the girls last week, I felt like a failure. However, when I left this week, I felt so much more sure of myself. Just like the first time around, I was respectful and receptive to the students' needs. What was different this week, however, was that they were willing to let me in. They may have still been guarded, but they trusted me enough to let me help them make personal art. I know that some students just are not ready to let you help them. They may open up in the future, but as of now, they just are not. I believe that when I return to the girls, I will be better equipped to give them the confident teacher they deserve. I will try my absolute hardest to make them excited about my lesson. If they like it, that is fantastic. If they are still unsure, I will keep trying.
>
> (Ostrowski, 2012)

The beauty of this reflection highlights the underlying goal of the art education program: To graduate art educators who accept all children, regardless of their labeled differences, as worthy of a robust, rich, and creative art curriculum, and to prepare them for the challenges of teaching incarcerated and at-risk youth.

Model 2: Lisa Kay

> [A]rt making is often deeply personal, the visual notes I created made me more aware of my personal interactions with the student, rather than just an observer of their behavior.
>
> (Albright, 2005)

It is important for pre-service teachers to develop compassion, empathy, and tolerance in working with all students, but especially when teaching students who have experienced psychological trauma. One way to understand the impact of trauma is to engage in self-reflection, to examine our own personal experiences with traumatic events. The creation of visual notes is one model that uses arts-based research for preparing art teachers for teaching children exposed to trauma.

The Visual Notes Project

Visual notes are miniature works of art. Visual note making is a creative arts approach that combines art-making and self-reflection (Kay, 2013; Leavy, 2015). Visual notes are a method of investigating encounters with pre-K-12 students who have experienced adversity, and to examine personal experiences and feelings about one's teaching practice. The art work and writing become a permanent record of thoughtful, aesthetic insights and new understandings which can inform one's teaching practice.

In one metropolitan university, pre-service teachers are asked to function as arts-based researchers as they created visual notes to document their own experiences and classroom encounters during their student teaching semester with pre-K-12 students who have experienced a range of adverse experiences, including trauma. Pre-service teachers are provided an arts-based research kit that includes: simple art supplies (pre-cut 4" × 6" paper and matt board, mixed collage media, a glue stick) and instructions for the assignment. The instructions are to create at least four 4" × 6" visual field notes outside of class and write creative reflections (free prose and poetic reflections) as a method of interrogation about their experiences.

To introduce this process, pre-service teachers are guided during class in a short progressive relaxation exercise followed by guided imagery. They are asked to close their eyes, only if they are comfortable, and to consider their personal experience with trauma, disability, or illness. "How have you been affected personally by trauma, disability, emotional disturbances, or physical illness? What do you recall? What can you remember about your experiences? How have they impacted you? In what ways have your

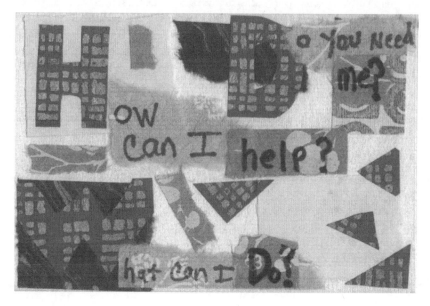

Figure 20.1 "Visual Note: 'How can I help? Do you need me? What can I do?'"

experiences shaped you into the person you are today?" After spending a
few minutes with the thoughts and the images that came to mind, they are
asked: "What do you see? What details do you remember? Colors? Smells?
Sounds? Is there anything you associate with your memory of this experience?" When they are ready to open their eyes, the students are invited to
use the art materials table to give visual form to their experience(s) and to
reflect about their art work on the back.

After completing the art-making process, the class discussed the art
work, shared their experiences, and talked about their feelings related
to working with students who have had traumatic stressors and events.
One female student's visual note and reflections is a powerful example
of this process:

On the back of her visual note, she wrote that she feared appearing as
if she were "too concerned, don't do enough, if I do too much, if I do it
all wrong, if I make it worse. I don't know how to ask, because I don't
want you to think that I think you aren't capable." This example illustrated
how creating visual notes and reflecting helped this pre-service art teacher
became aware of her personal interactions, understood the potential impact
of her actions, and empathized with her student's experiences.

A clinical diagnosis or a description of trauma or the difficulties a student has experienced can be impersonal and characterize the student from
a detached perspective. However, visual notes with written reflections provided a more humanistic response. As was explained:

[T]he act of developing a visual response to working with a student requires creative thought . . . since art making is often deeply personal, the visual notes I created made me more aware of my personal interactions with the student, rather than just an observer of their behavior. The visual notes also made me aware of the powerlessness I felt in regards to being able to help them . . . or how to determine if, and when they needed help. The visual notes helped me to get in touch with my own feelings about the students' particular situations, and that helped me forge a more empathic approach to interacting.

(Albright, 2015)

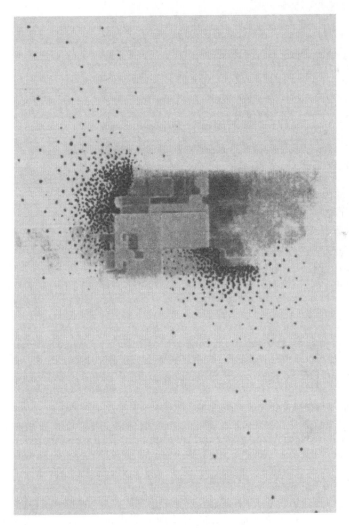

Figure 20.2 "Visual Note: Pieces Tiny Work"

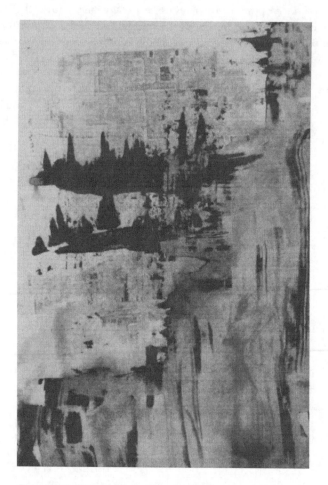

Figure 20.3 "Visual Note: Tiny Forests"

Another pre-service art teacher explained that the lines and shapes of her visual notes intertwined on paper as did her relationships with her students. In the making and reflecting, she better understood her own emotions and placed herself in the student's position, which assisted her in developing the best approach to work with her students.

As an artist and educator one graduate art education student explained that by "putting my hand to the paper and layering information and materials onto the surface," she engaged in what John Dewey called "flexible purposing." John Dewey defined flexible purposing as the "ability to shift direction, even to redefine one's aims when better options emerge in the course of one's work" (as cited in Eisner, 2002, p. 77). The Visual Notes Project was a method for pre-service students to independently problem-solve and think critically about their encounters with students and their work.

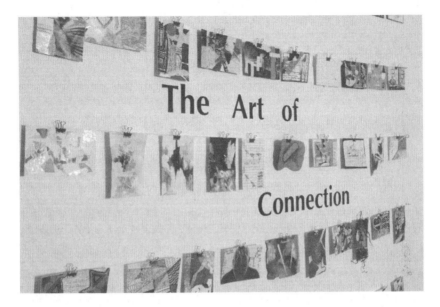

Figure 20.4 "Group Exhibition"

Collectively, the pre-service teachers shared their art work and reflections with each other throughout the semester, discussing issues and concerns that surfaced and what they were learning about their students and themselves. Often, connecting with their own losses and traumatic experiences helped them develop empathy for their students. This arts-based process helped them express themselves and relate better to their students.

At the culmination of their student teaching experience, the pre-service teachers co-curated a group exhibition where others could witness their art work and growth as art educators.

Through the Visual Notes Project, pre-service teachers developed compassion, empathy, and tolerance. They connected with their students, expressed their feelings, and reflected on their teaching experiences. They discovered new ways of seeing themselves and their students through art and, in the process, were changed.

Model 3: Lynne J. Horoschak

Stress is bad for children. It's associated with health problems, school failures, and youth delinquency. But the arts can help children reduce and manage their stress. The arts can be especially important in inner-city neighborhoods plagued by violence and where the resulting stress can be particularly damaging to children.

(Creedon, 2011)

Professors of the art education faculty at a college in a major city must be sensitive to the needs of the children in city public schools. Too many students are living in violent households and neighborhoods. Often one parent is incarcerated, children have seen loved ones victimized, and more students than can be imagined are living in emergency housing shelters. Living in the stress of a crisis situation increases the risk of severe anxiety and depression in homeless youth (National Coalition for the Homeless, 2008). Faculty who are experienced in teaching in urban public schools and are keenly aware of the challenges presented to teachers. Thus art education majors are taught strategies to best meet the needs of children who may be in crises. The art of being present and listening to children cannot be overstated.

Establishing trust, says Gracenin (1994), is important because a youth's behavior of acting out against authority can be used to mask deeper fear of insecurity or failure. Paying attention to what causes behaviors and what they are communicating, can give the teacher insight into understanding and, in turn, deliver the proper response.

As a Cooperating Teacher

As an experienced art teacher in the public schools, it was my privilege to mentor many student teachers. They arrived eager and excited to get to work. It was my responsibility to capitalize on their enthusiasm and model best practices in teaching art to children in an urban community so they would be well prepared to teach wherever the job market led them.

The art class schedule included teaching 800 different children a week, with seven classes of children with special needs, and four classes of inclusion. Initially, their responsibility was to watch, listen, ask questions, and pay attention to details: "What occurred before Andrew got up and hit Henry? Why was there confusion when handing out four different colors of paper? Why isn't Erin cleaning up her space? Why didn't the teacher speak to Ernie when he left his seat and went to the window? What is causing Jamie's unusual antagonistic behavior?" Paying attention to students' roles in class dynamics, which differ with each class and from week to week, is crucial in understanding and delivering successful art lessons. The pre-service teachers realized that they would be dealing with much more than art supplies, age-appropriate lessons, assessments, and administrative mandates. It was a little daunting for a pre-service teacher, but after the first few days she or he was anxious to get started leading the class.

We are dealing with children coming from all imaginable circumstances. As art educators, we must be sensitive to their needs and know that, through art, we can help the child explore, take risks, and discover in a safe and welcoming place.

When a combative, argumentative, and disruptive student is transferred into an otherwise responsive and enjoyable class, the class can become a room full of hostile students as they verbally arm themselves against the new student's jeers and insults. An experienced art educator will want this student to create successful art projects and help her or him engage positively with their peers and the teacher. Strategies that I try to teach pre-service educators are: private conversations, "good work" notes home to Mom, and an "I need your help" talk. Sometimes these work and sometimes they do not. I also want them to know that identifying the child's story, the reasons that precipitate negative behavior, has usually helped me work with a student. And on "bad days," I may allow the student to sit alone and not work on the project. Pre-service teachers can learn through trial and error, ways of modifying a child's behavior, and while it takes time and persistence to work with a student, the payoff is extraordinary. They experience firsthand the difficulties a student from a negligent foster home or a home that has been disrupted with violence can exhibit. Obviously, every student is different and every student brings with them their own story. When the story impacts their learning, it is our responsibility to use every means at our disposal to support the child.

Special Populations Course

It became clear from my experience with pre-service teachers that higher education was not preparing our art educators to meet the needs of children who were experiencing trauma in their lives and those with disabilities. In 1996, I developed the Special Populations course, which is required for pre-service teachers at a local college. This course is taken the semester before student teaching. Here, the students teach children with special needs under the supervision of a certified art educator. Initially, the students are hesitant and a bit fearful; afraid they will make a mistake and cause irreparable harm to a child; however, within the first 20 minutes all fears vanish when they realize the children won't break and are eager to engage in making art. The instructor for this class said,

> We know that consistency offers a sense of security and stability when all else feels out of control. What our Special Populations class teaches is the training that new teachers need to offer stability, by setting up a classroom culture that is constantly safe and accessible to all who enter. Routines are set in place from day one, and adaptive tools are offered in a way that doesn't single any one child out, but rather assures all that they will always get what they need. Once a child feels safe expressing themselves, the river of communication comes flowing through the art making process.
>
> (Lauren Stichter, 2015)

Teaching children with various disabilities and from all socio-economic classes builds confidence and skills that are necessary for a successful pre-service experience. This semester of discovery and effective planning, teaching, and assessing art lessons begins to prepare the pre-service teacher to work with children of all abilities and from all circumstances. This class equips the student to identify and teach to the strengths of each child.

One pre-service teacher, Carley, taught a 7-year-old child whose mother had passed away just weeks earlier. The child began having a difficult time getting along with her peers as she thought they were making fun of her and bullying her. Carley credits her experience in Special Populations in helping her relate to the child. It taught her the importance of flexibility, staying on task, classroom management, and the art of identifying the uniqueness of each child, helping her empathize with this child. In addition, she exhibited the student's art work, which gave the student a feeling of accomplishment and celebration.

Celeste, a student teacher, was assigned to a classroom with an experienced and capable cooperating art teacher who was scheduled to teach his first class of students with special needs. Because of the Special Populations course, Celeste was prepared and able to model for him ways to redirect the students to success by formulating her words and actions in a way which encourage them to shift their focus. She gave specific, positive feedback on their artwork—this lesson was clay robots—and asked the students what else they could do to make their robot unique. Encouraging a student to circulate around the room to see what their classmates were doing could often redirect a child's thought process. Having taken the Special Populations course gave her a practical understanding of how to relate to students.

Student Teaching Seminar

During their pre-service field experience, students met weekly with the faculty of the Student Teaching Seminar. They discussed the challenges and successes they had experienced in their field placement. Conversation starters included: "What makes the art lesson relevant to the students? How can directions be simplified so all feel confident in following them? What strategies are used so the child with a learning disability is not singled out? How do you raise the confidence of a child who is only used to failure? How is the art displayed? Celebrated?"

From this experience, the faculty and pre-service teachers compiled a short list of classroom wisdoms that are passed on to incoming pre-service art educators.

Classroom Wisdom from Pre-Service Art Teachers for Pre-Service Teachers:

1   Wait for quiet. Many student teachers, anxious to begin, will start motivating their class before they have their attention. Without their attention, it is likely that the noise level will rise and lack of attention will increase.

2 Be consistent in the way students enter the art room. If students enter the room in a rowdy manner, you will likely struggle with classroom management.

3 Teach relevant and age-appropriate lessons with adaptation for children with special needs. The best way to have effective behavior in the classroom is to have lessons that are relevant to the students' lives. Research your school and its population. Adapt lessons for the child with a disability. Know the students you teach.

4 Repeat answers after your student answers. Sometimes not everyone hears the responses. Repeating also gives emphasis to correct or interesting responses. Hearing the answer twice is a way to emphasize the answer.

5 Call on people who don't have their hands raised. Using this methodology keeps all the students tuned in. This is not a means to catch or embarrass a child. Give the student ample time to respond, eight seconds wait time, so they have the opportunity to share their thoughts on your open-ended question. A secret code can be used with children with a disability so you know when they have the answer.

6 Establish a teacher presence. Use your voice to engage students and maintain order. This is not to suggest that your voice needs to be loud, rather firm and effective. The pre-service teacher needs to let the children know she or he is always in the room and in charge.

7 Know art specific mnemonics, such as ROYGBIV. (Colors of the rainbow: Red, Orange, Yellow, Green, Blue, Indigo, and Violet.)

8 Be savvy about art media. Know your art supplies. Oil pastels are not chalk pastels. There is a difference between media and medium.

9 Be busy during prep time. Prep time is not a free period. It is preparation time. Mounting work to be displayed, readying supplies for the next classes, marking art work, planning lessons. Know what needs to be done and do it.

10 Promptness. Be early and stay late.

Stopping Time with Art that Heals

The children's art and writings in . . . *I Never Saw Another Butterfly . . . Children's Drawings and Poems from Terezin Concentration Camp, 1942–1944* (Volavkova, 1993) clearly illustrate the power that art has to transport a child from unspeakable trauma to a place where the hardships can be relieved. Chaim Potok in his Foreword to the book quoted from the Memoir of Raja Englanderova, a member of the art class organized by Mrs. Brandeis at Terezin Concentration Camp: "I remember Mrs. Brandeis as a tender, highly intelligent woman, who managed—for some hours every week—to create a fairy world for us in Terezin. . . . [A] world that made us forget all our surrounding hardships, which we were not spared despite our early age" (Volavkova, p. xx). We as art educators must remember that we have the power and responsibility to create a safe and nurturing environment for all of our students.

Model 4: Donalyn Heise

> Art is used to help students reframe adversity to see possibility instead of despair.
>
> (Heise, 2014, p. 29)

This model defines community engagement and describes how one urban university is using this model within a framework of resilience theory to better prepare art educators for meeting the needs of students exposed to trauma.

Many colleges and universities integrate a community component into teacher preparation courses. Community engagement, often referred to as service learning, civic engagement, engaged scholarship, or participatory research, builds on John Dewey's theory of interaction of knowledge and skills with experience. In 1996, Ernest Boyer challenged higher education institutions to connect the rich resources of the university to the community in an effort to address societies' most pressing needs. The result was an emphasis on discovery, and integration of discovery with application (Calleson et al., 2005). Bringle, Hatcher, and McIntosh (2006) define service learning as a course-based, credit-bearing educational experience that gives students the opportunity to participate in organized community activity and reflect on the experience. By this definition student teaching can be considered community engagement. However, combined with a resilience framework, community engagement can be extended to include a collaborative model that contributes to the well-being of individuals and communities exposed to psychologically traumatic events.

Art teacher preparation programs traditionally include studio courses and methods courses addressing art education pedagogy. Courses encompass necessary topics such as curriculum development, task analysis, instruction and assessment strategies, behavior management, and classroom organization. Field experiences in K-12 classrooms give pre-service teachers opportunities to practice teaching. But meeting the needs of all students in diverse classrooms, especially students who have experienced trauma, remains a challenge. As a university professor and student teacher supervisor, I witnessed pre-service teachers who reported apprehension about teaching in urban schools. Many felt ill-equipped to engage students, often citing students who were disrespectful and inattentive. I recognized a gap between pre-service teachers and the students they were about to teach. Most of my university students grew up in a middle-class environment and attended private or suburban schools. Many had little insight into the context of the lives of children who attend public school in a city that is ranked one of the poorest in the nation. Some of their future students have experienced homelessness at some point in their lives; some have family members who are or have been incarcerated. Many of the children have experienced violent crime in their short lives; and some are dealing with the challenges of poverty.

This prompted an immediate course redesign to better prepare teachers to meet the needs of all students. I wanted them to realize that all children deserve good teachers. A community engagement component was embedded prior to student teaching that bridged theory to practice. It emphasized the importance of understanding the context of the children's lives to best address needs, learning styles, and preferences. Pre-service teachers were assigned the task of designing and implementing an art program in a school or community center. Course objectives included understanding the positive impact the arts can have on youth who may have experienced trauma; designing and implementing effective arts-based programs that foster positive development in children; and creating models for evidence-based arts education practice to resolve issues important to individuals, families, groups, neighborhoods, and communities, such as positive youth development, building resilience, and violence prevention. The course was structured around five main components:

1   research/best practices,
2   collaborative process,
3   design/implementation,
4   critical reflection/evaluation, and
5   dissemination.

Each will be discussed below.

Research/Best Practices

The course began with a review of relevant research and best practices on topics such as understanding the effects of trauma, teaching with poverty in mind, positive youth development, resilience theory, and community engagement. Each pre-service teacher researched a topic, and shared key components with their peers. This provided insights as to the challenges they may face teaching in public schools where the majority of students have experienced psychological trauma.

Pre-service teachers learned that exposure to trauma such as neglect, abuse, or violence can create roadblocks to learning. Referring to the literature provided insights to dealing effectively with students exposed to trauma. For instance, students who have experienced trauma may have trouble with trusting someone new and may act out in class. As Benard (2011) states, "hurt people hurt people." He advocates an asset or strengths approach to foster resilience, as opposed to a deficit model. A deficit model uses labels such as delinquent, deviant, dysfunctional (Krovetz, 2007).

An asset approach recognizes and celebrates the strengths and assets an individual employs that helps them persevere in times of trauma. For instance, being resourceful, persistent, maintaining a positive outlook, and having a sense of humor can be assets when living in crisis.

Resilience theory provides a framework for working with children who have experienced trauma. Pre-service teachers discussed how some people seem to bounce back quickly after experiencing adversity, while others struggle with long-term effects. After reviewing related literature, they learned that a resilience framework does not focus on reducing risks, but rather increasing protective factors believed to foster resilience. A list was made of protective factors that art teachers might address in a classroom situation, such as ability to see multiple perspectives of a problem, vision for the future, resourcefulness, persistence, and having a sense of purpose. Additional factors included having at least one person who believes in you and supports you, and pride as a result of mastering artistic processes.

Theory and research revealed that children living in poverty often exhibit behaviors such as chronic tardiness, lack of motivation, inappropriate behavior, use of profanity, and disrespect of others (Jenson, 2009). Children living in poverty experience greater chronic stress more often than do their more affluent counterparts. Students may appear to be either out of control, showing an attitude, or lazy. But these behaviors are actually symptoms of stress disorders—and distress influences many behaviors that influence engagement. Distress affects brain development, academic success, and social competence (Evans, Kim, Ting, Tesher, & Shannis, 2007).

Research suggests that children experiencing trauma can show cognitive problems, including short attention spans, high levels of distractibility, difficulty monitoring the quality of their work, and difficulty generating new solutions to problems (Alloway et al., 2009). Lower socio–economic status can also affect outlook and attitudes, and is sometimes associated with viewing the future as containing more negative events than positive ones (Robb, Simon, & Wardle, 2009). Many children who struggle cognitively either act out (exhibit problem behavior) or shut down (show learned helplessness). Suggested strategies included building trust between teacher and student, reducing stress by making the learning environment a safe space to learn, creating learning that is fun, and engaging in multisensory learning experiences.

Art teachers can expand students' learning in ways that differ from methods used in other classrooms. Art lessons are problem-based, interactive, and encourage creativity in an environment that encourages risk-taking. Art teachers can focus on affirming and reinforcing students' efforts. Teachers can guide a student to recognize when she or he is making a strong choice and to cultivate a positive attitude. They can teach their students that their brains can change and grow.

Collaborative Process

Based on what was learned through review of research, a community engagement model was developed to extend learning, bridge theory to practice, and contribute to the body of knowledge in the field. Reciprocal relationships were created with students, faculty, and community partners who all collaborated as co-learners, co-teachers, and co-generators of knowledge. Consistent with the model proposed by Felten and Clayton (2011), pre-service art teachers created mutually beneficial relationships that explored a multitude of learning outcomes for all participants. Throughout this process, pre-service art teachers developed greater understanding of the importance of shared vision and shared leadership. Recognizing that persons most affected by a change effort are the ones who need to be a part of the decision-making and that leadership exists among all participants involved, pre-service art teachers facilitated collaborative models with a community partner. Planning meetings were conducted with the community staff and sessions were held with the youth to be served, in an effort to gain deeper insights into the students they serve, and to create an appreciation for the power of art for children exposed to psychological trauma.

They particularly focused on listening more than talking, learning from community partners and students, and creating shared vision and shared leadership. A culture of respect was emphasized. All participants were considered producers of knowledge instead of passive recipients. Pre-service art teachers abandoned the model of doing "for" and substituted the mindset of engaging "with" community.

Design/Implementation

Pre-service art teachers were given the task of designing a meaningful community art program for children exposed to trauma that utilized the therapeutic properties of art education and honored the creative process over product. Sites for implementation included working with children in homeless shelters, adolescents who were victims of sexual violence, and children of incarcerated parents. Art lessons focused on strengthening at least one of the protective factors of resilience, such as problem-solving, mastery, sense of purpose, vision for the future, self-awareness, or empathy. Thematic, integrated lessons focused on the four artistic processes of create, connect, respond, and present. In addition, they were to collaborate and create a plan for dissemination.

The art lessons used individual strengths and assets as a source of ideation. For example, students brainstormed things they do when they are stressed. The list included tasks such as listening to music, talking to a friend, or praying. They then created symbols for these activities and included the images in their art work. Lessons linked art to life and were interdisciplinary in nature, thereby connecting art to other subjects. In addition, teacher candidates discussed how the program connected theory to practice, students to students, and teacher candidates to community. They felt these connections increased social bonding and encouraged a positive learning environment characterized by respect, trust, growth, cohesiveness, caring, support, and challenge. Finally, connections were made in creating shared visions and shared values.

Consistent with the four artistic processes of the new visual arts standards, students were given opportunities to create, present, respond, and connect. Art was created using a variety of media and processes, and each lesson had a different theme or focus. In addition to making art, students had opportunities to respond to works of art representing a variety of cultures, to talk about art, and to reflect on their own art-making efforts. Students also worked collaboratively with pre-service teachers in selecting works to exhibit in the community. They engaged in dialog about how to prepare and present works of art. A community art exhibit was coordinated as well as electronic slide presentations.

Critical Reflection/Evaluation

Being a critically reflective practitioner is one of the professional teacher standards.

Prior to implementation of their designs, pre-service teachers shared their thoughts on pressing issues for teaching. One shared, "The parents don't even care enough to attend parent-teacher conferences, much less get involved in their children's education." Another stated, "When I hear them speak rudely to another or act out, I know they must experience that at home."

After research and implementation, their opinions changed as they realized the impact trauma can have on children. When asked about how their understanding of the context of students' lives affect curriculum and instruction, they replied, "After I realized that some of my students have experienced homelessness or are living in poverty with few material possessions, I stopped giving homework that required they purchase supplies or bring objects from home. I now use a re-envision, reuse, repurpose model for art-making, where I have boxes of found objects to stimulate creativity." Another pre-service art teacher revealed enhanced understanding of the context of students' lives:

> I am reluctant to require that a parent or guardian provide assistance on a homework assignment now that I realize so many are working more than one job, and some single moms are riding city buses for three hours a day to get to and from their low-paying job. So now I make the classroom a safe space for creative risk-taking, making it so engaging that students don't even realize they are learning.

As the implementation of the designs progressed, pre-service art teachers engaged in weekly reflections and ongoing discussions with peers. Weekly reflections allowed documentation of details while the information was still fresh in the minds of the candidates.

These reflections revealed a change in pre-service art teachers' perspectives as a result of participating in the community engagement model. At the beginning of the semester, pre-service teachers assumed they would be assigned a placement, then required to create an art lesson that they would teach to the students. One pre-service teacher commented, "I thought we were doing outreach to share what we know about art, and for them to benefit from our expertise. I had no idea how much I would gain and learn from them." Another shared, "I now have a better grasp of what true collaboration looks like, I now realize the difference between 'doing for' as opposed to 'doing with.'"

Responses also revealed teacher growth and increased competence in motivating young people. For instance, one pre-service teacher said, "Initially, upon approaching the idea of teaching this age group I felt very lacking in my ability to be an effective teacher." Afterwards, "My eyes were opened to an age range of children that normally I am not exposed to. I feel much more comfortable and confident in my abilities as a future teacher as a result of teaching at the community center." Another said, "I learned that each child comes to the center with a different story that might not be comfortable for the child to expose. Trust is crucial and I made a special effort to get to know the students on a personal level, asking about their school, their families, hobbies, and pets. I also offered personal stories about myself in an effort for them to see me as a real person they could open up to. I believe in this sense if a child feels connected with me or the group they are more likely to be motivated and participate."

Pre-service teachers felt that they benefitted as well as the community partners and the youth involved. One shared, "This program was an example of people coming together of different races, ages, and backgrounds, which is always a positive thing. An example was shown that we really can learn about each other and enjoy ourselves despite our differences."

Some pre-service teachers offered advice to others teaching art in a school or after-school setting, recommending that they "make it fun." That seems like a given, but it really is not. If I had not been told to make it fun, I would have hyper-focused on the instructional time rather than the fun time. Young students learn best when they are having a good time. I think we can say that about most adults as well.

Another pre-service teacher reflected on how they felt the youth benefited:

> I think the students learned about human rights and historical art without even realizing it. This is something that amazes me about teaching. As teachers we have the ability to plant seeds in our students without them even knowing it. They think they made a book about their family, but in reality they learned about a working community and demonstrated an understanding of one. They think they made a cool peace sign poster, but when they go home they will tell everyone about how people walk around with signs to make a point.

When asked how the pre-service art teachers felt the collaboration benefited the community at large, one responded,

Many of the lessons were targeted to community, environment, and cultural heritage, and these topics seemed to resonate even with this young age group. This subject matter when presented in a fun and creative way will stay with them and they will share their new knowledge with their families and the community around them. Pride in heritage and community makes for a brighter, more hopeful future for these students. The strong sense of community already apparent among these students, I feel, was strengthened due to the lesson content as well as a growing comradery from interaction outside the normal class setting.

Upon completion of the program, each participant also completed an engaged scholarship report. In addition to the demographics of the population served, the report described instructional strategies and highlighted ways the preservice teachers benefited from the collaboration, as well as how they felt the students and community at large benefited. Evaluation was guided by the following inquiry: "What impact did the community engagement model with a resilience framework have on the professional growth of art teacher candidates?" Evaluation consisted of observations, focus group interviews, and data gathered in the teacher candidate's weekly reflections and final reports.

Dissemination

Dissemination included traditional means, such as lectures and presentations on college campuses. Participants (pre-service art teachers, students, and community partners) brainstormed alternative ways to disseminate the successes of this community engagement effort. Ideas included a community art exhibition, sharing at civic meetings, articles in the newspaper and school newsletters, and sharing insights at professional education conferences.

A final group discussion resulted in a list of suggestions for future art-based community collaborations that are also applicable in a traditional art classroom.

- Provide opportunities for meaningful participation.
- Include students and community partners in planning and decision-making.
- Change the role of student as recipient and teacher as one who imparts knowledge, to both functioning as collaborators and co-learners.
- Challenge everyone to contribute to their fullest capacity.
- Link learning to real life and help students believe that what they do really matters.
- Make learning fun!
- Shift focus from deficits to a strengths- or asset-based model.
- Treat each other with respect.
- Encourage experimentation and risk-taking.
- Provide care and support.
- Remain flexible.

- Emphasize effort, growth, and motivation over compliance and minimally acceptable behavior.
- Emphasize cooperation and caring, celebrations and positive assets.
- Encourage reaching out to get and give help when needed.
- Talk to parents and staff and tell them what you like about their kids.
- Use art to celebrate sources of joy and strength.

Concluding Thoughts

Many of the students we teach have experienced a psychologically traumatic event or will experience trauma in the future. Knowing that stress from living in crisis can affect academic success demands, we continue to find ways to meet their needs. Trauma from natural or man-made disasters, violence, or poverty is a complex problem that requires a systemic effort. Parents, teachers, administrators, school counselors, and community members each have a role to play. This model suggests art teacher preparation as a part of this worthy effort. Using art to articulate individual strengths and assets, and to celebrate sources of joy, may strengthen protective factors believed to foster resilience and thus promote effective learning.

Ten Teaching Tips

1. Provide opportunities for pre-service educators to teach in alternative settings to provide experience in planning, implementing, and critically reflecting on effective instruction to meet the needs of students living in trauma.
2. Create an organized, structured, respectful learning environment with clear expectations.
3. Link theory to practice by building on the good work of others.
4. Use a collaborative model that engages peers, lead teachers, and students in all stages of planning and implementation.
5. Emphasize the importance in active listening, compassion, and empathy.
6. Consult professionals in your school when concerned about a child. Art teachers are not licensed art therapists, therefore we can listen and affirm while providing a safe space for artistic creation, but do not try to counsel or diagnose.
7. Design curriculum that is playful and relevant.
8. Use big ideas or themes to allow all students multiple entry points to engage in the content and processes of art.
9. Focus on resilience and help students to see the possibility within adversity.
10. Use all your resources to learn about your students so that you can design appropriate curriculum and instruction.

Notes

1 The importance of these rules cannot be understated. The initial emphasis for the pre-service educators is that these restrictions are for their personal safety during their teaching. While this is clearly part of the reason, the greater concern is for the safety of the students, student peers, and staff. These materials could be used by the students to do harm to themselves, and protection of the students is paramount.

2 See also Chapter 17, Art and Youth Who Are Incarcerated.

References

Akins, T. (2000). Simply sacred. In D. Fehr, K. Fehr, & K. Kiefer Boyd (Eds.), *Real World Readings in Art Education: Things Your Professors Never Told You*, pp. 99–105. New York: Falmer Press.

Albright, J. Personal conversation with Lisa Kay on June 1, 2005.

Alloway, T. P., Gathercole, S. E., Kirkwood, H., & Elliott, J. (2009). The cognitive and behavioral characteristics of children with low working memory. *Child Development, 80(2)*, 606–621.

Ayers, W. (1998). An unconditional embrace. *Teaching Tolerance, 13(2)*.

Benard, B. (2004). Resiliency: What we have learned. WestEd. Retrieved from wested.org/resources/resiliency-what-we-have-learned.

Boyer, E. L. (1996). The scholarship of engagement. *Bulletin of the American Academy of Arts and Sciences, 49(7)*, 18–33.

Bringle, R. G., Hatcher, J. A., & McIntosh, R. E. (2006). Analyzing Morton's typology of service paradigms and integrity. *Michigan Journal of Community Service Learning, 13(1)*, 5–15.

Brooks, J. G., & Brooks, M. G. (1993). *In Search of Understanding: The Case for Constructivist Teaching*. Alexandria, VA: Association of Supervision and Curriculum Development.

Cahan, S., & Kocur, Z. (2011). Contemporary art and multicultural education. In *Rethinking Contemporary Art and Multicultural Education* (pp. 3–13). New York: New Museum.

Calleson, D. C., Jordan, C., & Seifer, S. D. (2005). Community-engaged scholarship: Is faculty work in communities a true academic enterprise? *Academic Medicine 80(4)*, 317–321.

Creedon, D. W. (2011). Fight the stress of urban education with the arts. *Kappan Magazine*, March.

Dewey, J. (2007). *Experience and Education*. New York: Simon and Schuster.

Eisner, E. W. (2002). What the arts teach. In *The Arts and the Creation of Mind*. New Haven: Yale.

Evans, G. W., Kim, P., Ting, A. H., Tesher, H. B., & Shannis, D. (2007). Cumulative risk, maternal responsiveness, and allostatic load among young adolescents. *Developmental Psychology, 43(2)*, 341.

Felten, P., & Clayton, P. H. (2011). Service-learning. *New Directions for Teaching and Learning, 128*, 75–84.

Gracenin, D. (1994). Reaching and teaching the homeless. *Education Digest, 59(6)*, 37.

Gude, O. (2004). Postmodern principles: In search of 21st century art education. *Art Education, 57(1)*, 6–13.

Heise, D. (2014). Steeling and resilience in art education. *Art Education, 67(3)*, 26–30.

Humphrey, D. (2013) Personal communication with Juliann B. Dorff.

Jensen, E. (1998). *Teaching with the Brain in Mind*. Alexandria, VA: Association of Supervision and Curriculum Development.

Jensen, E. (2009). *Teaching with Poverty in Mind: What Being Poor Does to Kids' Brains and What Schools Can Do about It*. Alexandria, VA: Association of Supervision and Curriculum Development.

Kay, L. (2013). Visual essays: A practice-led journey. *International Journal of Education through Art, 9(1)*, 131–138.

Krovetz, M. L. (2007). *Fostering Resilience: Expecting All Students to Use Their Minds and Hearts Well*. Thousand Oaks, CO: Corwin Press.

Leavy, P. (2015). *Method Meets Art: Arts-Based Research Practice* (2nd edition). New York: Guilford Press

Ostrowski, M. (2012) Personal communication with Juliann B. Dorff.

Robb, K. A., Simon, A. E., & Wardle, J. (2009). Socioeconomic disparities in optimism and pessimism. *International Journal of Behavioral Medicine, 16(4)*, 331–338.

Romanic, K. (2013). Personal communication with Juliann B. Dorff.

Sedar, D. (2012). Personal communication with Juliann B. Dorff.

Shribman, D. (2001). *I Remember My Teacher*. Kansas City: Andrews McMeel Publishing.

Sloan, D. (2012). Personal communication with Juliann B. Dorff.

Stichter, L. (2015). Personal communication with Lynne J. Horoschak.

Volavkova, H. (Ed.) (1993) . . . . *I never saw another butterfly* . . . *Children's drawings and poems from Terezin Concentration Camp, 1942–1944*. Potok, C. Foreword (p. xx). New York: Schocken Books.

Walker, S. (2001). *Teaching Meaning in Artmaking*. Worcester, MA: Davis Publications.

21 Community-Based Art Programs, Collaborative Partnerships, and Community Resources for At-Risk Students

Laura Bailey Saulle, Joseph Lagana, Robin Crawford, and Barbara Duffield

Homeless Children's Education Fund

"Can you picture the turtle?" the storyteller asks a group of 6- and 7-year-olds who are sitting cross-legged in a circle. For the last 20 minutes, the children have clapped, sung, and pantomimed along with the storyteller's tale of a kindly old man who befriends a magical turtle. "Close your eyes and try to imagine what the turtle looks like," the storyteller instructs, closing her own and lifting her hands to her brow, a gesture the children copy reflexively. "I can see him!" shouts a little boy. "Good! Now keep that image in your mind, and when I say so, we're going to go over to the table where we have all kinds of materials for each of you to create your own turtle." The students race to the art table, and a colorful chaos ensues as two dozen small hands commence tearing, layering, and gluing bits of paper to make their turtle collages.

This scene is a snapshot of the summer program at Sojourner House, a housing facility for homeless, dual-diagnosed women and their children in Pittsburgh's East End neighborhood. The storyteller, award-winning children's author Sydelle Pearl, is one of a dozen artists, performers, musicians, and writers who use their talents to enrich the lives of children through out-of-school programming run by the Homeless Children's Education Fund (HCEF). Inspired by research that demonstrates the positive impact of arts training on cognitive development, HCEF collaborates with local artists to develop highly engaging art programs for youth who reside in homeless housing agencies throughout Allegheny County, Pennsylvania.

Background

Founded in 1999 by Dr. Joseph Lagana, a longtime educator and school superintendent on the verge of retirement, HCEF was created to provide educational opportunities for children and youth experiencing homelessness. The organization's founders were troubled by the disparity in educational outcomes between homeless youth and their stably housed peers, and were motivated to raise awareness within the local community to establish support for this underserved population. The shelter community of Pittsburgh represented HCEF's first major partnership. Recognizing that most family shelters and transitional housing facilities in the Pittsburgh area lacked any suitable space for children to study and work on homework assignments, HCEF raised money and in-kind support from the Pittsburgh business community in order to establish Learning Centers on the premises of 11 homeless housing centers. HCEF worked closely with the staff of these agencies to design each Learning Center; all were equipped with computers, educational software, a library of books, and child-friendly furniture. Once built, the Learning Centers were operated by the staff of each agency with support from volunteers and tutors trained by HCEF.

In 2004, the fund began issuing small, seasonal "mini-grants" to its partnering housing agencies to provide field trips and on-site learning activities. Around the same time, HCEF invited these housing agencies to form a support network known as the "Community of Learners." The network began meeting on a quarterly basis to share best practices from the mini-grants and Learning Center initiatives, as well as to learn about educational resources in the community. For HCEF staff, the meetings generated insight regarding the needs of families and presented an opportunity to work collectively to develop new program ideas for the Learning Centers.

Integrating the Arts

Several factors influenced HCEF's decision to create an enrichment program focused on the arts. By the early 2000s, HCEF found that the Learning Centers had become a powerful gathering place for families. As one social worker wrote to HCEF about her agency's Learning Center:

> We call our learning center the Happening Place. The books are widely used by our moms and children. They are borrowed daily from the library and upon returning them, both moms and children are enthusiastic. The children, some with the help of their moms, are reading the books, learning colors, numbers, and even body parts. The children tell us of different places they read about and imagine what it would be like to visit there in person. . . . The moms are so excited when they see what their babies can accomplish.

An evaluation of family supports within Pittsburgh's homeless housing community by Peter Miller and James Schreiber (2009) of Duquesne University, who collected survey and focus group data from 139 parents, indicated that parents perceived the Learning Centers to be effective academic supports (78% of parents indicated that these services were "very helpful") and that

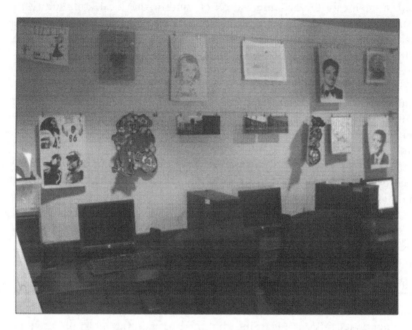

Figure 21.1 "Art work from the Andy Warhol Museum's on-the-road program
           brightens the Learning Center at Open Arms in Homewood,
           Pittsburgh, Pennsylvania"

the Learning Centers were highly used (60% of parents stated that they and/
or their kids used the Learning Center two or more times per week):

> Mothers and agency staff members alike resoundingly indicated that
> the after-school Learning Centers that are located within a number of
> residential homeless agencies in Allegheny County are highly effec-
> tive resources for students. . . . Without leaving the confines of their
> residential agencies, children can gain access to school supplies, com-
> puters, advanced online learning software, academic tutors, cultural
> enrichment activities, and adult supervision. . . . Parents and staff, in
> fact, almost universally lauded these in-house centers as some of the
> most fundamentally important factors in their school-age children's
> daily lives.

Meanwhile, research was emerging on the arts and their potential to have a
positive impact on disadvantaged youth, especially those with a background
of traumatic life experiences such as domestic abuse, peer violence, and sudden or chronic homelessness. Participation in high-quality arts programs was
shown to have an empowering effect on youth, as well as positive implications for their social-emotional, cognitive, and academic development.

At the same time that brain researchers and educators were extolling the many benefits of the arts, public schools were being forced to shutter or reduce many arts programs due to widespread budget cuts. Low-income school districts, which serve the highest numbers of homeless students, were the most impacted by these reductions. In an unfortunate "Catch-22," disadvantaged youth, who stood to gain the most from exposure to the arts, were also the least likely to have access to such opportunities.

Despite its modest size, Pittsburgh is known for its rich, interconnected arts community. By the early 2000s, HCEF had begun tapping into this network, frequently inviting representatives of local museums and arts organizations to attend meetings with the homeless housing community. Initially, this was done to encourage shelters to think about the arts when planning educational field trips for their clients. However, a number of arts organizations, in particular the museums, were also starting to promote alternative, "on the road" programs. These mobile programs brought high-quality instruction into schools, day-care centers, and boys' and girls' clubs—either in conjunction with a field trip or as a stand-alone program. Compared to field trips, these activities were relatively inexpensive and provided more hands-on content. In additional, mobile arts programs often worked closely with classroom teachers, tailoring activities to complement a particular lesson or to suit a particular group of learners. HCEF and the homeless housing providers saw potential in these mobile programs as a practical and cost-effective way to connect youth to meaningful arts experiences on an ongoing basis. With many families making regular use of the HCEF Learning Centers for tutoring and access to technology, creating an arts-based program seemed to be a natural next step.

An opportunity for HCEF to test this concept presented itself in Pennsylvania's Educational Improvement Tax Credit (EITC) Program. In 2001, Pennsylvania was the first state to award tax credits to businesses that contribute to Education Improvement Organizations (EIOs), groups that offer innovative learning opportunities that supplement the traditional academic programs offered by public schools through use of specialized focus, instruction, or materials. More than 300 Pennsylvania organizations qualify as EIOs, including numerous museums, mentoring agencies, family centers, libraries, after-school programs, and youth-serving foundations. There is great incentive for corporations to give to such organizations. Businesses receive tax credits equal to 75% of their contribution, or if the company makes a two year commitment of giving, then the tax credits equal 90% of their contribution up to $750,000 in tax credits per year.

In 2007, HCEF submitted a successful application to the Pennsylvania Department of Community and Economic Development, the agency that oversees the EITC program, and launched a shelter-based enrichment program. Through the program, known by the acronym CAPE (Customized Accelerated Programs for Enrichment), HCEF developed partnerships with several of Pittsburgh's leading arts and cultural organizations to provide summer learning activities within homeless housing agencies. EITC contributions enabled HCEF to contract with these organizations, covering the cost of instruction and materials so that neither families nor the housing agencies would be required to pay a program fee in order to participate. The CAPE program focused on three major objectives:

- Stress Reduction: Providing a healthy outlet for stress by tapping into children's sensory and kinesthetic skill sets.
- Increased Self-Esteem through Skill Building: Giving children opportunities to take pride in discovering new interests and developing skills in activities that are not found in the course of a typical school day.
- Family Bonding: Creating meaningful opportunities for children to spend time learning and creating together with their parents.

With minimal funding in the first year, the CAPE program began as a small-scale initiative and has expanded steadily over subsequent years. In 2007, the program reached 175 children at eight housing agencies through a series of week-long summer camps, one taught by a master storyteller and another led by the Pittsburgh Dance Ensemble. By 2012, CAPE had grown into a year-round program with over 450 children participating in shelter-based workshops taught by eight contracted partners, seven of which offered arts-based programs. Partnering arts organizations included the Andy Warhol Museum; Art Expression, Inc.; the Institute for International Arts and Languages; Saturday Light Brigade Radio; and the America's Arts and Music Crossroads Center; as well as numerous independent artists.

When choosing art programs to serve as CAPE providers, HCEF looks for individuals and organizations that have the agility and experience necessary to adapt programming to suit different situations, age groups, and age ranges—often on the fly. Workshops must be flexibly designed to fit a variety of different types of housing agencies. Short-term emergency and domestic violence shelters focus on the exploratory and therapeutic aspects of expressive arts programs. Given the steady turnover of clients every 30 to 60 days in these shelters, the workshops are less formalized and more aimed at providing a creative respite from the extreme stress children endure during situations of family crisis. Transitional and permanent supportive housing agencies, which have relatively stable populations by comparison, use CAPE programs for their therapeutic qualities but also as opportunities for youth to develop a particular skill set. These programs can last weeks or months, may include a curriculum of lessons that build progressively over time, and often culminate in a final performance, exhibition, or publication

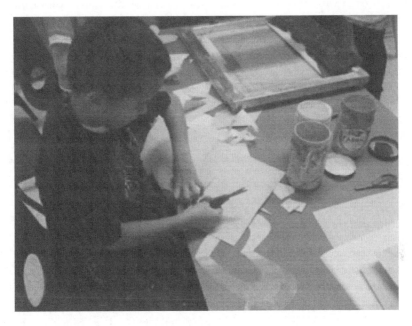

Figure 21.2 "A child creates an original screen-print during a workshop led by the Andy Warhol Museum."

to showcase the youth's creative accomplishments to parents and siblings. HCEF serves as the facilitator between housing agencies and CAPE providers, interviewing both parties to determine what sort of program will be most beneficial, overseeing the scheduling process, and monitoring program outcomes and data collection.

Partnership with Art Expression, Inc.

Art Expression, Inc. is a not-for-profit organization that facilitates positive socialization with children through expressive art activities in an after-school setting. Art therapy is not performed during sessions, but components of art therapy are used to guide students toward developing self-esteem, problem-solving skills, frustration tolerance, and social skills. Rather than critiquing student work from an aesthetic standpoint, a certified art therapist engages children in group discussions that explore their affective experience working with a given medium. In this way, the workshops are designed to expose children to new materials and processes in a non-judgmental way that encourages emotional awareness and supports creative risk-taking.

In the spring of 2012, HCEF partnered with Art Expression to adapt their school-based program for application in a shelter setting with mixed age groups. HCEF identified two transitional housing agencies to host a series of Art Expression workshops as part of their existing after-school and summer programming. Prior to conducting the workshops, Art Expression and HCEF staff visited each location for a consultation to familiarize housing agency staff with the program objectives and methodology, as well as to become acquainted with the housing agencies' current demographics. Each participating housing agency then hosted six 90-minute workshops over an eight-week period. At the end of the session, parents, children, and housing agency staff were asked to comment on what the workshops meant to them.

As the following example demonstrates, the workshops were successful in engaging not only children and adolescents, but often their parents as well. Art therapist Cheryl Silinskas describes a project in which parents and children used paper doll templates to create a "body map of stress":

> Some of the children needed help in defining how they felt and how to draw it, using symbols. Most everyone was able to display their work and talk about it. [One father] noticed headaches or feeling pressure like a band around the head, as an indication of stress. Some of the girls noticed stomach aches, flutters, nausea, associated with feeling anxious, scared, or overwhelmed. The women and older boys tended to notice muscle aches in their backs, necks, shoulders, or legs. Some of the younger children drew circles on their stomachs and pelvises, indicating stress about potty training or finding a restroom in time.

After the drawings were shared and discussed, the art therapist guided the children and parents through a discussion about ways that people respond to the physical symptoms of stress. Reflecting on the activity, one child wrote, "If you have a tummy ache it can be stress. I learned to tell my parents so they can help fix it." A parent reflected that "even the kids feel stress—in the stomach, in the head." In a related activity, the art therapist used the children's "free-time" drawings to further expand on the discussion about coping with stress:

> Some of the older students asked if they could create dragons and monsters. So I asked those who needed direction for their art to draw a monster that breathed an emotion or emotions, like a fire-breathing dragon. A few asked for instruction on "making a monster to wear," like a mask. . . . Some of them had the idea that their monster could help eat or stomp out their stress. We talked about disarming our fears by being silly or by focusing on positive emotions.

As a condition for hosting an Art Expression program, the housing agencies were required to designate a staff person who would co-facilitate each workshop alongside the art therapist. The active participation of housing agency staff yielded its own benefits, enriching their professional skill sets and offering new ways to think about working with children. The child development specialist at Womanspace East Transitional Housing, Inc. described her experience as a co-facilitator as an "eye-opener":

> I had to let go of my ideas about appropriate boundaries and let Cheryl dictate when things were out of control or just part of [the art-making process]. Watching how she used art to help the students develop their process of overcoming frustration and [developing] patience was an eye-opener. I also learned from this process that the end result wasn't the point—it was the process—and that flexibility was really refreshing and took a lot of pressure off of me, and more importantly the kids.

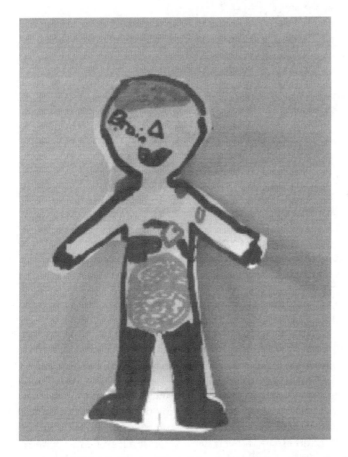

Figure 21.3 "'Body Maps of Stress' drawn by children during the Art Expression program at Family Promise in Crafton, Pennsylvania"

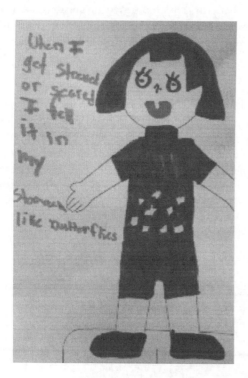

Figure 21.4 "'Body Maps of Stress' drawn by children during the Art
Expression program at Family Promise in Crafton, Pennsylvania"

Robin's Art Story: Robin Crawford

A First-Person Account of The Maker's Clubhouse, a Church Sponsored After-School Program in Pittsburgh

For the past three years, I have been working with inner-city students in grades K through five. I make my way weekly to the east side of the inner city of Pittsburgh to serve as a leader during an after-school program. The program services 35 students separated into small groups based on age and grades. The students attend the program three times a week for about two and a half hours per day.

My classroom assignment was art. This is a passion I have shared with children over the past 40 years. The students would come to my creative classroom to explore art, science, and engineering projects. Creative opportunities were also built into assignments: self-expression, free drawing, paper collages, pop art, cartoon strips, recyclable race car designs, and much more. It was refreshing to observe and experience the kids' excitement about creating and making something with their hands. Day in and day out, the students came with the same exciting energy, eager to start the day's project.

There were students who were unsure of what was happening but were willing to participate in the daily process of creating with their hands. Many of the students lacked creative opportunities. Inner-city students struggle with imagination. They have become accustomed to following others' instructions. It's a challenge for them to come up with their own ideas, especially the students in the community I work with. This presented challenges for many of the children to be able to imagine and dream a design that can come to life. They believe that this is out of their reach. Students would express their frustration by stating things like "I can't!" When encouraged that they can do it and reassured that there is no right or wrong way, the students began to create with an openness and amazement. As the weeks passed, students began to catch the idea that coming into the art classroom allows them to experience and explore the creative process. They were able to follow directions but struggled to imagine and create ideas of their own.

A select few were able to come up with creative ideas and create. They would always express joy, excitement, and vision flowing through the young child. Their excitement freed them to be creative and imaginative. What a joyful time for me to witness the beginning of the creative process. The creative process is an opportunity for students to begin to think about what else they could create. To provide a time and space for students to imagine is a gift for them. It opens their mind to begin to think of new ideas to create not only art but also other areas of life.

At the beginning of the fall 2013 program session, the program manager asked if I would lead a science station one day a week. This station was designed to expose students to science topics. I said, "I'm not a science teacher." I lacked the skills I needed to take on the challenge. Because of this I thought that I would not be capable of delivering a quality experience for the children we served. I felt unprepared and incompetent in this area of study, and most certainly I would be taking a risk if I accepted this opportunity. I thought, I don't even remember all of what I had learned in grade school, and what are they teaching the children in school today? I said yes to the teaching of the science projects and thought, well the challenge is on. I incorporated art into the science lessons and this reduced my anxiety around teaching the lessons. We successfully completed science projects that covered topics such as chemical reactions, engineering design, logic, and earth science. I took the challenge in my stride. As I taught the students, I was reminded of some of the science I had been taught years ago. The students were sparked with excitement to learn science and art which led to the implementation of our STEAM station (science, technology, engineering, art, and math) being taught three days a week. In looking back on this experience, I realized the importance of taking forward steps with my own growth in order to move the children forward in their educational and personal growth.

STEAM Challenge: Wonder Turner

Objectives: In this lesson, students will create a thaumatrope or wonder turner and learn about optical illusions.

Materials (per student): Straws, circle templates (two per student), markers, scissors, stapler, and pencils.

Preparation: Place all materials for the students on the table before beginning the lesson.
Procedure:

"For today's lesson, we will create a simple toy called a wonder turner. Does anyone know what a wonder turner is?" (Some students have completed this project before.)

"A wonder turner was a very popular toy in the past. Before we create our wonder turners, let's talk about how the toy will work. Has anyone ever heard of what an optical illusion is? Let's break down these two words: 'optical' is related to our sight. So that means it is something related to what we see with our eyes; 'illusion' is something that is likely to fool you. That means we may see something but it may not really be there or exist in the way that we see it. We will talk more about this after we create our wonder turner."

Directions:
Plan: Select a design.

1   "Think about what you would like to place on each circle. BE CAREFUL how you place the words or pictures on each of the circles. If you would like a bird in a cage, be sure to place the bird in the location that matches the center of the cage."
2   Create: "Take some time to draw and color your two images. Cut out the circles and staple them to the straws."
3   Test: "Twirl your wonder turner in your hands to view your optical illusion."

Questions:

1   What did you draw and why?
2   What was the most challenging?
3   How could you improve your design if you had more time?
4   Ask a few students to share and demonstrate their toys.

Engineering Design Process

Students were introduced to another example of creative learning, known as the Engineering Design Process (EDP). This focuses on allowing students to be creative while learning problem-solving skills. They were taught the five steps of EDP which are imagine, plan, create, improve, and ask. The students learned that engineers are people who find and solve problems, and that anything created to solve a problem is a technology. The students were introduced to the problem: How can we maintain a healthy environment? The creative process challenge was to create a toy car out of recycled materials like bottles, caps, cardboard boxes, used compact discs, plastic containers, and other everyday items that would normally be tossed into the trash.

At first, the students struggled with the idea of what they were being asked to do and learn. But to help them along the process, I would repeat over and over again what I wanted them to learn, providing different examples of the lesson but allowing the students to come up with their own creative problems to solve. This step helped the students, and from this place of understanding they rose to the challenge of creating a plan and implementing the steps of the design process. Excitement grew and joy was expressed among the team members just like a light had been turned on. "Ok I got it" (smile). Now they were off and running with solving the problem of creating a toy car that represents protecting the world's environment from harm. Over six weeks, students learned that by using recycled materials they were helping to create a healthier environment in our world; they understood the importance of protecting the environment that they live in; and they gained new problem-solving skills that will serve them for life.

It was the moment when one of the students handed me a note that read, "Thank you Ms. Robin for art!" I thought, yes, this is what it is all about! When you have shared your love for creative expression and it touches another's life, then what more is there? It is a precious gift given to the student while being received by the instructor.

It opens the door for endless possibilities for the children, who have discovered a gift inside themselves, a place that screams for freedom of self-expression. As the students become very excited over the discovery of his or her gift to create, more of the creative imagination kicks in and a flow of ideas fills the mind. An overwhelming sense of joy takes center stage in the hearts of the students. A desire to create more just grows as time moves on. One is able to create very satisfying works of art.

Artist Residencies

Another approach HCEF takes to provide children and adolescents with access to the arts is to apply an "artist residence" model. Working closely with individual artists as well as arts organizations, HCEF has developed numerous programs that bring visual artists, performers, writers, and musicians into shelters and transitional housing facilities to teach their crafts and mentor youth in their own creative endeavors. These programs can occur in short bursts or over an extended period of time.

Christine Bethea, a Pittsburgh-based quilter, eco-artist, and entrepreneur completed a week-long residency at a summer camp at a permanent supportive housing agency in 2012. The artist taught youth about the history of quilts as both an art form and a traditional commodity, showing examples of different quilt designs and types of fabrics. Throughout the week, students worked on their own quilt squares, which would later be stitched together to form a community quilt for the children's Learning Center. The campers were divided into two groups based on age. The younger children were given blunt plastic needles and simplified instructions, while the older youth were challenged to work with traditional tools and more sophisticated techniques. A summer camp teacher who observed the activity reflected on the value of the activity for the children who participated:

> I believe that it gave them an opportunity to see the benefits of spending a week working on one project. They were able to see the value in revisiting a work of art to add details and refinements. I think this process helped them build confidence in their own abilities and allowed them to see how taking time on something over a long period of time can make a great result. . . . Not only that but they learned practical skills like basic sewing, and stitching on a button as well.

Other artist residencies funded by HCEF have included Sydelle Pearl, a notable children's author and storyteller; The Schmutz Company, a group of artists specializing in puppetry and digital animation; poet-musician Shawnee Lake; and visual artist Sara Beck Sweeney. Through these in-house programs, children are afforded the opportunity not only to make art work or write stories, but also to interact with professional artists who make their living through creative work. For older youth, who are beginning to envision a future career for themselves, this can have a powerful impact on their sense of what is possible. One arts organization that works with HCEF, America's Arts and Music Crossroads Center, teaches entrepreneurial skills for aspiring artists. Shawnee Lake, a jazz musician and writer from the center, conducted an artist residency at Auberle's Movin' On program for teenage boys transitioning into independent living. During the five months of her residency, Ms. Lake mentored the young men twice a week as they wrote stories and raps, but also took time at each session to tutor the youth in math, teach basic business skills, and help them prepare for their GED exams. As a successful performer, she was able to speak convincingly of the importance of literacy and numeracy in managing the business side of her art career.

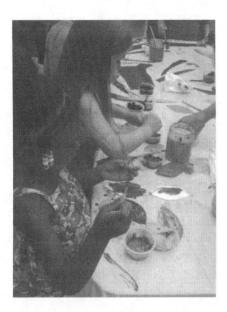

Figure 21.5 "Children create a group painting with Pittsburgh-based painter
Sara Beck Sweeney during summer camp at Sojourner House
MOMS in Pittsburgh, Pennsylvania"

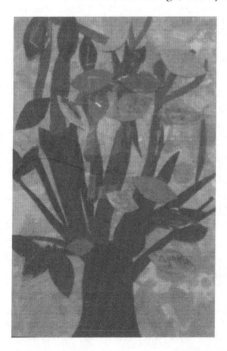

Figure 21.6 "Children create a group painting with Pittsburgh-based painter
Sara Beck Sweeney during summer camp at Sojourner House
MOMS in Pittsburgh, Pennsylvania."

Outcomes and Next Step

HCEF measures the impact of the CAPE program through surveys and interviews of parents, students, and homeless providers. In a survey conducted in 2013, 100% of participating homeless providers felt that the CAPE program delivers a high-quality service that supports their organizations' missions that their housing agencies could or would not otherwise provide for youth. Comments from housing agency staff emphasize that, for many students, the CAPE program provides an opportunity for children to explore new activities and techniques that they would not otherwise have access to:

> I feel that the CAPE programming has been a highlight for many of our children while attending our program. The children are constantly asking when the next "Hip Hop Day" will be. The families are always thankful that their children have the opportunity to take part in activities that they are unable to involve them in themselves. I have also observed how the children really absorb the materials learned during programming.
>
> Child Development Specialist, Womanspace East
> Transitional Housing, Pittsburgh, Pennsylvania

> The children have been exposed to activities that they may not have had the opportunity to experience otherwise. They have enjoyed the programs and look forward to the next time they come. I feel that the workshops have helped the children build self-esteem and have helped them learn that there is more available to them that they would like to pursue outside of Sisters Place
>
> Child Development Specialist, Sisters Place
> Transitional Housing, Inc., Clairton, Pennsylvania

> Sarah at Saturday Light Brigade Radio (SLB) was a wonderful instructor. She did a superb job encouraging the kids to explore something new and make it very interesting and accessible at the same time. She also went above and beyond her role as an instructor and invited us to visit the SLB studio during our visit to the Children's Museum. . . . The experiences the students have had from recording sounds to building radios to recording spots for the radio show have been great learning experiences.
>
> Family Support Specialist, Sojourner House MOMS
> Permanent Supportive Housing, Pittsburgh, Pennsylvania

The next iteration of the CAPE program will focus on developing arts programs specifically geared to young children (birth to age 5) and older youth (ages 18 and above, commonly referred to as "unaccompanied homeless youth"). These "bookend" populations are often overlooked by

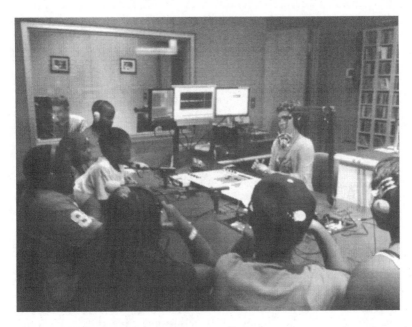

Figure 21.7 "Middle school students visit the Saturday Light Brigade Radio studio in Pittsburgh, Pennsylvania"

the educational system, in part because the McKinney-Vento Homeless Assistance Act does not mandate educational services for preschoolers and older youth who have dropped out of school. Fortunately, this is beginning to change in Allegheny County. In the last two years, numerous work groups have formed to study these underserved populations, including the Pennsylvania Task Force on Homeless Education and an Unaccompanied Youth Coalition composed of law-enforcement officers, youth advocates, and outreach workers. As these groups collaborate to assess the needs and whereabouts of these young people, more opportunities are emerging to provide programs and services, including those rooted in the arts.

Arts Partnerships across the United States

The Homeless Children's Education Fund's CAPE initiative is not the only program of its kind in the United States—yet creative programs for youth experiencing homelessness are not universally available, either. In a 2011 article entitled "The Art of Creating Stability: Homeless Children Find Confidence, Trust and Expression through Arts Programs," published in the Institute for Children Poverty and Homelessness's *Uncensored* magazine, Carol Ward writes:

Programs that attempt to positively impact the lives of homeless children and teens can be found in a few major cities, super-sizing the less formalized "arts and crafts" sessions offered in some shelters and homeless outreach facilities. Options run the gamut, from painting and drawing to theater to music and dance. A few are formalized "teaching" programs but most just seek to provide a creative diversion and a bit of therapy for some of society's most vulnerable children. The art programs can also fill an educational gap caused by the pullback by most school districts in art education.

(Ward, 2011, pp. 8–11)

Most art programs for children experiencing homelessness are relatively new on the non-profit scene and tend to be found in large metropolitan areas with significant homeless populations. Organizations like ArtBridge (Houston), Project Create (Washington, D.C.), and Art Start (New York City) were established in the 1990s following the homelessness crisis of the 1980s. From 1982 to 1988, New York City saw a staggering increase in its number of homeless families—from under 1,000 to over 5,000 in less than a decade (Nunez & Sribrick, 2013). As more family shelters and transitional housing agencies began opening their doors in American cities throughout the late 1980s and 1990s, serving as one-stop shops for services like counseling, food assistance, and job training, a number of artists and educators began to realize both the need and the opportunity for arts programming to serve the youngest shelter residents.

A Reason to Survive (ARTS)

The ARTS program gained the national spotlight in 2012 when the film *Inocente* received an Academy Award for best documentary short. The film, which follows the story of a 15-year-old artist experiencing homelessness, shows how Inocente's participation in ARTS shapes her creative and personal development. ARTS provides outreach to at-risk youth in the San Diego area through a continuum of programs that are influenced by Maslow's Hierarchy of Needs[1] (ARTS, 2013). According to the organization's website, the first stage of programming, called HEAL, focuses on Maslow's levels of safety, love, and belonging by engaging children in therapeutic art activities that help them reduce stress and develop trust in adult mentors. The second phase of programming, INSPIRE, corresponds to Maslow's esteem level and is designed to help youth build skills in their medium of choice over a longer period of time. The final phase, EMPOWER, deals with self-actualization and provides one-on-one mentorships, portfolio development, internships, and scholarships to older youth who demonstrate special aptitude and motivation to pursue the arts. Programming is housed in the 7,000-square-foot Pat D'Arrigo ARTS Center, which includes studio and performance spaces for youth to explore visual arts, dance, theater, music, and digital media, as well as a gallery that displays art work by students and their teachers. A compelling component of ARTS is its Van Go Transportation initiative, which provides door-to-door transportation to students who would otherwise be unable to access the Pat D'Arrigo ARTS Center. Van Go eliminates one of the most significant barriers that prevents unstably housed children from participating in community arts opportunities.

Art Start

Art Start, a New York-based organization, takes advantage of the city's rich artistic landscape to leverage support for its youth programs, partnering with organizations as diverse as the Museum of Modern Art and Bronxnet Television (Art Start, 2013). Art Start offers both in-house arts programming for children aged 5 to 18 residing in homeless shelters, as well as an Emerging Artists-in-Residence (EAR) program, which gives opportunities to aspiring artists ages 17 to 20 to develop their artistic talent into a viable career path. According to the organization's website, artists-in-residence must commit up to 20 hours per week for six months and participate in a schedule of coursework, paid internships, project creation, and exhibitions.

The EAR program also provides residents with a transportation stipend and career counseling. The questions asked on the residency application form are indicative of the everyday challenges faced by young, aspiring artists who are homeless: Do you have internet access on a regular basis? What was the most recent difficult situation you encountered? (Examples: Getting lost on the train; you needed materials but you didn't have the money to purchase what you needed; or maybe you had a performance but you had to baby-sit your sister.) Once they complete the residency program, EAR alumni may continue to participate in the program as mentors to the incoming cohort of residents.

AlyKat, an 18-year-old who completed an EAR dance residency in 2013, wrote on her blog:

> Becoming a master of the EAR program is like a dream. Being able to continue another 6 months with the Art Start program and developing my craft even more and being able to help the new students get off to a start is something I never thought will happen. The EAR program . . . allows me to volunteer and develop upon my craft.

Although these programs display a diversity of instructional methods and areas of focus—ranging from therapeutic play to career-oriented internships—one factor they all have in common is the use of art-making as a means of youth empowerment. Today's art programs for homeless youth emphasize active participation in the artistic process, as opposed to merely observing or appreciating the art of others.

Shooting Back

The belief in the transformative power of art making is perhaps best described by Jim Hubbard, an award-winning photojournalist who founded Shooting Back, an organization that teaches photography to young people. While on assignment to document the lives of Washington D.C.'s homeless in the 1980s, Hubbard began to share his camera with his young subjects. In Hubbard's words, equipping young people with cameras enabled them to "shoot back" as "experts of their lives rather than subjects of a professional's work" (Hubbard, BIO, 2013). The resulting black-and-white photographs yield only occasional hints that they were taken by children. In one, a police officer looms in the foreground with his back to the camera and his upper body out of frame, the lens sharply focused on the various weapons and keys hanging from the officer's belt—a child's eye view of authority. Most of the images are of other children—children playing outdoors, embracing siblings and parents, or pictured alone and deep in thought—largely eclipsing the motels, graffiti-covered walls, and non-descript streets that make up the backgrounds. Hubbard's young collaborators capture a striking range of emotion and human expression in subjects both young and old, evoking the notion that people are impacted, but not defined by, homelessness (Hubbard, Shooting Back, 2013).

The American Almanac of Family Homelessness

The Institute for Children, Poverty, and Homelessness (ICPH) has provided the following information about The American Almanac of Family Homelessness (The American Almanac of Family Homelessness, 2013).

With family homelessness still on the rise after the "Great Recession" and resources failing to meet demand, homeless services budgets must strike a more equitable balance between homeless families and single adults. Despite the fiscal challenges the field faces, there is still great potential to decrease family homelessness. Many national, state, and local efforts have proven successful in helping homeless families attain stability and self-sufficiency. Although homelessness looks different across the country, researchers, policymakers, advocates, service providers, and other stakeholders can share data and evidence-based practices in order to alleviate family homelessness as effectively and efficiently as possible.

The Almanac is a comprehensive guide to family homelessness in the United States, a go-to resource for newcomers and experts alike. Published by the ICPH, the Almanac offers original, in-depth analysis of demographics, barriers to services, policies, and service systems at the national, state, and local levels. It:

- Investigates the needs of not only homeless parents but also children and unaccompanied youth.
- Uses data from national, state, and local agencies, including data acquired through the Freedom of Information Act.

- Draws on interviews with government officials, service providers, advocates, and researchers across the country.
- The "Issue by Issue" section presents the lay of the land of homelessness at the national level. First, it explores the challenges that homeless families must negotiate, ranging from unemployment to domestic violence. Then, it examines homeless families' safety net, investigating both homeless services and mainstream benefits.
- The "State by State" section's 51 articles—one on each state and the District of Columbia—highlight unique local challenges and solutions; demonstrate the interconnections among public, private, and non-profit efforts to end homelessness; and present common benchmarks across states.
- The "Ideas in Action" section provides examples of successful, innovative funding strategies and early childhood and after school programs at the national, state, and local levels.

Over the past decade, federal funding for programs targeting chronically homeless single adults has increased, and the number of single adults accessing shelters has fallen. Homeless parents and their children have not yet received the same level of attention or resources, and family homelessness has grown. A greater understanding of the homeless family population across the country and a stronger commitment to addressing the unique challenges they face are urgently needed.[2]

Programs for Homeless Children and Youth

National Association for the Education of Homeless Children and Youth

The National Association for the Education of Homeless Children and Youth (NAEHCY) provided the following information about its programs. It was established in 1989 to ensure that children and youth experiencing homelessness receive equitable and excellent educational services in public schools across the country. NAEHCY connects educators, parents, social workers, advocates, service providers, and researchers to ensure school enrollment, attendance, and overall success for children and youth whose lives have been disrupted by the lack of safe, permanent, and adequate housing. NAEHCY accomplishes its goals through education, partnerships, and advocacy.

NAEHCY's programs connect members to peer support and learning opportunities through an annual conference, content-specific member committees, and regular updates on issues and practices affecting homeless children and youth. These programs also strengthen professional practice networks by making available timely information on best practices for McKinney-Vento activities, ensuring that homeless students of all ages are able to access a quality public education.

Further, NAEHCY's programs provide information to the public, the media, and public officials that increase awareness of educational and other needs of homeless children and youth. This information is critical to NAEHCY's advocacy program. By making available reputable, unbiased information on public policies, programs, and emerging issues affecting homeless students, NAEHCY serves as an advocate for effective action. NAEHCY's informational role also provides critical support for advocates across the country as they work to see that the needs of homeless students are addressed by federal, state, and local government.

Finally, NAEHCY's annual conference is unique; it is the only national conference dedicated to improving the education of homeless children and youth. It provides a showcase of best practices in education and homeless service provision from across the country, equipping participants with skills and strategies to ensure that every child and youth experiencing homelessness is successful. NAEHCY is committed to continuing its national leadership in equitable and excellent education for homeless children and youth.

SchoolHouse Connection: Barbara Duffield

Education is a critical strategy both for addressing child and youth homelessness and for preventing it from reoccurring in the future. Yet, homeless children and youth face unique barriers in accessing early childhood, pre-K-12, and post-secondary education.

SchoolHouse Connection (SHC) is a national organization working to end and prevent homelessness by ensuring that homeless youth have access to educational opportunities from early childhood through post-secondary education. SHC engages in a variety of activities, including federal and state legislative advocacy, technical assistance to schools and communities, grassroots partnerships and collaboration, and a youth leadership and scholarship program. While the organization is relatively new (founded in 2016), SHC's team has over six decades of experience working on child, youth, and family homelessness.

SHC works to strengthen protections and resources for children, youth, and families who are experiencing homelessness. SHC's federal policy advocacy includes early care, pre-K-12 education, higher education, and housing and homeless assistance. SHC's state advocacy program, "Building Teams for Change," works to achieve lasting, state-level policy changes and to improve the lives and futures of young people experiencing homelessness.

SHC is one of four anchor institutions (including Civic Enterprises, America's Promise Alliance, and the Institute for Children, Poverty, and Homelessness) in a national campaign to improve education and life outcomes for homeless youth. The campaign will significantly raise the profile of youth homelessness among the most influential education policy-makers across the country.

SHC's technical assistance activities include webinars, regular "Q&A" sessions with educators and service providers, state and local trainings, and tools for the effective implementation of early care and educational policies and practices. SHC publishes a comprehensive e-newsletter approximately twice a month, highlighting resources, events, research, and guest perspectives, and maintains an active social media presence on Facebook and Twitter.

SHC also operates a Youth Leadership and Scholarship Program which provides scholarships and support to youth who have experienced homelessness to ensure their completion of a post-secondary education program. The program offers young people meaningful opportunities as Young Adult Leaders to take leadership roles as advocates to address the systemic barriers facing homeless youth.

Ten Teaching Tips

1 Go mobile! Family shelters and other homeless agencies are often eager to bring in outside art programs to engage their youth.

2 Network with nonprofit leaders in your community—many of them are enthusiastic about partnering with schools and have access to private foundation money to support joint programs.

3 Challenge your classroom students to create an arts-based service-learning project, such as painting a mural at a local shelter or collecting art supplies for youth in need.

4 Expose your student to artists who have dealt with adversity. Discuss how their artwork reflects both their struggles and their inner resilience.

5 Create opportunities for homeless youth to feel the pride and satisfaction of sharing their own art work in public.

6 When teaching in a shelter or residential setting, be mindful and respectful of the agency's goals, expectations, and boundaries.

7 Seek out scholarships for homeless students to attend afterschool and summer art programs in the community. Many museums and arts organizations have money set aside for low-income students, but they may not publicize it—so don't be shy about asking!

8 Transportation assistance is critical to youth gaining access to community-based art programs. Talk to your district's homeless liaison about options for your students.

9 Find ways to involve parents in art programming, whether at school or in the community.

10 For older homeless youth who aspire to have a career in the arts, provide concrete guidance and mentoring to help them visualize a path to success—and to deal with challenges along the way.

Notes

1 In 1943, Abraham Maslow wrote "A Theory of Human Motivation." Visualizing a pyramid, Maslow defined five human needs: Beginning at the top of the pyramid is self-actualization (achieving one's full potential, creative activities); following downward is esteem (prestige, feeling of accomplishment); loving/belonging (friends, relationships); safety (security); and lastly (or most important of all), physiological needs (food, water, warmth, rest).
2 The American Almanac of Family Homelessness is available online in a variety of formats. To receive a print copy (while supplies last), email: info@icphusa.org.

References

ARTS (2013). What we do. Retrieved December 4, 2013 from http://www.areasontosurvive.org/about/whatwedo.

Art Start New York City (2013). Programs. Retrieved December 4, 2013 from http://art-start.org/programs-2/.

Hubbard, J. (2013a). BIO. Retrieved December 4, 2013 from: http://www.jimhubbardphoto.com/about-jim-hubbard.

Hubbard, J. (2013b). Shooting back, images, homeless children. Retrieved December 4, 2013 from shootingback.net.

Institute for Children, Poverty and Homelessness (2013). *History of Poverty and Homelessness in New York City*. Retrieved December 4, 2013 from http://povertyhistory.org/about.

Maslow, A. (1943). A theory of human motivation. *Psychological Review, 50(4)*, 370–396.

Miller, P., & Schreiber, J. (2009). Educating homeless children in Allegheny County: An evaluation of families, agencies and services. *Retrieved on* June 30, 2017 from http://www.alleghenycountyanalytics.us/index.php/2009/05/29/.

Nunez, R. da C., & Sribrick, E. G. (2013). *The Poor Among Us: A History of Poverty and Homelessness in New York City*. Institute for Children, Poverty, and Homelessness.

Ward, C. (Summer, 2011). The art of creating stability: Homeless children find confidence, trust and expression through arts programs. *Uncensored*, 8–11.

22 The Deep Joy of Teaching Art to Students Who Have Experienced Trauma

Lynne J. Horoschak

For 36 years, I taught art in the School District of Philadelphia and loved almost every minute of it! I enjoyed some tremendous emotional highs that were followed by lows. I cried in frustration, not knowing how to calm a potentially volatile situation or understand a student's belligerent behavior. But I kept showing up. Soon those frustrating times of "I can't," "I won't," "I messed up," "you can't make me," and paint where it shouldn't have been, slowly gave way to exhilarating times when students enthusiastically responded to projects, couldn't wait to come to art, and thought that the art room was definitely the best place in the school.

Here, I have written some of the strategies and beliefs that made my art classroom a place where students of all abilities found success. I worked with children in poverty; children whose second language was English; children who had never been to school until the age of 9; children with all types of disabilities, including cognitive, emotional, and physical; and children who had suffered psychological traumas in their young lives.

With all the differences students brought into the classroom, and with all the struggles that weighed on them, the art room became the great equalizer. There were no reading levels; they were all on the same art level. To the best of my ability, I worked to model best practices of kindness and respect for my students and, in turn, they taught me many life lessons, the good with the difficult. When an art teacher cultivates an atmosphere of respect and acknowledges everyone's worth, it has a way of overflowing into the school community. In my room, I worked to listen carefully to the children's voices.

This is not always easy when one is hurrying around the room tending to 33 children who are typically developing—if there is such a thing as a typical child—as well as an additional five who have autism or other special needs. But it can be done. The teacher must convey a passion for what he or she is doing, which includes the subject matter and the children. Each student needs to feel that the process and product of their art-making is respected and admired. This doesn't have to take much time. What it does take is working to get to know each student and making that child feel successful. This can't always be accomplished during the excitement of a lesson, but opportunities present themselves.

A chat in the lunchroom with a particularly shy child, or before school with a student who seems to be in need of extra attention, can make all of the difference in the behavior or attitude of a child who does not feel like a worthwhile part of the class. I found that asking a student who was "acting out"—we all know what acting out means, right?—what I had done to make her upset with me was usually enough for the student to realize that I wasn't the cause of the anger; I was the one getting the brunt of it. When I kept my requests personal by using "I" and "me," it made a difference in our relationship. A quick couple of words as a reminder to this student when entering my room the next class period was often enough to disrupt the potential of unwanted behaviors.

As art teachers, we teach children over several years, giving us the opportunity to have an impact in their lives, to see them grow over time in confidence, and to be a steady presence in their lives when there may not be any other such person.

Students with immeasurable problems and struggles come through our classroom doors. Some of these problems and struggles are deeply rooted and held closely to the chest, while others are more obvious, like autism. With some children, we may never know the challenges that they face daily. We work with what we do know: Behavioral defenses are triggered by fear, real and perceived. Avoidance, blaming, attacking, rudeness, and non-responsiveness are some of the behaviors that we observe. Art is a means to begin to break down those barriers of fear. Encouraging risk-taking in the safe space of the art room can build confidence, which can be transferred to other aspects of children's lives.

These students who add meaning to our lives, who challenge us to challenge them, and then respond in hundreds of different ways, all make us aware of the responsibility we have as their teachers. How we respond to their fears is the key to establishing a positive relationship in which they can relax their defenses. Learning how to find the child behind the defense and actively engage him or her in relevant art lessons can only happen if we care to take the time and energy to build a relationship. This may take years, and it usually does.

My first teaching experience was in North Philadelphia where the art room became a place where students voluntarily arrived at 8:00 in the morning as I was getting my materials ready for the 9:00 class and the day. It was a safe place, a warm place, and a place where they felt valued. A place where they could speak their minds, share their dreams, and have someone who listened. There were certain times I could meet their needs, and sometimes their needs were greater than I or the art room could provide. But the art room, with its policies of "no wrong answers to open-ended questions," "we can fix anything," and "take-that-risk" attitude, encouraged the self-expression that links self-confidence to success. In the art room, reproductions that depicted art from all over the world—realistic to non-objective, sculpture, prints, fabric art, ceramics—hung on the walls and were periodically changed. In addition, the art that the children were currently working on was displayed. This was not only to show the diversity of art and often to start that age-old discussion of "What is art?" but also to be a constant reminder to the students that there are as many ways of making art as there are people. Each person makes his or her own marks as only he or she can; you are the only one who looks like you and can make marks like you—so celebrate and make art! Anyone entering my school couldn't help but notice framed original art hanging in the lobby, created by the students currently in attendance at the school. This was evidence of a thriving, thoughtful, active, and enthusiastic art program! It said unequivocally that art was included and vital to the education of these children. The hallways that led to the office and classrooms had art that was matted—not stapled to a piece of paper: Would you want staples in your watercolor painting?—from children in all grades and of all abilities. Beautifully written and illustrated signage explaining the origin and process of the art work was hung next to the pieces to serve as teaching moments for all who walk by. Many parents exclaimed to me that they learned more by "reading the walls" in my elementary school than they had all throughout their own schooling.

Not only does the public display of the children's art beautify the school, but it also assures the children that their work is treasured and appreciated. Art teachers have told me that they couldn't hang art in the halls because the children would vandalize it. That never happened in my school, which had the same population as those schools a few blocks away. Making sure that every child has a piece hung in the hallway at least once during the school year is not an easy task. To make sure this happened, I would hang an entire class's art, attempting to get each child's art mounted and exhibited. The art of the children with special needs was matted and included among those of typical children, often generating disbelief from faculty and staff: "Anna did this?" What a great way to shine a spotlight on the abilities of all of our children. The exhibiting of the students' work spread throughout the community. Parents asked if I could put children's art in the windows of a temporarily vacant shop, in the local bank, library, and post office, which I gladly did. Getting the art into the community raises awareness of the quality of the art work from children, and advocates for art in the schools. This takes extra work and was well worth the effort.

In order to foster a climate of trust and risk-taking, not only between teacher and student but also between student and student, the students must feel safe. In many of our schools, this is not easy. Too often, the rules of the street are transferred into the classroom, causing physical fighting, verbal disagreement, and an overall feeling of chaos and uncertainty. I have no fool-proof answers, I am sorry to say. And as with all students, one solution does not work in every circumstance. I will tell what I found helpful and you, as art teachers who know your student population, can adapt as you see fit.

Please know that the first step is to learn who your student population is. How do you do that? Ask questions of the students, the staff, and faculty who have successful classrooms. You can easily recognize the teachers who are organized, creative in their teaching strategies, and whose students want to come to school. Ask them how they organize, reward, and run their classrooms. Ask parents of difficult children what they suggest as modifications for behavior; this helps to create a relationship with parents, who truly want their children to succeed. Talk to the parents about how they can help their child at home. Work toward a partnership. Talk to the student one on one; build a relationship here, too. Seeing the difference in a child when he or she is not trying to impress his or her peers is usually seeing a different student. Remembering that someone loves that student always helped me recognize the goodness that the child may so desperately be trying to conceal. When they know you like them for who they are—for the goodness they are—you have another student in your corner. This takes time and then more time. It usually involves time before and after school, giving up your lunch to talk with students, or perhaps, having lunch with some special students of the day. It may entail taking a group to an art museum on a weekend.

One of the most important inroads to establishing a positive relationship is visiting the home of a child. Setting up a time and date with a parent and perhaps walking the child home on that day, is seen as the teacher taking the time and trouble to invest in the education of the student. In some areas, it is advisable to visit a home with another teacher or staff member and keep the conversation on the steps of the home. The point is to reach out; to show you care by going the extra mile.

Establishing routines contributes to the well-being of the classroom. The students' anxiety is lessened when they know what to expect, what is coming next, and that they will get a heads-up when a time limit is imposed. A consistent routine includes how students enter the room, the procedures for motivation and class discussions, handing out supplies, working on the project, and transitioning from working to collecting supplies and cleaning up. These are all vitally important processes to make sure everyone feels comfortable as part of the art room community.

After teaching for five years, I took a maternity leave for six months. The woman who was to substitute for me wisely took the initiative and visited the school before I left. I reviewed the schedule, where the supplies were kept, what projects the children were doing, and how the children washed their hands in a bucket, which I supervised, since we didn't have a sink in my room. (After traveling for years, having a room was a step up!) Three days into maternity leave, I received a call from the woman. She was crying. "How do you get them in their seats?" Never did I think to explain that crucial point to her. If you can't get them in their seats, you can't have meaningful lessons and dialogue. So I explained what I learned; after much trial and error, I might add.

This is the strategy of seating the students, as I explained to my substitute. The children were brought to my art room by the classroom teacher. I greeted them at the door, expressing my delight in seeing them, and telling them about the exciting art they can expect to make today. The desks were arranged in groups of four, no art tables—classroom desks. I ushered the first four children into the art room, praising them for how beautifully they were walking to their desks, and saying it loud enough for all the children in the line to hear. From the door, I could see the children in the art room and the children in line. When the first four were seated, I ushered in the second group of four to sit at the next table, again praising them for how well they were entering the room. After all the children were seated, I continued praising and went right into the lesson at hand. I never stopped talking. Transitions are often very difficult, and when there is down time, things you don't want to happen have a way of happening. I would immediately launch into the motivation and a demonstration of the lesson, which helped keep their attention, because often it was a project they had requested. There were no supplies on their tables or within their reach. Hands would get busy fiddling with whatever was available and now was not the time for fiddling. When we were ready to begin the lesson, I chose helpers to pass out supplies and always said why—for example, "Anthony did a great job of quietly entering the classroom today. I would like him to pass out the glue." You can always find something nice to say to a student: "Margaret, thank you for that pretty smile. Please pass out the scissors." Getting the students engaged as quickly as possible is essential.

A few days later, my substitute teacher called to say things were much better. She let the children know that Mrs. Horoschak was interested in hearing about their great artistic creations. And yes, she got them in their seats. Following the routine that they were used to helped them adjust to the newness of another art teacher. As I grew in experience, many of these strategies were adapted to fit into the new ways I conducted lessons, and many continued to serve me well throughout my career.

Keeping them engaged was my responsibility. Is the project relevant to their lives? Is it age appropriate? Are there adequate, adapted materials and strategies for children with learning differences? Do children who might need extra help know how and where to get it? Throughout the lesson, I talked. I praised students with specific remarks, all loud enough so the formative assessment was heard by all, and therefore kept all on track. Often with an eye toward clean-up, I would say that, "James is working so well that I might have him collect the trash." Part of the constant talking strategy was to make sure that the 33 children in the room remembered that I was there. The students were always given a five-minute warning before it was time to clean up. Some needed a timer because the visual representation of time worked better for them. After we counted down the last ten seconds to clean-up, I would ask certain people to clean up, loudly enough so the class knew who was in charge of what. I would say, "Four people are out of their seats cleaning up and that's all who I want up." Sponges for wiping off desks were wrung out by me and handed to a table wiper. From where I was standing, I could also see the children at the sink. (This was after I ended up in a room with a sink.) Children love to play in water, but now was not the time, so I would have a sink monitor (a coveted position!) who counted to ten and handed a paper towel to each student. After clean-up, when there was one minute left, we would review the objectives of the lesson with some quick questions, stand and jiggle our bones, then line up.

When I first began to teach in the 1970s, all children with special needs received Individual Educational Programs (IEPs) and were in self-contained classrooms. I had no idea what a learning disability was, nor did I have a clue about how to work with children who were diagnosed with a disability. It became clear that the act of doing—of creating—of working hands on and celebrating the outcome was the way all children flourished. Trust me, I didn't always succeed. I was unschooled in the reasons behind the behaviors of the children with learning disabilities, emotional and behavioral disorders, and attention deficient/hyperactivity disorder. Trial and error, mostly error, was the school that educated me. I realized that art, with its visual cues and clear step-by-step instructions, led to a tangible product. Success! So many children came into my art room never having experienced the feeling of a successful moment in school. They were the "dumb" ones; everyone in the school knew it, and so did they. Realizing that they could succeed in art class and that their work was celebrated was an enormous first step in raising their self-efficacy. Because most of the children are visual learners, seeing the sample product before they began was important to them—to see where they were going. I would make art projects and pin them to the board behind my desk. I always made the art project with the materials the students would use. This let me experience what the child would; maybe these papers would stick together with my Elmer's Glue, but with the library paste in my room, not so much. Because I always used the supplies the class would be using, I once, out of habit, painted watercolors over some scribbled crayon to make sure the crayon would resist, but it didn't. The crayon was covered up. The district had changed their vendor, and wax crayons were not delivered in my order. If I hadn't done this quick exercise, the children's art from an entire period would have been hidden. This process of making an exemplar also let me know if there were any difficult steps the students might encounter, so I knew to make it easier. The children would see my projects hanging on the board and ask if they could make this one or that one: It was a wonderful motivator and it happened by accident, because I displayed my examples.

During those first years of teaching, happy accidents did occur and continued throughout my teaching experience. Experiencing success paved the way for the children to experiment on their own, to branch out with little guidance from me, with the exception of specific words of praise: "Your choice of pushing that shape off the paper was a terrific one!"

Empowering children with choices goes a long way. A choice that the child, and you as the art teacher, can live with helps the child feel that he or she has some control. I gave students two choices when it came to behavior modification: Do you want to sit on the stool (which I provided for students who needed downtime) to give yourself a chance to regroup, or do you want to continuing working? If the choice was to regroup, after a short minute I would ask if the child wanted to return to work, and they almost always did. When it came to choosing a color of paper for a background, I offered the students many colors. It's amazing how many choices you can offer during one class period. Soon the choices will make the student artists more independent.

It was during my first week of teaching that I had an "ah-ha" moment. I was teaching a sixth-grade class for the first time. The classroom teacher was in the back of the room marking papers—and his presence kept the children well behaved and attentive. For me, it was a get-to-know-each-other session. I was telling a little about myself and asking them to say a bit about themselves. We were from two different worlds: I grew up in a tiny rural town in Pennsylvania and they were growing up in the inner city of a huge urban area. As a young teacher, I was eager to see how we connected. During the conversation, in referring to a type of movement, I said, "It is like an ocean." I saw the teacher's head pop up with a little smile on his face while there were blank looks on the faces of the children. I realized that the metaphor meant nothing to them. If you have never experienced the roar and crashing waves of an ocean, that language doesn't work. Another lesson learned; know your students. If you aren't teaching to the relevance of their lives, there will be no connection and no learning. That inappropriate metaphor, however, had rich rewards: We went to the ocean, cast plaster footprints in the sand, gathered living plants and organisms from the ocean waters and beaches, and drew the sound and smell of the waves. After that exciting trip, "like an ocean" made a lot of sense.

During my second year of teaching, I learned a lesson the hard way. Clifton was his name. He was in a fourth-grade class and was very quiet, painfully shy, and uncommunicative. During an art lesson, I leaned over to Clifton and whispered that I would hang his art work in the hallway outside of his room because he was doing such a good job. During class the following week, Clifton was more withdrawn than usual—and here I thought we were making strides. Finally, at the end of class, he buried his head in his arms and whispered, "You didn't hang up my drawing." I was as devastated as Clifton! I learned an important lifelong lesson. Make absolutely certain that you follow through on what you say. Of course, I did hang up his drawing and made a personal apology to Clifton and a public apology to his class, telling them that I had made an error. From that day forward, if I made a special "hanging art pact" with a student, I would draw a star on the back of the work. I realized that I had the power to "humiliate or humor, hurt or heal," as Haim Ginott says (1972, p. 15). It was a valuable lesson to learn, and I learned it at the expense of a child's trust. Fortunately, children are forgiving, and Clifton and I re-established the trust between us.

Learning to pick my battles was a lesson that took me a while to learn. Initially, I wanted the entire class of 33 students to give me their undivided attention when I was motivating. I would actually interrupt myself to tell a student to pay attention or stop humming or whatever behavior I thought needed redirecting. As I grew in experience and wisdom, I learned that children bring the challenges they faced at home and with their peers to school. I was taught by the students that they came to school hungry, that mom didn't come home last night, and the 8-year-old was responsible for getting her siblings of 6 and 7 years old dressed and to school. Through conversations with children, I became aware of the responsibilities placed on many of the children and the toll that poverty took in preventing absolute attention in class. A child cannot listen and contribute to a class discussion if he or she is hungry or doesn't know who will be at home when he or she arrives after school. My attention shifted to student-directed lessons, involving them in activities that would allow them some fun, releasing them from their problems and concerns, and that would provide them with the experience of knowing that they could achieve, once their bellies were full. It took me a while to understand why so many students wanted to give their art work to me rather than take it home. I was told more than once, "Mommy would throw it away." I promised the children that I would treasure their work, and I did, and they knew it.

I learned early on that reflection was an important part of teaching—maybe as important as being organized and preparing materials before a lesson. Taking the time to intentionally recall the happenings from the day informs the next day and the next. Jotting down what comes to mind in a journal or on a legal pad helps solidify the thoughts, and therefore the actions. It helps to make sense of various behaviors and notice where patterns occur. Are the transitions bumpy and creating problems? Do the students need some calming time after recess? What went well? What didn't go well and why? What happened before an incident? How could I change the climate so the class would go well? What was beyond my control, and what could I do to make the best of the situation? It was about me learning to recognize when unacceptable behavior was about to occur and stop it with humor when possible. Leaving a "window open" so the student could gracefully back through it without losing face is an important strategy to master. It takes practice. I could tell when a child did something he was not supposed to by the guilty look on his face, even if I hadn't seen the action. So a little sad face from me was all that was needed to know that we connected and the behavior was behind us. It was my job to keep the climate positive. It was about me learning to recognize the triggers of unacceptable behaviors—the students and my own. As Haim Ginott writes:

I have come to the frightening conclusion that I am the decisive element. It is my personal approach that creates the climate. It is my daily mood that makes the weather. I possess tremendous power to make life miserable or joyous.

(1972, p. 15)

Devon (pseudonym) transferred into my school in February of his fourth grade. He was combative, argumentative, and a disruption in the room. An otherwise responsive and enjoyable class was turned into a room full of hostile students as they verbally armed themselves against Devon's jeers and insults. At this time, I was an experienced art educator, teaching in higher education, and giving presentations at the national level. I was sure that I would be able to meet Devon where he was and, with the incentive of successful art projects, help him to engage positively with his peers and me. I tried private conversations, the "good work" notes home to Mom, the "I need your help" talk; I pulled out all I knew, to no avail. After a few weeks of losing the battle of engagement, I spoke with his teacher to see what she knew about his history. It seemed that his father, a police officer, had been found guilty of illegally selling guns and was incarcerated. The harassment from the neighbors was so difficult for the family that they moved mid school year to escape. Knowing the reason behind the behavior made for a whole new strategy. In a quiet time outside of art class, I talked with Devon about this difficult situation and made a pact with him. I would do everything I could to make him successful in the art room, and when he did not want to work, he could go to a designated place in the room and sit with the choice of looking at books or doing nothing. Annoying the other students was not a choice. For the most part, this strategy worked very well. We continued to have some moments, but overall, Devon made art and the class in general thrived.

The trauma this boy was going through contributed to his disruptive behavior, and no wonder. Identifying the reason that precipitates negative behavior has usually helped me work with a student, and this was no exception. Now, the personal conversations with Devon before school had substance and we could better understand one another. Most art days, he would work and create art that was meaningful to him and on the "bad days," he could keep to himself and was excused from the project. His classmates welcomed the change and were not concerned when he was allowed the day off.

Every art teacher learns, through experiencing the trial and error of finding a way to modify the behavior of a child like Devon, that it takes time and persistence to work with a student and the payoff is extraordinary. They experience firsthand the difficulties a student from a negligent foster home or a home that has been disrupted with violence can exhibit. Obviously, every student is different and every student brings with them their own story. When the story impacts their learning, it is the teacher's responsibility to use every means at his or her disposal to support the child.

Most of us don't have the budget to buy all we might like to have, so asking parents to send in their discarded odds and ends became a practice of mine. At the beginning of each year, I would send home a list of supplies we could use in the art room. Buttons, yarn, odd pieces of lace and cloth, egg cartons, toilet paper and paper towel rolls, and the list went on and on, as you can well imagine. After a while, the list of materials didn't need to go home, as it became a culture in the school community to send stuff and things to the art room. I received a huge box of ping-pong balls, which the first-grade children used for bodies of fantasy bugs when they were studying insects in their classrooms. The fifth-graders used them in their moveable sculptures. Once, a parent showed up with a large woven hamper, which we ended up breaking down and using the bamboo slats for weavings and sculptures. I never turned down any donated supplies, although it did take me months to think how we could use a hamper! Each morning, I would find Styrofoam plates stacked outside of my classroom door that the children collected from the school cafeteria—except on those days when pancakes with syrup were served. These we used for many projects, from printmaking to a palette for paint.

One day, the parent of a student stopped by with a huge box of socks—single socks. He was a sock salesman and these were the samples that were now out of season. There were enough socks to keep us busy making all kinds of things, including sock puppets. One of my students, Annie, who was 8, had autism and was nonverbal, created a sock puppet. After putting on the ears, eyes, and finishing touches, she stuck her hand in the sock and said to her puppet, "Hi, Annie." This nonverbal child spoke to her puppet! It was the first time she'd said a word, and it was in art class. After that, as we passed in the hallway, she took great delight in saying in a deep, rough-sounding voice: "Horschak!" Leaving out the "o" from Horoschak was fine with me! Hearing her voice always made me smile.

I taught children with severe and profound impairments (SPI) who would be classified as Life Skills Students (LSS) today. Some children with physical disabilities also experience psychological trauma, and yet these children taught me the value of laughter. Some children were wheelchair bound, some had tracheotomy tubes, and some were fed through their bellies. Often, their reflexes were arbitrary; arms could jerk without warning. And yet, with the severity of the disabilities, we would laugh, sometimes at ourselves and sometimes with the children. Sarah, with a sneaky grin on her face, would toss paintbrushes so I would have to pick them up. Since I had never worked with LSS children, the para-educators taught me much about their lives and illnesses. It was clear they loved the children and what they were doing. As Doris M. Guay writes, "As a role model for students . . . para-educators can show enthusiasm, a delight in learning, and an acceptance and positive attitude toward meeting challenges" (2014, p. 200).

Sometimes art teachers are the ones whom the students trust with their concerns and struggles. Maybe it is because we encourage a safe classroom environment, maybe it is the compassionate personalities of art teachers, or maybe for many reasons of which I am unaware—but students do seem to trust us. Emily Smith (2013) reports, through her research, that there are seven strategies that mediate symptoms in middle school students with emotional/behavioral disorders:

1 clear choices in art projects and seating location;
2 relationship of trust with teachers;
3 buddy system among peers;
4 instructional humor;
5 timed teacher checks;
6 teacher-modeling; and
7 hands-on learning.

Intentionally implementing these strategies into the classroom routine will improve behaviors and result in students focusing on the task at hand.

Art soothes the soul. One 6-year-old at the end of art class, which was the last period of the day, whispered to me as she was putting on her coat, "My Daddy lost his job and we don't have any food." That sent me to the nurse to ask her to contact the family to see if it was okay if I gave them food from a food cupboard. I didn't want to offend. Not only was it okay—it was welcomed. The child's mother said she used to be in a position where she could help others and now she needed help. A few months later, the father got his job back and all was okay.

When Sandra's grandmother died and she was sent to school crying with no outlet for her grief, the principal brought her to the art room, where she spent the day painting crying faces. Even the flower in a painting was crying.

One of my most memorable students was a fifth-grader of Russian descent, Sergey, who was 12 years old and recently arrived in this country via Israel. He had lived there with his father, who evidently decided that Sergey was more trouble than he could bear, so the father sent him to his mother in Philadelphia. Sergey arrived mid-year and ready for trouble. He was bigger and older than our other students and soon established himself as the leader of all that is trouble: stealing cars, endless fighting, playing hooky, and cutting classes when he was in school. But he always attended art class. He never missed a day. He was a talented draftsman and had a strong sense of color. His work was imaginative and beautifully executed; however, he never kept one picture. They were always left for me. Finally, his behavior reached the point of no return and the principal, who was at his wit's end, told him not to come to school, to take off the last week of school. And Sergey did just that and thanked the principal by leaving a stolen car on our playground. During that last week before summer vacation, Sergey would sneak into school and come to the art room. The art room was a safe place for him where he could succeed. He would stay a few hours, working constantly, with beautiful results, and leave as abruptly as he came. I talked with his mother about enrolling him in an art camp and continued to search for him in the streets of the neighborhood during the summer. I never found him, nor did his mother follow up on art camp. I lost this one to the streets and eventually to prison.

One day, a new student came into the art room with his second-grade class. The students in the class clamored, "Where will he sit?" I asked Keith to sit at a table with three other children. Instead, he sat on the floor at my feet. The children were amazed, and I kept on with our motivational discussion as Keith stayed on the floor at my feet. When the time came to begin the art-making, I asked Keith to sit with Deborah, my student teacher, to do his self-portrait. That's when I noticed that he was very thin and had three large scars on his neck. He told Deborah that his name was Keith, but she could call him Tony. She replied that she liked the name Keith and would call him that. While the children in the class drew their heads filling up the paper, he drew his very small. The following week in class, I called on him and said that I'd forgotten his name, wondering if I would get Keith or Tony. He said, "It doesn't matter. I'm nobody." At the age of 7, he was nobody. Tears welled up in my eyes. "You are somebody," I said. "You have a name." We began the work of empowering Keith in believing he was somebody. Deborah saw him a few days later in a corner store and said, "Hi, Keith!" His face lit up! "You remembered my name" he exclaimed. And they crossed the road to school hand in hand. It is the little things that can have the greater impact. When a child has been abused and moved from abuser to abuser, is it any wonder that having a name that is his own and to be recognized by that name would make his day? Fortunately, Keith was placed in a foster home where he received the love and nourishment he deserved. Through your actions and words, let your students know you love what you are doing. Have fun. Be playful. Know that your sense of humor will disarm more potential for inappropriate behavior than anger. When the students are engaged in learning, the prospect of acting out is limited. When I realized that kinesthetic learning had a prominent place in the art room, I loosened up my "stay in your seat" policy, which resulted in more student-to-student learning, active conversations about the art-making, and more creative ideas. Watching 25 kindergarten children become the stars in Van Gogh's *Starry Night*, moving around the art room, flashing their starlight each in their unique way was a beautiful sight.

There was an excellent kindergarten teacher who could not bring herself to touch the insides of a pumpkin, but she wanted her students to experience creating a jack-o-lantern. So I did it. It was a perfect, tactile way to demonstrate positive and negative shape. The cut-out triangle for the eye was a positive shape and the space it left was a negative shape. I was talking about this with 5-year-olds. You never know what is going to stick—so always teach to high standards. The following day, a mother of one of the kindergarten children told me that her son had demonstrated positive and negative space using the bubbles in his bath. You never know what is going to make an impact on a child.

The social studies curriculum in my school assigned a culture to each grade. The second grade was to study Ancient Greece. At that time, there were no materials on a second-grade reading level for the teachers to use, so they were spending a good deal of time translating the text from higher-level books to an appropriate level for their students. And they complained a lot. Because good teachers don't like whining and would rather seek solutions, the five second-grade teachers and I decided that we would have the children write a book on Ancient Greece—that way it would be on their level. What a way for the children to learn; to write and illustrate a book. Each classroom was assigned a chapter to write, and during art the students illustrated their chapter. I found an editor who wanted to give back to the community, and she and a graphic artist generously edited and printed the book for us. Our Home and School Association paid for the color printing. When the beautiful books came in, we celebrated with cookies and juice and gave gifts to the editor and graphic artist. Each child received a book. The additional books were used the following years to teach Ancient Greece.

There are many incidents that happen in the world that affect the children—for instance, 9/11. How did I talk about that tragedy? I couldn't pretend it didn't happen and have the students go on with the regular projects of the day. The children knew what had happened. They heard the adults in their houses talk about it and saw images of the destruction on television. I thought hard about this, decided that I would discuss it with the classes to see what they knew, and led a discussion about the bravery of the police and fire fighters. It was to these brave people that we drew pictures of gratitude. The children decided that we should give them to our local police and fire fighters.

As difficult as it might seem at times, teachers have to park their personal troubles at the door. If you can't park them, take a day off and do yourself and the children a favor. I learned this the hard way. I went to the funeral of the son of a dear friend and went back to work in the afternoon. My emotions were raw and both the children and I had a terrible afternoon. I was short-tempered, and they didn't know why. I knew that my emotions were getting in the way of my rational behavior. I yelled at a first-grade student, and that's when I knew that I needed a time out. Yelling never solves anything. I have been known to count out loud to ten when I am feeling on edge. There is always someone in the class who says, "Uh-oh, she is counting to ten," which relieves the tension, and the class realizes they are stepping over the loudness barrier.

When my nephew died of crib death, I was out of school for a number of days. It's appropriate for children to know that teachers suffer loss. The faculty told the children of my loss. On my return, the children were kind and generous with their comfort. Actually, as I came in the building, a little unsure how I would handle the day, a first-grader came running up to me. Rooting through her book bag, she took out a drawing and handed it to me saying, "Finally, you're here! I've been waiting to give this to you!" I knew the day would be just fine!

The children with disabilities were included in most aspects of school life. They ate with the other children in the cafeteria during lunch, went to recess, went to assembly programs, and were included in art, gym, and music. The typical children were used to seeing children with disabilities walking in the hallways and sitting by themselves in the cafeteria. But there wasn't the kind of interaction among the children so they could get to know one another, except in specialized subjects like art. During these classes, all the students would intermingle and learn from and about one another. Once, there was a program in the auditorium. The older children with autism were making some sounds, and a couple of boys from a fifth-grade class started to make fun of them. This class had no interaction with the students with autism in any subject. Their teacher asked if I would have these boys in my classroom to help out when the children with autism had art. I thought that was a wise move on her part. The boys came, and I assigned each of them to help a child. They got to see the abilities of the children with autism, to see beyond the autism—to see the person. Another strategy I used to integrate typical children was to have them help prepare supplies for some of the art classes for children with disabilities. Some children could not cut out shapes, so that fell to the children who could. The typical children helped the children with special needs and enjoyed seeing the art with its many variations produced using the pre-cut shapes for a City in the Rain project. Typical children were also given the responsibility of taking the children to and from the school bus. Bringing the students together inside and outside of the classrooms helps both the typical child and the special needs child.

One student with autism, Shaun, spent each lunchtime in the art room. He would hurriedly eat the same Skippy smooth peanut butter on white bread sandwich, cut in triangles, and dash to the art room, conveniently located next to the cafeteria. Shaun would get the drawing he was working on, a fresh Sharpie marker, and take himself to the back of the room where an empty table was located. Covering a reproduction with acetate, he would meticulously trace over it, making decisions as to what would be traced and what would be left out. The fifth-grade classes in the art room during his lunch marveled at his patience, tenacity, and artistic judgment. Having Shaun in the room with the typical fifth-grade class helped the children to get to know someone with autism and his abilities.

I learned not to underestimate the importance art has for children with disabilities, especially if they are nonverbal. I was scheduled to teach a class of 8-year-old children with autism at 9:00 on a Wednesday morning. There was an assembly program to which we were invited. My plan for the art lesson was to read *Where the Wild Things Are* (Sendak, 1963) and have the children create paper bag puppets of Wild Things. However, with the assembly beginning at 9:15, I decided I would only read the story to them, then reread it the next week and make the puppets. They arrived and, after greeting each child with a good morning and asking for their good morning in return, we began. I read the book and, as I read, I encouraged them to become wild things: to roar their terrible roars, and gnash their terrible teeth, and roll their terrible eyes, and show their terrible claws. And they did each to the extent of their own participation. Then it was time to go to the auditorium for the assembly. We seated the children in the last row. I stood behind them, just in case one of them exhibited inappropriate audience behavior. For the first ten minutes of the performance, the children seemed to be absorbed. Then Pat, the classroom assistant, whispered to me that a child, Peter, was crying. He was right in front of me, and I looked down at him. Sure enough, tears were running down his cheeks. He was making no sound, just weeping. I quickly took him into the hallway, and I asked this child who was just beginning to talk, "Peter, what's the matter?" He looked directly into my eyes, which autistic children rarely do, and through his tears in a very pained little voice he said, "Art." He wanted art—not this assembly. To hear from him that this art class was so important that he silently wept because it was denied him was a powerful message. I was so touched by his emotion, and he was a child not expected to exhibit emotions, that I left the rest of the class in the capable care of the classroom assistant and my student teacher and took a smiling Peter back to my room to make art!

Too often, students with special needs are placed in an inclusive classroom and they don't benefit from that inclusive environment. However, there are instances when it is helpful for all concerned, typical students and students with special needs. If I received my class schedule at the beginning of a school year and noted that a class would have special needs children included, I would go to that class and tell them that I chose them to help me with these students whom I loved. I described how the children with disabilities might act and speak, and explained how I expected the class to respond. I asked for children who would help me by having the special needs students sit at their tables. Never was there any hesitation to help, and indeed, help they did. Telling the class what to expect, what I expected of them, and asking for their help made for an easy inclusion of the children with disabilities. Some students had the job of clearing a path for wheelchairs; others made sure that their friend had the proper supplies, keeping them gently on track and praising the work being completed.

I called my students artists because that was who they were. I made sure they knew from the time they stepped into my classroom that everything they created was unique because they were unique. They were the only person in the whole world who could make that mark. Everyone looked different and everyone's marks were different. We celebrated that uniqueness every day.

Make sure you celebrate your successes, no matter how small. Sometimes we get so bogged down with our challenges that we miss seeing our successes. Pay attention when Evan sits in his seat and works for three minutes, which is an increase of a minute from last week, and celebrate. Make sure that Evan participates in your celebration. Take your art classes out of the art room. Only making art in the art room tells the student that art is stagnant and only happens in Room 108. Push the boundaries of your lessons. Go and make rubbings from textures in the schoolyard. Draw the 100,000 dandelions that are blossoming in the grass in front of the school. Draw with chalk on the sidewalks. Trace around shadows cast by bicycles in the early morning. Collect natural objects to use in a weaving.

We know that the arts have the power to influence lives. Art gives the student an alternative to the negative influences that daily bombard our children. As Dennis Creedon says, "The arts not only build our brains, they insulate them from our stressful urban environments" (2011, p. 36). Having a well-structured arts program enhances the emotional well-being of children and readies them for learning, as it reduces stress and negative behaviors (Teplin et al., 2002). As art educators, we experience the success students have in the art room, although they may be failing in other areas of the school. We need to actively seek ways to embed the arts into the curriculum for all children, most certainly including those with special needs like Annie who finally spoke. To paraphrase Aristotle, we are called to be where our deepest joys meet the world's greatest needs.[1] My deep joy of teaching art has met the world's need to educate children. My hope is that you, too, will share your greatest joy with the needs of the world and all of our children.

Note

1 Aristotle. "Where your talent and the needs of the world cross; there lies your vocation."

References

Creedon, D. W. (2011). Fight the stress of urban education with the arts. *The Kappan, 92*(6), 34–36.

Ginott, H. (1972). *Teacher and Child: A Book for Parents and Teachers*. New York: MacMillan.

Guay, D. (2014). Clarifying roles for para-educators in the art room. In B. Gerber & D. Guay (Eds.), *Reaching and Teaching Students with Special Needs through Art*. Alexandria, VA: National Art Education Association.

Sendak, M. (1963). *Where the Wild Things Are*. New York: Harper & Row.

Smith, E. (2013). An analysis of how the art environment can mediate the symptoms associated with emotional and behavioral disorders (p. 60) (unpublished master's thesis). Moore College of Art and Design, Philadelphia, PA.

Teplin, L., Abram, K., McClelland, G., Dulcan, M., & Mericle, A. (2002). Psychiatric disorders in youths in juvenile detention. *Archives of General Psychiatry, 59*, 1133–1143.

Index

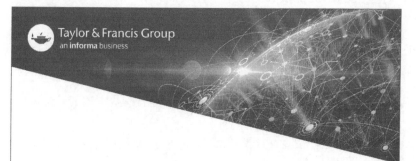